MOLECULAR EXERCISE ONCOLOGY

Molecular Exercise Oncology breaks down the cellular and molecular mechanisms underlying the benefits of different types of physical activity—from aerobic and resistance exercise to simple daily activities—including key scientific findings that provide insights into the foundational concepts of modern exercise oncology, revealing exercise as a potent tool throughout the cancer continuum.

This book uncovers the evidence underpinning primary cancer prevention, how physical activity and exercise can improve treatment outcomes, reduce secondary recurrence risk and enhance quality of life (QoL). With practical resources and pedagogical features, this text serves as an accessible and engaging key text to support student learning and to redefine the way exercise as medicine is perceived, in that every step counts in the battle against cancer.

For students studying sport and exercise science, clinical exercise physiology and exercise as medicine, for researchers in the field and for clinicians working with patients, *Molecular Exercise Oncology* offers invaluable insights into the latest findings in physical activity, exercise and cancer, with additional perspectives on the cellular and molecular basis of exercise as medicine.

Mhairi A. Morris, PhD, is a Reader in Exercise Oncology at Loughborough University, UK, where she teaches cancer biology and conducts research into the obesogenic breast cancer microenvironment using novel 3D co-culture models to explore the effects of exercise and endocrine-disrupting chemicals on breast cancer growth and metastasis. Mhairi is a two-time recipient of the Eric Reid Methodology Award and has received numerous awards for her innovative teaching methods in cancer biology, including gamification and VR technology. She earned a PhD in tumour virology at the University of Birmingham in 2009 and pivoted her research focus to exercise oncology in 2017 after joining Loughborough University. Outside of academia, Mhairi is a certified Les Mills Dance™ and BodyJam™ instructor, teaching four classes a week. Dance has become an integral part of her life, combining her enthusiasm for exercise with her academic pursuits.

MOLECULAR EXERCISE ONCOLOGY

Mhairi A. Morris

Routledge
Taylor & Francis Group
NEW YORK AND LONDON

Designed cover image: Getty Images

First published 2027
by Routledge
605 Third Avenue, New York, NY 10158

and by Routledge
4 Park Square, Milton Park, Abingdon, Oxon, OX14 4RN

Routledge is an imprint of the Taylor & Francis Group, an informa business

ISBN: 978-1-032-84170-0 (hbk)
ISBN: 978-1-032-84168-7 (pbk)
ISBN: 978-1-003-51151-9 (ebk)

DOI: 10.4324/9781003511519

Typeset in Sabon
by Apex CoVantage, LLC

To my students (past and present)

You are the reason I do what I do. Your curiosity and energy inspire me every day.

To my daughter

For you, I aim higher.

To my dancers

Thank you for dancing with me. Movement really is *medicine!*

And to my husband—my rock

Thank you for standing beside me, believing in me, carrying the load for me.

CONTENTS

FIGURES

TABLES

BOXES

PATIENT VIGNETTES

PREFACE

This book was born out of a growing recognition that movement matters in cancer care, not just as a preventive tool, but as a meaningful intervention throughout the whole of the cancer continuum, from diagnosis and treatment through to survivorship and palliative care. Over the past decade, the field of exercise oncology has seen significant advances, driven by epidemiological data, mechanistic insights and clinical application. Yet, much of this knowledge remains siloed across subdisciplines or is inaccessible to those who need it most: The general public.

The aim of this book is to bring clarity to a complex and rapidly evolving field. It is written for students, clinicians and researchers alike, with the hope that it will serve as both a foundational text and a catalyst for further research and action. In particular, it seeks to bridge the gap between cellular and molecular understanding and the practical realities of prescribing and implementing exercise in cancer care.

My path to completing this book has been shaped by many conversations, collaborations and late-night writing sessions. I am grateful to those who have contributed their insights, encouragement and expertise along the way. Most importantly, I am inspired by the individuals who have battled with cancer, reminding me of the strength and resilience that movement can help to restore.

AI DISCLOSURE

Throughout the development of this book, I used ChatGPT (version GPT-4o, developed by OpenAI) as a writing assistant to support a variety of non-substantive but valuable tasks. Specifically, it helped me with:

1. Structuring and restructuring content (e.g., organising sections, deciding where material best fit within chapters)
2. Brainstorming and refining ideas for figures (no figures were created with AI)
3. Clarifying or cross-checking interpretations of scientific concepts or statements in research articles
4. Enhancing clarity and precision in phraseology and sentence construction
5. Verifying key claims aligned with the conclusions of referenced studies
6. Generating draft titles and captions for figures, as well as drafting "Test Your Understanding" questions and answers
7. Helping adapt patient vignettes based on anonymised survey responses to ensure clarity, readability and sensitivity

All intellectual content, conceptual framing, interpretation of data and final decisions remain entirely my own. I reviewed, edited and approved all content where AI assistance was used to ensure it met academic, ethical and disciplinary standards. No text was reproduced directly from AI output without review and significant modification. Absolutely no text was "cut and paste" from AI output either.

1

INTRODUCTION TO PHYSICAL ACTIVITY, EXERCISE AND CANCER

1.1 Why this book, why now?

Cancer is now the leading cause of death in high-income countries, and the second leading cause of death globally, with over 18 million new cases and 10 million deaths in 2023 (1). Despite significant advances in screening, diagnosis and treatment, disease incidence continues to rise, making cancer one of the most pressing global health challenges of our time. As populations age and lifestyle-related factors continue to accumulate, these numbers are projected to rise in the coming decades. Meanwhile, emerging evidence mounts, revealing a stark picture of the significant role of lifestyle factors in cancer risk and progression, with an estimated 50% of all cancers thought to be preventable through making dietary and lifestyle changes (2). Among these, physical activity and exercise have been shown to not only reduce primary cancer risk but also improve patient outcomes at every stage of the disease process. As such, exercise is increasingly being recognised as a potential therapeutic modality in its own right.

The concept that movement could play a role in cancer care is not new but has gained traction in recent decades as the body of evidence grows. While exercise has long been recognised for its role in prevention and recovery in cardiovascular and metabolic disease, its application in cancer only began to emerge in the 1990s. Since then, the field has expanded rapidly, with hundreds of studies demonstrating the benefits of physical activity and exercise across a wide range of cancer types and treatment settings (3–7). This book is written in response to this growing body of evidence and a clear need to deepen our understanding of why and how exercise

DOI: 10.4324/9781003511519-1

works at a biological level. Within the following chapters, this book will explore the mechanisms by which exercise influences cancer growth and recurrence, how signals from muscle, metabolic processes and the immune system interact in the tumour microenvironment (TME), and how this knowledge could be used to inform better, more personalised exercise prescriptions. This book aims to bridge that gap, bringing together current research on the molecular and cellular effects of exercise in the context of cancer, grounded in both preclinical and clinical evidence. It is designed for students, clinicians and early-career researchers who are curious to understand how exercise might shape the future standard of cancer care.

1.2 What is cancer?

The term "cancer" is an umbrella term for more than 200 distinct but related diseases, characterised by the uncontrolled growth and spread of abnormal, rogue cells that arise from a dysfunction in the tightly regulated processes that control cell growth, division and death. Oftentimes, these dysfunctions arise from an accumulation of genetic mutations and epigenetic alterations. Sometimes these mutations are inherited predispositions, but more commonly, they are acquired over time in response to environmental exposures, lifestyle factors and random errors in deoxyribonucleic acid (DNA) replication. In addition to being a genetic disorder, cancer is also an immunological disease. While mutations in oncogenes, tumour suppressor genes and DNA repair mechanisms can drive malignant transformation, it is faulty immune surveillance that allows these abnormal cells to evade detection and destruction. This interplay between genetic instability and immune evasion is central to cancer development and progression (8).

In 2000, Hanahan and Weinberg famously outlined the "Hallmarks of Cancer," a conceptual framework that has become central to the field (9). These hallmarks, common to all cancers, include traits such as sustained proliferation, evasion of anti-growth signals, resisting cell death, replicative immortality, the growth of new blood vessels (angiogenesis) and invasion and metastasis. In subsequent years, the framework was expanded to incorporate additional hallmarks and enabling characteristics such as avoiding immune destruction, deregulating metabolism and promoting inflammation (8,10).

While survival rates have improved in many high-income countries due to early detection methods and better treatments, the number of people living with and beyond cancer, often referred to as cancer survivors, is also increasing. However, lower-income countries bear a disproportionate burden of late-stage diagnoses and limited access to care, emphasising the importance of prevention and early intervention to reduce the global burden of cancer.

One of the most striking statistics is that between 30–50% of cases are preventable, since many cancers are linked to modifiable risk factors, including tobacco use, an unhealthy diet, obesity, physical inactivity, excessive alcohol consumption and exposure to infectious agents and environmental carcinogens (2). Of these factors, physical inactivity and excess body fat are among the most significant risk factors, contributing not only to cancer incidence but also to poorer outcomes after diagnosis. Understanding what cancer is and how lifestyle factors such as exercise can influence its development is essential. The remainder of this chapter and book will explore this link in detail, starting from population-level observations, then moving towards cellular and molecular mechanisms.

1.3 Defining physical activity, exercise and sedentary behaviour

To understand the role of movement in cancer care, it is essential to first define the terms physical activity and exercise, which are often used interchangeably but have distinct meanings in both research and clinical practice.

Physical activity refers to any bodily movement produced by skeletal muscles that results in energy expenditure. This includes a wide range of activities such as walking, gardening, household chores, occupational tasks and recreational pursuits. By contrast, exercise is a structured, planned and repetitive form of physical activity performed with the objective of improving or maintaining one or more components of physical fitness, such as strength, endurance or flexibility.

In the context of cancer care, both physical activity and exercise are beneficial. However, understanding the distinction is important when designing, evaluating and prescribing interventions. Informal physical activity, such as light walking or standing breaks, can help reduce sedentary behaviour (SB) and support overall health, while structured exercise programmes may be more targeted towards improving treatment tolerance, physical function and long-term survivorship outcomes.

A useful framework for tailoring physical activity and exercise interventions is the FITT principle, which stands for Frequency, Intensity, Time and Type. This model provides a structured approach to exercise prescription:

- Frequency: How often activity is performed (e.g., days per week)
- Intensity: How hard the activity is (e.g., light, moderate, vigorous)
- Time: Duration of each session (e.g., minutes per bout)
- Type: The mode or form of activity (e.g., aerobic, resistance, flexibility)

The FITT principle enables clinicians and researchers to adjust exercise prescriptions according to individual needs, goals and treatment phases. In cancer care, this flexibility is particularly valuable, as patient capacity and tolerance may vary widely across the continuum, from diagnosis and treatment to recovery and long-term survivorship.

Framing physical activity across the cancer continuum underscores its diverse applications and benefits. During primary prevention, regular movement reduces the risk of developing cancer through favourable effects on metabolic health, inflammation and hormone regulation. In prehabilitation, structured activity can improve physical and psychological readiness before surgery or systemic therapy. Throughout treatment, exercise helps mitigate side effects such as fatigue, deconditioning and anxiety. In the rehabilitation phase, it aids in restoring function, muscle mass and confidence. Finally, in secondary prevention, regular activity contributes to reduced recurrence risk and improved quality of life (QoL) in survivorship.

By embracing both structured and incidental movement, physical activity becomes a versatile and accessible tool: One that can be adapted to the needs, abilities and preferences of each individual across their cancer journey.

1.4 The emergence of exercise oncology

The idea that exercise could play a meaningful role in cancer care is relatively new. While the benefits of structured exercise programmes for chronic diseases such as coronary artery disease and heart failure were firmly established in the 1960s and 1970s, exercise was not considered part of routine cancer care for several more decades. The first formal investigations of exercise as therapy in people with cancer did not appear until the late 1980s, and even then, publications remained sparse until the late 1990s, when interest began to accelerate (Box-out 1.1).

For many years, exercise in cancer care was viewed primarily as a tool for symptom management: A way to reduce fatigue, maintain strength and improve emotional wellbeing. However, over the past decade, evidence has shifted the field towards viewing exercise as a potential therapeutic adjunct. Observational studies demonstrate associations between higher physical activity levels and improved prognosis, including lower recurrence and mortality in breast, colon and prostate cancers (11). Preclinical studies offer compelling mechanistic insights into the effects of exercise on immune function (12). As the field continues to expand, there is growing recognition that exercise may need to be tailored more precisely, reflecting tumour type, treatment stage and individual patient characteristics. The field of exercise oncology has therefore evolved from a supportive rehabilitation strategy into a scientifically grounded, mechanistically plausible adjunct to modern cancer care.

BOX-OUT 1.1 TIMELINE OF KEY RESEARCH MILESTONES IN EXERCISE ONCOLOGY (7)

1960s–1970s: Exercise becomes standard of care in cardiovascular rehabilitation, establishing a model for structured exercise prescriptions in chronic disease management.

Late 1980s: First small-scale trials explore the feasibility of exercise during cancer treatment. These early studies emphasise safety and tolerability.

1990s: Gradual increase in observational and interventional studies. Exercise viewed largely as supportive therapy to counteract treatment-related fatigue and deconditioning.

Early 2000s: Rapid growth of exercise-oncology research. Systematic reviews begin to show consistent improvements in QoL, fatigue, and physical function during and after treatment.

2010s: Emergence of mechanistic research exploring immune, metabolic and hormonal pathways. Preclinical models demonstrate direct tumour-suppressive effects of exercise.

Late 2010s–2020s: Exercise oncology recognised as an emergent subdiscipline of oncology, with hundreds of trials across prevention, treatment, survivorship and palliative care.

1.5 The role of physical activity and exercise in cancer prevention, treatment and survivorship

Physical activity and exercise play varied roles across the cancer continuum. The effects are not confined to a single phase but extend from prevention through to long-term survivorship, offering benefits that are physiological, psychological and functional. Understanding this broad spectrum of influence is central to appreciating the clinical and public health relevance of exercise in cancer care.

1.5.1 Primary prevention: Risk reduction across cancer types

A substantial body of epidemiological evidence supports the association between regular physical activity and reduced risk of developing several common cancers, including breast, colorectal, endometrial, kidney, bladder, oesophageal and stomach cancers (13) (see Chapter 2). These protective effects are believed to be mediated by improvements in insulin sensitivity, reductions in systemic inflammation, regulation of sex hormones, and maintenance of healthy body weight. Even modest increases in activity levels can yield meaningful reductions in cancer risk, reinforcing the message that all movement counts.

1.5.2 *Prehabilitation: Preparing the body and mind for treatment*

Prehabilitation refers to the period between cancer diagnosis and the initiation of treatment: A window of opportunity to enhance physical and psychological resilience. Structured exercise during this time can improve cardiorespiratory fitness, muscle strength and functional capacity, leading to better surgical outcomes, reduced treatment-related complications and shorter hospital stays. In addition, prehabilitation can improve emotional readiness, helping patients feel more in control at a time of uncertainty (see Chapter 7).

1.5.3 *During treatment: Preserving function and managing symptoms*

Engaging in physical activity and exercise during chemotherapy, radiotherapy or immunotherapy can help preserve muscle mass, cardiovascular function and energy levels. Randomised controlled trials (RCTs) have shown that exercise during treatment reduces cancer-related fatigue, maintains physical function, improves mood and enhances QoL. While individual tolerance may vary depending on treatment type and side effects, even light activity, when feasible, can offer substantial benefit. Importantly, exercise during treatment is safe and does not increase adverse events when appropriately prescribed and monitored (see Chapter 7).

1.5.4 *Post-treatment rehabilitation: Restoring strength, resilience and quality of life*

After treatment, many individuals face lingering side effects such as fatigue, neuropathy, reduced mobility and psychosocial challenges. Physical activity is core to rehabilitation, supporting the restoration of strength, endurance, balance and confidence. Exercise also plays a role in managing long-term effects such as weight gain, bone loss and metabolic dysfunction. Furthermore, regular activity post-treatment is associated with improvements in mental health, self-efficacy and social reintegration (see Chapter 7).

1.5.5 Secondary prevention: Reducing recurrence and supporting survivorship

Physical activity may also influence cancer outcomes beyond the treatment phase. Evidence suggests that higher levels of post-diagnosis physical activity are associated with reduced risk of recurrence and improved overall and cancer-specific survival in several tumour types, including breast, colorectal and prostate cancers (11,13). Survivorship guidelines now emphasise the importance of maintaining regular activity as part of a healthy lifestyle. By supporting immune function, modulating inflammation and improving metabolic health, exercise contributes to long-term resilience and disease control.

Together, these stages illustrate the importance of physical activity and exercise in the continuum of cancer care, where movement serves not only as a preventive strategy but also as an active component of treatment, recovery and survivorship.

1.6 Scope and structure of this book

This book is structured to guide readers through the scientific foundations, practical applications and future directions of physical activity and exercise in cancer care. Each chapter builds on the last, offering insights from epidemiology and cellular biology, through to clinical practice and public health messaging. While no prior expertise in molecular biology or oncology is required, this book assumes a basic familiarity with human physiology and scientific reasoning. It aims to be both an accessible entry point and a detailed reference, suitable for reading cover to cover or for dipping into specific chapters. Below is a brief overview of what each chapter covers.

1.6.1 Chapter 2: The evidence behind exercise versus sedentary behaviour and cancer

This chapter examines the epidemiological data linking physical inactivity with increased cancer risk and explores how regular physical activity can reduce incidence and improve survival. The chapter also considers behavioural and environmental contributors to sedentary lifestyles.

1.6.2 Chapter 3: The cellular response to exercise in cancer

This chapter explores how exercise influences the TME, including immune activation, vascular remodelling and changes in cancer stem cell behaviour. It also highlights the cellular adaptations that underpin the anti-tumour effects of exercise.

1.6.3 Chapter 4: The molecular basis of exercise in cancer

This chapter delves into intracellular and extracellular signalling pathways affected by exercise, including a detailed breakdown of the key myokines and exerkines involved. It also considers actionable strategies for increasing physical activity participation.

1.6.4 Chapter 5: Types of exercise and their benefits

This chapter compares aerobic, resistance and endurance, everyday physical activities and mind-body therapies, outlining their respective benefits for people living with and beyond cancer. It applies the FITT framework to different exercise modalities and patient needs.

1.6.5 Chapter 6: Differential effects of exercise intensities

This chapter investigates how varying intensities of exercise, from low to high, affect the immune system, tumour biology, inflammation and fatigue. It highlights clinical and preclinical evidence supporting both moderate- and vigorous-intensity training.

1.6.6 Chapter 7: Frequency and length of exercise bouts

This chapter reviews the evidence on optimal dose, frequency and length of exercise for cancer prevention and survivorship. It also discusses how short, accumulated bouts can deliver meaningful physiological effects and improve adherence.

1.6.7 Chapter 8: Exercise guidelines and recommendations

This chapter summarises international physical activity guidelines for people with cancer, from diagnosis through to survivorship. It gives consideration to personalising, adapting and implementing exercise prescriptions across settings and populations.

1.6.8 Chapter 9: A new perspective on exercise and cancer

This chapter synthesises the book's core themes, reinforcing the message that every move counts. It reflects on future research directions and calls on clinicians, researchers, students and advocates to be part of the movement for change.

1.6.9 Chapter 10: Additional resources

This final chapter provides additional materials and practical resources for students, educators and clinicians.

This structure is designed to support both linear reading and topic-specific exploration. Whether the reader is seeking to understand the molecular mechanisms of exercise, looking for practical guidance on prescribing activity, or preparing to teach the next generation of exercise oncologists, each chapter offers accessible and evidence-informed content grounded in current best practice.

1.7 Introducing the core message

At the heart of this book lies a simple but powerful message: Sit less, move more. This guiding principle reflects decades of research showing that physical activity, of almost any kind, can support health, resilience and recovery in people living with or beyond cancer. Crucially, this message is not limited to structured exercise or high-intensity training. While these may offer specific physiological benefits, even small amounts of movement, accumulated throughout the day, contribute to improved outcomes. Breaking up prolonged sitting, taking short walks, engaging in light household tasks, or performing resistance exercises with minimal equipment, can all make a meaningful difference. However, it is equally important to acknowledge the barriers many people face. Fatigue, pain, limited mobility, mental health challenges, lack of time, access and support are all common concerns, particularly during and after cancer treatment. Recognising these challenges does not diminish the message; rather, it reinforces the need for compassionate, personalised and flexible approaches to physical activity promotion. Whether starting from a place of inactivity or building on an existing routine, any movement towards more activity and sitting less is a step in the right direction.

References

1. The Lancet: Cancer deaths expected to rise to over 18 million in 2050—an increase of nearly 75% from 2024, study forecasts | Institute for Health Metrics and Evaluation [Internet]. [cited 2025 Dec 1]. Available from: https://www.healthdata.org/news-events/newsroom/news-releases/lancet-cancer-deaths-expected-rise-over-18-million-2050-increase
2. Aicr, WCRF. Diet, nutrition, physical activity and cancer: A global perspective a summary of the third expert report. [cited 2025 Nov 14]. Available from: http://gco.iarc.fr/today
3. Courneya KS. Physical activity in cancer survivors: A field in motion. Psychooncology [Internet]. 2009 Apr [cited 2023 Dec 13];18(4):337–42. Available from: http://www.ncbi.nlm.nih.gov/pubmed/19306338

4. Friedenreich CM, Neilson HK, Farris MS, Courneya KS. Physical activity and cancer outcomes: A precision medicine approach. Clin Cancer Res [Internet]. 2016 Oct 1 [cited 2025 Nov 22];22(19):4766–75. Available from: https://pubmed.ncbi.nlm.nih.gov/27407093/
5. An KY, Min J, Lee DH, Kang DW, Courneya KS, Jeon JY. Exercise across the phases of cancer survivorship: A narrative review. Yonsei Med J [Internet]. 2024 Jun 1 [cited 2025 Nov 23];65(6):315–23. Available from: https://doi.org/10.3349/ymj.2023.0638
6. MCTiernan A, Friedenreich CM, Katzmarzyk PT, Powell KE, Macko R, Buchner D, et al. Physical activity in cancer prevention and survival: A systematic review. Med Sci Sports Exerc [Internet]. 2019 Jun [cited 2024 Nov 8];51(6):1252–61. Available from: https://journals.lww.com/00005768-201906000-00020
7. Jones LW, Alfano CM. Exercise-oncology research: Past, present, and future. Acta Oncol (Madr) [Internet]. 2013 Feb 17 [cited 2019 Dec 10];52(2): 195–215. Available from: http://www.ncbi.nlm.nih.gov/pubmed/23244677
8. Hanahan D, Weinberg RA. Hallmarks of cancer: The next generation. Cell [Internet]. 2011 Mar 4 [cited 2025 Dec 1];144(5):646–74. Available from: https://pubmed.ncbi.nlm.nih.gov/21376230/
9. Hanahan D, Weinberg RA, Yang Q, Goldstein AM, Tucker MA, Walker GJ, et al. The hallmarks of cancer. Cell [Internet]. 2000 Jan 7 [cited 2017 Aug 16];100(1):57–70. Available from: http://www.ncbi.nlm.nih.gov/pubmed/10647931
10. Hanahan D. Hallmarks of cancer: New dimensions. Cancer Discov [Internet]. 2022 Jan 1 [cited 2025 Nov 29];12(1):31–46. Available from: https://pubmed.ncbi.nlm.nih.gov/35022204/
11. Brown JC, Gilmore LA. Physical activity reduces the risk of recurrence and mortality in cancer patients. Exerc Sport Sci Rev [Internet]. 2020 Apr 1 [cited 2025 Nov 25];48(2):67–73. Available from: https://pubmed.ncbi.nlm.nih.gov/31913187/
12. Hojman P, Gehl J, Christensen JF, Pedersen BK. Molecular mechanisms linking exercise to cancer prevention and treatment. Cell Metab [Internet]. 2018 Jan 9 [cited 2024 Jan 26];27(1):10–21. Available from: http://www.ncbi.nlm.nih.gov/pubmed/29056514
13. Moore SC, Lee IM, Weiderpass E, Campbell PT, Sampson JN, Kitahara CM, et al. Association of leisure-time physical activity with risk of 26 types of cancer in 1.44 million adults. JAMA Intern Med [Internet]. 2016 Jun 1 [cited 2025 Nov 14];176(6):816–25. Available from: https://jamanetwork.com/journals/jamainternalmedicine/fullarticle/2521826

PART I

Exercise and cancer

2

THE EVIDENCE BEHIND EXERCISE VERSUS SEDENTARY BEHAVIOUR AND CANCER

2.1 Introduction

This chapter explores the contrasting roles of sedentary behaviour and physical activity in relation to cancer risk. Over recent decades, a growing body of epidemiological evidence has revealed that while sedentary lifestyles are associated with increased cancer risk, regular physical activity, including structured exercise, can play a protective role in both cancer prevention and survivorship. Before exploring the evidence base, it is important to clarify key terms used throughout this chapter (see Box 2.1). These distinctions are essential, as the terms are not interchangeable and will be used with precision throughout the book.

Sedentary behaviour, as defined by the Sedentary Behaviour Research Network, refers to any waking behaviour characterised by an energy expenditure ≤1.5 metabolic equivalent of tasks (METs), while sitting, reclining or lying down (1). Common examples include watching TV, playing video games, using a computer or smartphone (collectively known as "screen time"), as well as driving and reading.

Physical activity encompasses any bodily movement produced by skeletal muscles that requires energy expenditure. This includes a broad range of daily movements such as walking, cycling, wheeling, sports, active recreation, play, housework and gardening (2) (Figure 2.1).

Exercise is a subcategory of physical activity that is planned, structured, repetitive and purposefully focused on the improvement or maintenance

DOI: 10.4324/9781003511519-3

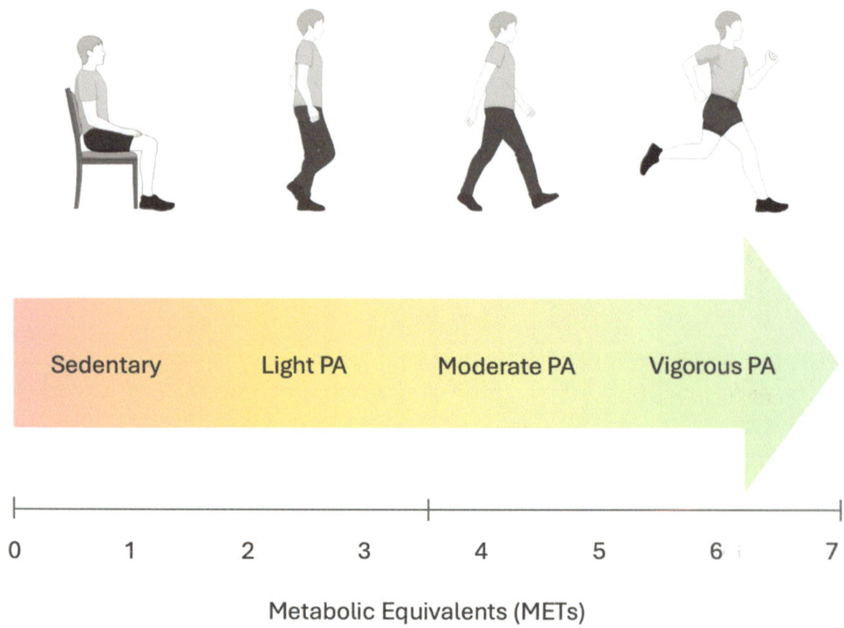

FIGURE 2.1 The energy expenditure continuum across physical activity intensities. This continuum illustrates the classification of physical activity based on energy expenditure measured in METs. Sedentary behaviour (≤1.5 METs) includes seated or reclining activities with minimal movement. Light physical activity (1.6–2.9 METs) involves low-effort movements such as slow walking or light play. Moderate physical activity (3–5.9 METs) encompasses more dynamic movement like brisk walking or active games, while vigorous physical activity (≥6 METs) includes high-intensity actions such as running or jumping. Understanding this gradient is critical for distinguishing between activity types in relation to health outcomes and cancer risk. Adapted from the Sedentary Behaviour Research Network (3) using Biorender.com.

of one or more components of physical fitness, for example, strength or cardiorespiratory fitness (2).

Understanding these distinctions is vital for interpreting the evidence presented in this book and the wider literature as a whole. Clear and consistent terminology helps to delineate the biological mechanisms, health outcomes and cancer-related implications associated with different types and intensities of activity.

BOX-OUT 2.1 KEY DEFINITIONS

Sedentary behaviour

Any waking behaviour performed while sitting, reclining or lying down, with an energy expenditure of ≤1.5 METs. Typical examples include TV viewing, screen use, deskwork, driving and reading.

Light physical activity

Activities requiring 1.6–2.9 METs. These involve gentle, low-effort movement such as slow walking, pottering around the home, light household tasks or casual play.

Moderate physical activity

Activities requiring 3–5.9 METs. These elevate the heart rate and breathing but still allow conversation, such as brisk walking, steady cycling, active games or water aerobics.

Vigorous physical activity

Activities requiring ≥6 METs. These substantially increase heart rate and breathing, such as running, fast cycling, aerobic dance or competitive sport.

Physical activity

Any bodily movement produced by skeletal muscles that increases energy expenditure. This broad term includes everyday movement (walking, cycling, wheeling), active recreation, sports, play and household or occupational activity.

Exercise

A structured subset of physical activity that is planned, purposeful and performed with the goal of improving or maintaining physical fitness (e.g., strength, flexibility, cardiorespiratory fitness).

Physical fitness

A set of attributes, such as aerobic capacity, muscular strength, endurance, flexibility and balance, that reflect the body's ability to perform physical activity or exercise.

MET

A standardised unit used to estimate energy expenditure. One MET reflects resting metabolic rate; higher MET values indicate greater intensity.

Sedentary time

The total accumulated time spent in sedentary behaviours across the day.

Physical inactivity

An insufficient level of physical activity to meet current guidelines. Importantly, a person can be physically inactive and still spend relatively little time sitting or vice versa.

Breaking up sedentary time

Interrupting prolonged sitting with brief bouts of standing or light movement. These short breaks can have independent metabolic and vascular benefits.

2.2 Understanding sedentary behaviour and cancer risk

It is well known that high levels of sedentary behaviour negatively impact health independently of other factors, including body weight, diet and physical activity (4–6). The World Health Organisation (WHO) identifies physical activity as critical to positive health outcomes for adults. These include reducing adiposity to support weight control, improving mental health by reducing anxiety and depression, and enhancing personal resilience to adverse life events (7). In a longitudinal study of 17,000 Canadian adults tracked over a 12-year period, those who spent most of their time sitting were more likely to die from all causes and cardiovascular disease (CVD), even after adjusting for confounding factors, such as age, smoking status and levels of physical activity (4). Evidence linking sedentary behaviour with cancer incidence and mortality comes from a recent umbrella review and meta-analysis. This study included 14 meta-analyses covering 17 cancer sites from 77 original studies and identified that sedentary behaviour was associated with an increased risk of developing six cancer types: Ovarian, endometrial, colon, breast, prostate and rectal cancers. This study also reported an increased risk of cancer mortality (8).

2.2.1 Prevalence of sedentary behaviour

Almost a third (31%) of the global population over the age of 15 is considered sedentary (6). The average duration of sedentary behaviour varies across global populations, with Koreans reporting the highest mean daily sedentary time at 8.3 hours, followed closely by Americans who spend an average of 7.7 hours engaging in sedentary behaviour (6). In Europe, 40% of leisure time is spent watching TV, equating to around 2.7 hours per day (9). In six low- and middle-income countries (China, Ghana, India, Mexico, Russia, South Africa), the overall prevalence of high sedentary behaviour was 8.3% (range: 7.1–9.7%). Higher sedentarism was associated with unemployment and urban residence (10). In the multi-ethnic Asian population of Singapore, 17% failed to meet the minimum physical activity guidelines, and nearly half (47.7%) spent ≥7 hours per day sedentary. Lower sedentary time was associated with older age and a primary-level education, while higher income, obesity and multiple comorbidities were linked with increased sedentary time (11).

Affluent populations have also been shown to spend a higher proportion of waking hours (≥70%) in sedentary behaviours (12). However, UK government data report that 70% of individuals living in the least deprived socio-economic areas are sufficiently active, and 20% engage in ≤30 minutes of moderate physical activity per week. In contrast, among those in the most deprived areas, just 55% are sufficiently active, representing a 15% difference (13). This lack of physical activity carries a large economic burden. In the UK, sedentary behaviour is estimated to cost up to £7.4 billion annually, including £0.9 billion to the National Health Service (NHS) alone (14).

Further disparities exist between genders and across ages. For example, women are consistently less active than men across all demographic categories, and perhaps unsurprisingly, older individuals are generally less active than younger adults. Nearly half of those over 75 engage in less than 30 minutes of physical activity each week, compared to only 20% of individuals aged 16 to 34 (13). UK Biobank data show differences in sedentary time by sex (female > male), education (did not attend college > did attend) and employment status, with employed men at highest risk for driving-related sedentary time (9). Numerous factors contribute to the rise in sedentary behaviour, including lack of available spaces for physical activity and exercise, increased sedentary occupations (e.g., office work) and increased screen time. These trends are summarised in Figure 2.2.

In summary, people face two overlapping challenges: (1) too little physical activity and (2) too much sitting. The overriding advice is to sit less and move more.

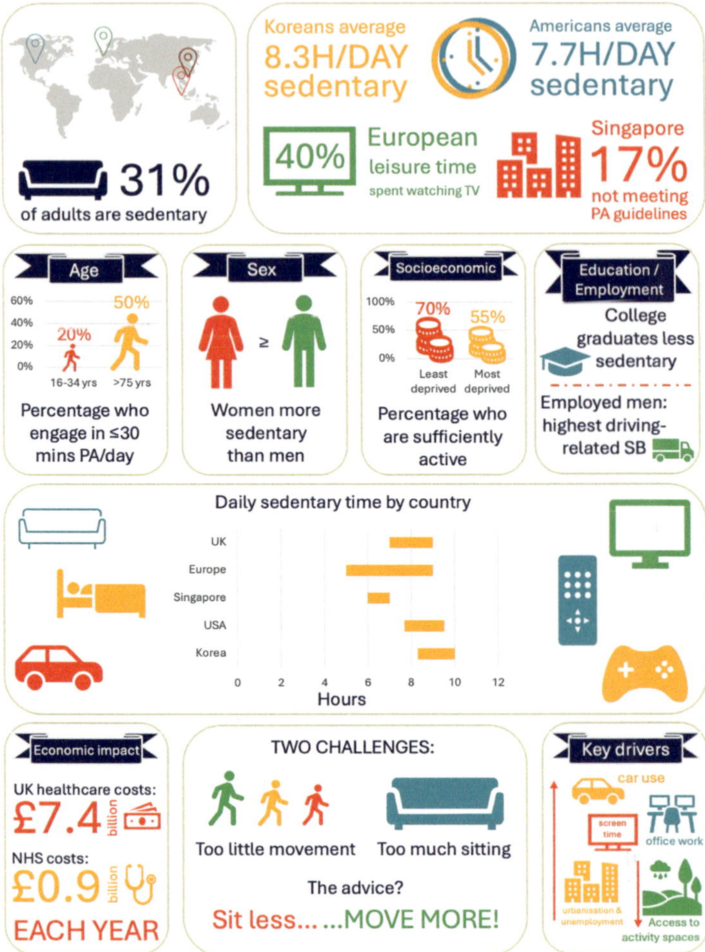

FIGURE 2.2 Global and demographic patterns of sedentary behaviour. This infographic summarises key trends in sedentary behaviour across global regions and demographic groups. Worldwide, nearly one-third of adults are sedentary, with substantial variation in daily sitting time across countries. Demographic disparities are evident: Women, older adults, people living in more deprived areas and those with lower educational attainment tend to spend more time sitting and are less likely to meet activity guidelines. Country-level comparisons highlight particularly high sedentary time in East Asia, North America and urbanised settings. These behaviours carry a significant economic burden, with UK sedentary behaviour estimated to cost £7.4 billion annually. Together, the data illustrate two overlapping public health challenges: Insufficient activity and excessive sitting, reinforcing the actionable message to sit less and move more. Data adapted from Sport England (2023), Park et al. (2020) and Patterson et al. (2018) (6,9,13).

2.2.2 Biological pathways linking sedentary behaviour to cancer

It is estimated that 30–40% of all cancers could be prevented through modification of lifestyle and environmental risk factors (15–18). Independent of physical activity status, sedentary behaviour has been shown to increase the risk of colon, endometrial and lung cancers (19). While physical inactivity and sedentary behaviour are often discussed together, they exert distinct effects on health. Prolonged sitting or low-energy postures alter systemic metabolism, vascular function and hormone regulation in ways that increase susceptibility to cancer. Many of these biological effects arise from metabolic dysregulation and chronic low-grade inflammation, both of which are key themes explored in more detail in Chapters 3 and 4.

2.2.2.1 Metabolic and endocrine dysregulation

Sedentary behaviour disrupts normal lipid and carbohydrate metabolism, largely through suppression of enzymes and transport proteins critical to metabolic homeostasis. For instance, inactivity reduces the activity of lipoprotein lipase (LPL), an enzyme that breaks down triglycerides in the blood, converting them into free fatty acids and glycerol for energy use. Reduced LPL activity contributes to metabolic dysfunctions, such as those observed in type 2 diabetes. In addition to raised levels of plasma triglycerides, lower levels of high-density lipoprotein (HDL) cholesterol and reduced insulin sensitivity are also observed (20,21). Moreover, low LPL concentrations are associated with hypertension, metabolic syndrome and coronary artery disease. Not only does sedentary behaviour reduce LPL blood concentration, but it also inhibits LPL activity in skeletal muscle tissue, signalling for impaired lipid metabolism (22,23).

In addition to reduced LPL activity, carbohydrate metabolism is also altered by sedentary behaviour through reduced expression of glucose transporter (GLUT) proteins in skeletal muscle (24). GLUT proteins are a family of membrane-spanning proteins responsible for the transport of glucose (and other nutrients) into the cells. The GLUT4 isoform, normally stimulated by insulin and exercise, becomes downregulated during periods of muscle inactivity, contributing to decreased glucose uptake and systemic insulin resistance (25–27). These metabolic disturbances are closely linked with cancer-promoting environments characterised by high circulating glucose, insulin and insulin-like growth factor-1 (IGF-1) (8).

Sedentary behaviour results in the loss of nerve supply to skeletal muscle, and this denervation in turn causes a reduction in both muscle GLUT4 content and insulin-stimulated glucose uptake (28), an effect that can be repaired with even very low-intensity exercise, as evidenced by studies in individuals with spinal cord injury—a population likely to exhibit high levels of sedentary behaviour (29,30). A plethora of systemic changes induced by sedentary behaviour are summarised in Figure 2.3.

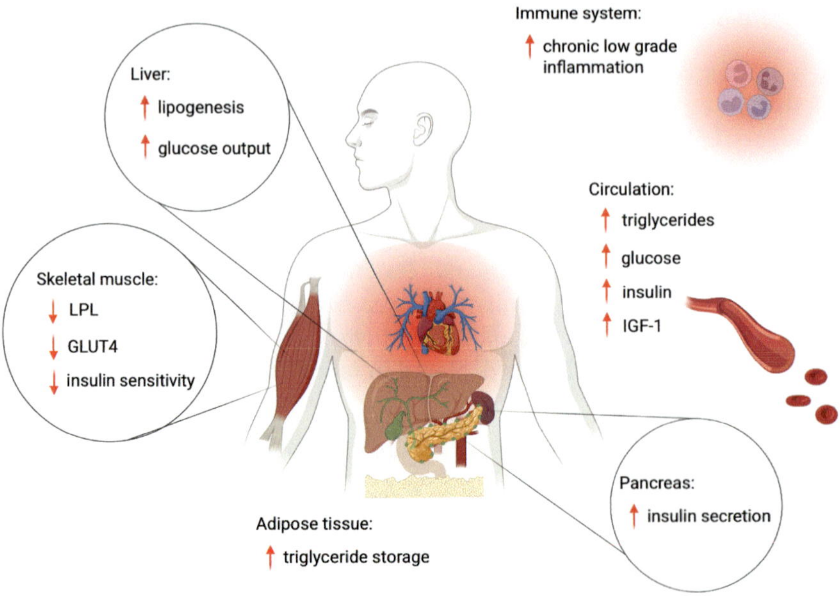

FIGURE 2.3 Systemic metabolic and endocrine consequences of sedentary behaviour. This figure illustrates how prolonged sedentary behaviour disrupts metabolic regulation across multiple organ systems, creating a systemic environment that favours cancer development. Muscle inactivity reduces LPL activity and downregulates glucose transporter-4 (GLUT4), leading to elevated circulating triglycerides, impaired glucose uptake and insulin resistance. These disruptions stimulate increased insulin and insulin-like growth factor-1 (IGF-1) signalling, with downstream effects on hepatic lipid metabolism, pancreatic hormone secretion and adipose tissue storage. Reduced skeletal muscle activity also contributes to poor vascular function and diminished shear stress, while altered immune cell signalling promotes chronic low-grade inflammation. Together, these metabolic, hormonal and inflammatory disturbances create a pro-tumourigenic milieu that increases susceptibility to cancers such as colon, endometrial and lung cancer. Created in Biorender.com.

2.2.2.2 Adiposity, hormones and cancer risk

Sedentary lifestyles contribute to increased adiposity, particularly visceral fat accumulation, which in turn alters systemic hormone profiles. In post-menopausal women, adipose tissue is a major site of aromatase activity, an enzyme which is involved in converting androgens to oestrogen (31). However, sedentary behaviour can also independently increase oestrogen levels, regardless of an individual's weight or BMI (32), suggesting that simply being active is not enough to counteract long sedentary periods. Oestrogen acts as a growth factor stimulating the proliferation of hormone-sensitive tissues such as the breast and endometrium, which in turn increases the risk of cancers in these sites. Furthermore, obesity and inactivity are linked with reduced circulating sex hormone-binding globulin (SHGB) protein, which binds freely circulating oestrogen, sequestering it away from its receptors. This in turn increases the availability of biologically active oestrogens and increases cancer risk (33).

Another pathway through which sedentary behaviour may elevate cancer risk involves the development of peripheral insulin resistance (34) and type 2 diabetes (35). These metabolic disturbances are characterised by increased circulating levels of insulin-like growth factor-1 (IGF-1) and blood glucose. Collectively, these factors promote cellular growth and proliferation, creating conditions that favour tumour development. Consequently, higher risks have been reported for several cancers, including those of the breast, endometrium, colon, liver, oesophagus, kidney and pancreas (36–39).

2.2.2.3 Inflammation and oxidative stress

Chronic, systemic low-grade inflammation, which is often observed in obese, overweight and sedentary individuals, is another independent risk factor for cancer. Reduced muscle contraction diminishes the release of anti-inflammatory cytokines (e.g., IL-10, IL-1Ra) and enhances the secretion of pro-inflammatory mediators from adipose tissue and immune cells. This shift towards a pro-inflammatory microenvironment drives DNA damage, oxidative stress and impaired DNA repair mechanisms, particularly in obesity-associated cancers such as those of the liver, colon and pancreas. Cancers develop from initiating events that involve irreversible DNA damage, for example, reactive oxygen species (ROS), but require a second round of stimulation (known as "promotion"), which can result from exposure to various chemical irritants or chronic inflammation. This induces cell growth and the recruitment of inflammatory cells, which in turn increase the production of ROS leading to oxidative DNA damage and reduced DNA repair. Normally, inflammation is self-limiting from the homeostatic production of anti-inflammatory cytokines following a spike in pro-inflammatory cytokines. However, chronic inflammation arises when initiating factors persist and the normal mechanisms for resolving inflammation fail (40). Together, these effects lead to an increased risk of developing various types of cancer, including endometrial, oesophageal, renal and pancreatic adenocarcinomas, hepatocellular carcinoma, gastric cardia cancer, meningioma, multiple myeloma, colorectal, post-menopausal breast, ovarian, gallbladder and thyroid cancers (41–43). These systemic biological effects of sedentary behaviour and cancer risk are summarised in Figure 2.4. See Chapter 4 for further discussion on inflammatory signalling and tumour-stromal crosstalk in the TME.

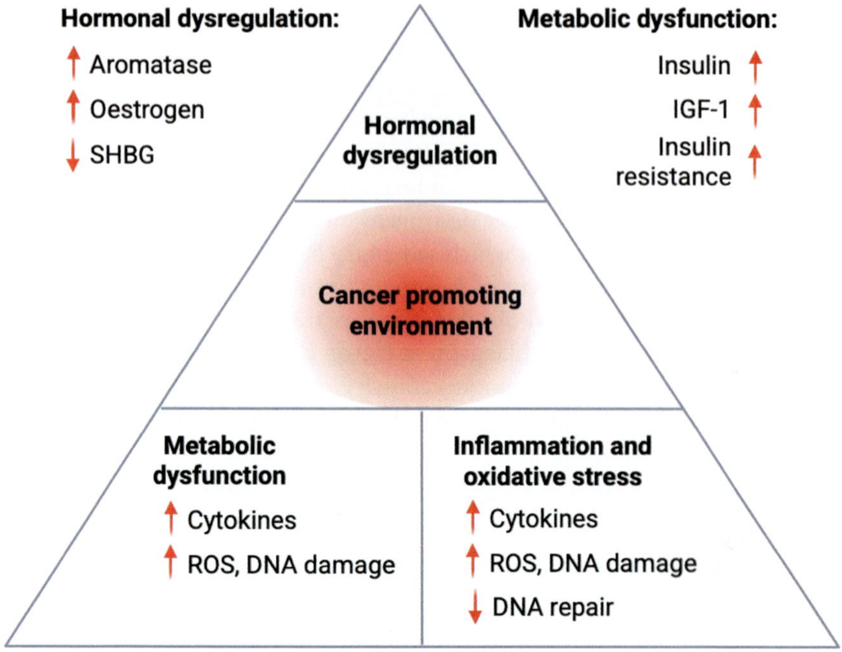

FIGURE 2.4 The biological effects linking sedentary behaviour to increased cancer risk. This figure illustrates three interconnected biological pathways through which sedentary behaviour contributes to a cancer-promoting internal environment. Hormonal dysregulation arises from increased aromatase activity in adipose tissue, elevated circulating oestrogen and reduced sex hormone-binding globulin (SHBG), all of which enhance the availability of bioactive sex hormones that stimulate growth in hormone-sensitive tissues. Metabolic dysfunction is characterised by insulin resistance, raised insulin and insulin-like growth factor-1 (IGF-1) concentrations, and associated downstream proliferative signalling. Inflammation and oxidative stress result from increased production of pro-inflammatory cytokines, higher levels of reactive oxygen species (ROS) and impaired DNA repair mechanisms. Together, these processes converge to create a systemic environment that favours cellular proliferation, DNA damage and tumour development across multiple organ sites. Created in Biorender.com.

See Chapters 3 and 4 for a detailed exploration of the biological mechanisms through which physical activity exerts its protective effects, including hormonal regulation, metabolic control and immunomodulation.

2.3 The protective role of physical activity against cancer

Physical activity is a well-established modifiable behaviour associated with a reduced risk of developing several types of cancer. This protective effect is observed across various demographic groups and activity domains, including occupational, recreational, household and transport-related activity. Importantly, physical activity can be accumulated across the lifespan or initiated later in life, with both approaches demonstrating protective benefits (19).

Large-scale epidemiological data suggest that regular physical activity may reduce the risk of developing several cancers by up to 30%, with most risk reductions ranging from 10–25% depending on cancer type (14,44). This protective effect does not differ significantly by sex or ethnicity and is particularly evident for certain cancers, including breast, colon and endometrial cancers. While observational data dominate this area, the sheer volume of consistent findings (over 500 studies as of 2020) supports the robustness of this association (19).

Despite this, there remain challenges in defining the optimal type, domain and volume of physical activity for cancer prevention and current evidence is still limited on how the association between physical activity and cancer varies by cancer type. Measurement approaches differ across studies, and while dose-response relationships are observed, precise thresholds for risk reduction remain difficult to quantify. Nonetheless, the evidence base continues to expand, and the role of physical activity in cancer prevention is now widely endorsed by public health agencies worldwide (45,103,104).

2.3.1 Epidemiological evidence linking physical activity to cancer risk

Physical activity is most strongly associated with reduced risk of colon, breast (particularly post-menopausal) and endometrial cancers. Moderate evidence exists for cancers of the bladder, oesophageal adenocarcinoma and cancers of the gastric cardia, with limited or emerging evidence for ovarian, pancreatic, renal and lung cancers (see Table 2.1 and Figure 2.5). The limited evidence for lung cancer is partly due to residual confounding factors from smoking (19). A small number of studies suggest a possible increased risk of melanoma among highly active individuals; however, this is likely due to increased UV exposure from time spent outdoors engaging in physical activity rather than the activity itself (46).

Lifelong physical activity is most protective, but even those who become active later in life experience benefits. For example, post-menopausal women who increase their physical activity can reduce their breast cancer risk regardless of premenopausal activity levels (44). The magnitude of risk

TABLE 2.1 Summary of epidemiologic evidence for cancer risk reduction with physical activity

Cancer site	*Evidence strength*	*Risk reduction (%)*
Colon	Strong	20–30%
Breast (postmenopausal)	Strong	15–25%
Endometrial	Strong	20–30%
Bladder	Moderate	~15%
Oesophageal adenocarcinoma	Moderate	~20%
Gastric cardia	Moderate	~20%
Ovarian, pancreatic, renal	Moderate-limited	10–15%
Lung	Limited	Variable (confounded)
Prostate	Limited	Inconclusive

Data taken from Friedenreich et al., 2021 and WCRF, 2018 (19,45).

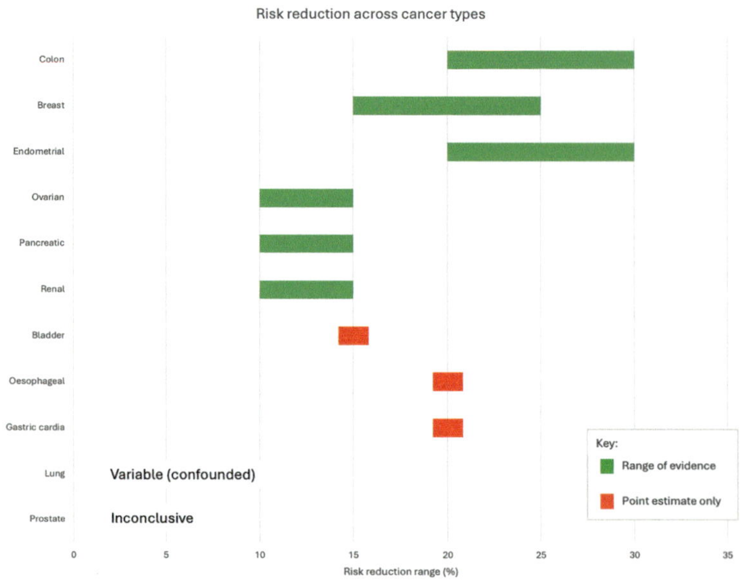

FIGURE 2.5 Estimated risk reduction associated with higher physical activity across cancer types. This chart summarises epidemiological estimates of the percentage reduction in cancer risk associated with higher levels of physical activity. Strongest protective associations are observed for colon, breast (post-menopausal) and endometrial cancers, with risk reductions typically ranging from 15–30%. Moderate protective effects are reported for cancers of the bladder, oesophageal adenocarcinoma and gastric cardia, while smaller or more variable effects (10–15%) are seen for ovarian, pancreatic and renal cancers. Evidence for lung cancer is limited due to residual confounding by smoking and current findings for prostate cancer remain inconclusive. Data taken from Friedenreich et al. (2021) and the World Cancer Research Fund (2018) (19,45).

reduction with higher levels of physical activity ranges from 10–25% for most cancers (44). Although a dose-response relationship can be observed between increasing levels of physical activity and specific cancer risks for several cancers, the methods for measuring and categorising physical activity levels vary across epidemiological studies, making it difficult to definitively conclude exactly how much physical activity is required to provide an effect. Moreover, there is insufficient evidence to identify specific links between which domain (e.g., leisure versus household) or type (e.g., aerobic versus resistance) of physical activity is required to reduce risk (47).

2.3.2 *Physical activity in the cancer care continuum*

In addition to reducing primary cancer risk, physical activity also plays a key role before, during and after cancer treatment. In the pre-treatment phase, a model known as prehabilitation (or "prehab") focuses on optimising patients' health to improve treatment outcomes (see Box-out 2.2). Prehab covers three key areas of health: 1) diet and weight; 2) physical activity and exercise; and 3) mental wellbeing (48). Originated from a military model of getting soldiers physically and emotionally ready for combat (49), prehabilitation is a model of care in rehabilitation. Evidence suggests cancer prehabilitation leads to better functional outcomes for patients and improves many important endpoints for surgery and cancer treatment (50).

Multimodal prehabilitation involves two or more interventions which may have cumulative or synergistic effects on health outcomes. Interventions could include any combination of the following: 1) aerobic exercise to maintain cardiorespiratory function or resistance training to prevent musculoskeletal deconditioning; 2) dietary interventions to combat disease-driven or treatment-related malnutrition, to support building muscular strength and conditioning, and to support the metabolic cost of exercise; 3) psychological interventions to reduce stress and anxiety; 4) lifestyle behaviour changes (e.g., smoking cessation, reduction in alcohol consumption); 5) optimising medications and treating underlying complications such as anaemia; 6) counselling to promote behaviour change to support adherence to interventions and establish self-management skills to empower patients to maintain long-term health behaviours (51,52).

Since its first appearance in the literature, the evidence supporting prehabilitation in cancer care has grown exponentially. The evidence base has developed primarily from colorectal, lung, gastrointestinal, prostate and haematological cancers (53–66). Exercise-based prehabilitation has been associated with improvements in physical function, shorter hospital stays, fewer complications and better QoL in patients with cancers of the digestive system (67). In prostate cancer patients, for example, prehab can reduce post-operative incontinence and the loss of muscle mass (68–71). In breast cancer, it can reduce the risk of treatment-induced lymphoedema and preserve functional capacity (65,66,72,73). While the majority of literature focuses on surgery, emerging data also support exercise prehabilitation before chemotherapy or radiotherapy (74–76). Systematic reviews show high feasibility (89.7%) and acceptability (87.7%) of prehabilitation interventions, with no significant adverse effects (63). While prehabilitation could become integral to healthcare plans for cancer survivors, it is intended to complement post-treatment rehabilitation, not replace it (77).

BOX-OUT 2.2 DEFINITION OF CANCER PREHABILITATION

"A process in the cancer continuum of care that occurs between the time of cancer diagnosis and the beginning of acute treatment and includes physical and psychological assessments that establish a baseline functional level, identify impairments, and provide interventions that promote physical and psychological health to reduce the incidence and/or severity of future impairments."—Silver & Baima, 2013 (78)

2.3.3 Physical activity and exercise during and after cancer treatment

Physical activity during treatment has been shown to mitigate several common side effects of cancer and its therapies, including fatigue, depression, cognitive changes, pain and sleep disturbances. It also improves physical functioning, cardiorespiratory fitness and bone health (79). The benefits of both aerobic and resistance exercise are discussed in more detail in Chapter 5. In brief, aerobic exercise has been shown to improve fatigue, anxiety and sleep quality (80–84), while resistance exercise can improve muscle mass, strength and chemotherapy tolerance (79,85–87). Importantly, patients do not need to engage in intense or prolonged exercise to see benefits. Even small increases in physical activity are associated with improvements in treatment response and overall wellbeing. For instance, relatively inactive patients are less likely to achieve optimal chemotherapy dosing compared with those who are physically active (88). Post-treatment rehabilitation is traditionally focused on improving QoL by improving physical functioning and independent living. As a result, this could contribute to the chronic problem of under-referral from oncology services (89–97) since oncologists are primarily focused on survival outcomes, rather than issues like cancer-related fatigue, chemotherapy-induced peripheral neuropathy and musculoskeletal dysfunction.

2.4 Long-term benefits of exercise for cancer survivors

Emerging evidence suggests that physical activity not only improves QoL during and after cancer treatment but may also play a role in reducing recurrence and slowing metastatic progression. A narrative review of 24 studies surmised that physical activity can regulate key steps in the metastatic cascade—the complex biological process through which cancer cells spread from the primary tumour to distant organs (98). In particular, moderate-intensity exercise has been shown to promote vascular normalisation, reduce endothelial permeability and enhance immune surveillance, thereby reducing opportunities for circulating tumour cells (CTCs) to establish secondary tumours (99). Exercise-induced shear stress and improved perfusion may help to stabilise the tumour vasculature, reducing hypoxia and the associated pro-metastatic signalling. Moreover, regular physical activity may enhance natural killer (NK) cell mobilisation and function, improving the body's ability to identify and destroy tumour cells in circulation (100). By contrast, in some contexts, high-intensity exercise may temporarily suppress immune function or promote stress hormone release, particularly if unaccustomed or performed without adequate warm-up, which may therefore facilitate tumour cell escape and survival (98). While the majority of these studies are conducted in mouse models and human data remain limited, these findings point to a protective effect of chronic, moderate-intensity endurance activity, particularly when undertaken consistently post-diagnosis. Observational cohort studies in breast and colorectal cancer survivors, for example, have linked higher physical activity levels with reduced risk of recurrence and cancer-specific mortality (101,102). Overall, chronic adaptations to moderate-intensity endurance exercise seem to be the most effective way to prevent metastasis. The mechanistic basis of these concepts will be explored in more detail in Chapters 3 and 4.

2.5 Conclusion

This chapter has explored the dual narrative of how sedentary behaviour and physical activity independently influence cancer risk, progression and survivorship. While sedentary lifestyles contribute to the development of several cancer types through metabolic dysregulation, inflammation, hormonal imbalance and impaired immune function, regular physical activity offers significant protective benefits, not only in preventing cancer but also in improving treatment outcomes and long-term survivorship. Epidemiological evidence supports a consistent association between higher levels of physical activity and reduced risk of cancers such as breast, colorectal and endometrial. Just as importantly, even small increases in activity, especially for those starting from a sedentary baseline, can yield meaningful improvements in QoL, treatment tolerance and functional capacity.

Yet, challenges remain. Sedentary behaviour is widespread and often socially and structurally reinforced, particularly in ageing, low-income and chronically ill populations. Despite growing awareness, many cancer survivors remain insufficiently active, with under-referral and poor access to rehabilitation services continuing to limit progress. Looking ahead, further research is needed to clarify the optimal types, doses and modes of activity for specific cancer populations, and to understand how exercise interacts with emerging therapies, such as immunotherapy.

Chapter 2 Test your understanding question bank

1. Define sedentary behaviour and explain how it differs from physical inactivity.
2. What MET categories classify light, moderate and vigorous physical activity? Provide one example of each.
3. Why is it important not to use the terms "physical activity" and "exercise" interchangeably when interpreting epidemiological evidence?
4. Summarise two major global patterns in sedentary behaviour. Which populations are most sedentary?
5. Describe two socio-economic or demographic disparities in physical activity or sedentary behaviour identified in the UK.
6. What evidence links sedentary time to increased cancer incidence or mortality?
7. List three biological pathways through which sedentary behaviour increases cancer risk.
8. Explain the role of lipoprotein lipase (LPL) in metabolic health and describe what happens to LPL during prolonged sitting.
9. How does reduced GLUT4 expression contribute to insulin resistance, and why is this relevant for cancer development.
10. Describe how adiposity and sedentary behaviour influence hormone levels in post-menopausal women.
11. Explain how chronic, low-grade inflammation contributes to carcinogenesis. In your answer, refer to ROS and DNA repair.
12. Outline how sedentary behaviour could elevate risk for both endometrial and pancreatic cancer, despite differences in tissue type.
13. Which three cancer types have the strongest evidence for risk reduction through physical activity, and what is the approximate percentage reduction?
14. Why is the evidence for physical activity and lung cancer risk reduction considered limited?

15. Despite measurement challenges, what overall conclusions can be drawn about the dose-response relationship between physical activity and cancer risk?
16. Describe how becoming physically active later in life can still reduce cancer risk. Provide one example from epidemiological studies.
17. Define "cancer prehabilitation" and describe its purpose within the treatment pathway.
18. Explain two ways in which moderate-intensity exercise may reduce metastatic progression after a cancer diagnosis.

References

1. Tremblay MS, Aubert S, Barnes JD, Saunders TJ, Carson V, Latimer-Cheung AE, et al. Sedentary Behavior Research Network (SBRN)—Terminology consensus project process and outcome. International Journal of Behavioral Nutrition and Physical Activity [Internet]. 2017 Dec 10 [cited 2024 Nov 8];14(1):75. Available from: http://ijbnpa.biomedcentral.com/articles/10.1186/s12966-017-0525-8
2. Dasso NA. How is exercise different from physical activity? A concept analysis. Nurs Forum (Auckl) [Internet]. 2019 Jan [cited 2024 Nov 8];54(1): 45–52. Available from: http://www.ncbi.nlm.nih.gov/pubmed/30332516
3. Tremblay MS, Aubert S, Barnes JD, Saunders TJ, Carson V, Latimer-Cheung AE, et al. Sedentary Behavior Research Network (SBRN)—Terminology consensus project process and outcome. International Journal of Behavioral Nutrition and Physical Activity [Internet]. 2017 Jun 10 [cited 2025 Nov 22];14(1). Available from: https://www.sedentarybehaviour.org/what-is-sedentary-behaviour/
4. Katzmarzyk PT, Church TS, Craig CL, Bouchard C. Sitting time and mortality from all causes, cardiovascular disease, and cancer. Med Sci Sports Exerc [Internet]. 2009 May [cited 2024 Nov 8];41(5):998–1005. Available from: https://journals.lww.com/00005768-200905000-00005
5. De Rezende LFM, Lopes MR, Rey-Lopéz JP, Matsudo VKR, Luiz ODC. Sedentary behavior and health outcomes: An overview of systematic reviews. PLoS One [Internet]. 2014 Aug 21 [cited 2025 Nov 14];9(8):e105620. Available from: https://pmc.ncbi.nlm.nih.gov/articles/PMC4140795/
6. Park JH, Moon JH, Kim HJ, Kong MH, Oh YH. Sedentary lifestyle: Overview of updated evidence of potential health risks. Korean J Fam Med [Internet]. 2020 Nov [cited 2024 Nov 8];41(6):365–73. Available from: http://www.ncbi.nlm.nih.gov/pubmed/33242381
7. WHO guidelines on physical activity and sedentary behaviour [Internet]. [cited 2025 Nov 14]. Available from: https://www.who.int/publications/i/item/9789240015128
8. Hermelink R, Leitzmann MF, Markozannes G, Tsilidis K, Pukrop T, Berger F, et al. Sedentary behavior and cancer–an umbrella review and meta-analysis. Eur J Epidemiol [Internet]. 2022 May 25 [cited 2024 Nov 8];37(5):447–60. Available from: https://link.springer.com/10.1007/s10654-022-00873-6
9. Patterson R, McNamara E, Tainio M, de Sá TH, Smith AD, Sharp SJ, et al. Sedentary behaviour and risk of all-cause, cardiovascular and cancer mortality, and incident type 2 diabetes: A systematic review and dose response meta-analysis. Eur J Epidemiol [Internet]. 2018 Sep 28 [cited 2024

Nov 8];33(9):811–29. Available from: http://link.springer.com/10.1007/s10654-018-0380-1
10. Koyanagi A, Stubbs B, Vancampfort D. Correlates of sedentary behavior in the general population: A cross-sectional study using nationally representative data from six low- and middle-income countries. PLoS One [Internet]. 2018 [cited 2024 Nov 8];13(8):e0202222. Available from: http://www.ncbi.nlm.nih.gov/pubmed/30096192
11. Lau JH, Nair A, Abdin E, Kumarasan R, Wang P, Devi F, et al. Prevalence and patterns of physical activity, sedentary behaviour, and their association with health-related quality of life within a multi-ethnic Asian population. BMC Public Health [Internet]. 2021 Dec 25 [cited 2024 Nov 8];21(1):1939. Available from: https://bmcpublichealth.biomedcentral.com/articles/10.1186/s12889-021-11902-6
12. Owen N, Sparling PB, Healy GN, Dunstan DW, Matthews CE. Sedentary behavior: Emerging evidence for a new health risk. Mayo Clin Proc [Internet]. 2010 Dec [cited 2024 Nov 8];85(12):1138–41. Available from: http://www.ncbi.nlm.nih.gov/pubmed/21123641
13. Active Lives | Sport England [Internet]. [cited 2025 Nov 14]. Available from: https://www.sportengland.org/research-and-data/data/active-lives
14. Physical activity: Applying All Our Health—GOV.UK [Internet]. [cited 2025 Nov 14]. Available from: https://www.gov.uk/government/publications/physical-activity-applying-all-our-health/physical-activity-applying-all-our-health
15. Kulhánová I, Znaor A, Shield KD, Arnold M, Vignat J, Charafeddine M, et al. Proportion of cancers attributable to major lifestyle and environmental risk factors in the Eastern Mediterranean region. Int J Cancer [Internet]. 2020 Feb 1 [cited 2025 Nov 14];146(3):646–56. Available from: https://pubmed.ncbi.nlm.nih.gov/30882889/
16. Parkin DM, Boyd L, Walker LC. 16. The fraction of cancer attributable to lifestyle and environmental factors in the UK in 2010. Br J Cancer [Internet]. 2011 Dec 6 [cited 2025 Nov 14];105 Suppl 2(Suppl 2):S77–81. Available from: https://pubmed.ncbi.nlm.nih.gov/22158327/
17. Poirier AE, Ruan Y, Volesky KD, King WD, O'Sullivan DE, Gogna P, et al. The current and future burden of cancer attributable to modifiable risk factors in Canada: Summary of results. Prev Med (Baltim) [Internet]. 2019 May 1 [cited 2025 Nov 14];122:140–7. Available from: https://pubmed.ncbi.nlm.nih.gov/31078167/
18. Whiteman DC, Webb PM, Green AC, Neale RE, Fritschi L, Bain CJ, et al. Cancers in Australia in 2010 attributable to modifiable factors: Summary and conclusions. Aust N Z J Public Health [Internet]. 2015 Oct 1 [cited 2025 Nov 14];39(5):477. Available from: https://pmc.ncbi.nlm.nih.gov/articles/PMC4606779/
19. Friedenreich CM, Ryder-Burbidge C, McNeil J. Physical activity, obesity and sedentary behavior in cancer etiology: Epidemiologic evidence and biologic mechanisms. Mol Oncol [Internet]. 2021 Mar [cited 2024 Dec 13];15(3):790–800. Available from: http://www.ncbi.nlm.nih.gov/pubmed/32741068
20. Yanagibori R, Kondo K, Suzuki Y, Kawakubo K, Iwamoto T, Itakura H, et al. Effect of 20 days' bed rest on the reverse cholesterol transport system in healthy young subjects. J Intern Med [Internet]. 1998 [cited 2025 Nov 14];243(4):307–12. Available from: https://pubmed.ncbi.nlm.nih.gov/9627145/
21. Hamburg NM, McMackin CJ, Huang AL, Shenouda SM, Widlansky ME, Schulz E, et al. Physical inactivity rapidly induces insulin resistance and

microvascular dysfunction in healthy volunteers. Arterioscler Thromb Vasc Biol [Internet]. 2007 Dec [cited 2025 Nov 14];27(12):2650–6. Available from: https://pubmed.ncbi.nlm.nih.gov/17932315/
22. Hamilton MT, Hamilton DG, Zderic TW. Role of low energy expenditure and sitting in obesity, metabolic syndrome, type 2 diabetes, and cardiovascular disease. Diabetes [Internet]. 2007 Nov [cited 2025 Nov 14];56(11): 2655–67. Available from: https://pubmed.ncbi.nlm.nih.gov/17827399/
23. Bey L, Hamilton MT. Suppression of skeletal muscle lipoprotein lipase activity during physical inactivity: A molecular reason to maintain daily low-intensity activity. J Physiol [Internet]. 2003 Sep 1 [cited 2025 Nov 14];551(Pt 2):673–82. Available from: https://pubmed.ncbi.nlm.nih.gov/12815182/
24. Tremblay MS, Colley RC, Saunders TJ, Healy GN, Owen N. Physiological and health implications of a sedentary lifestyle. Applied Physiology, Nutrition, and Metabolism [Internet]. 2010 Dec [cited 2025 Jan 17];35(6):725–40. Available from: http://www.nrcresearchpress.com/doi/10.1139/H10-079
25. Henriksen EJ, Bourey RE, Rodnick KJ, Koranyi L, Permutt MA, Holloszy JO. Glucose transporter protein content and glucose transport capacity in rat skeletal muscles. Am J Physiol [Internet]. 1990 [cited 2025 Nov 14];259(4 Pt 1). Available from: https://pubmed.ncbi.nlm.nih.gov/1699426/
26. Klip A, Pâquet MR. Glucose transport and glucose transporters in muscle and their metabolic regulation. Diabetes Care [Internet]. 1990 [cited 2025 Nov 14];13(3):228–43. Available from: https://pubmed.ncbi.nlm.nih.gov/2407478/
27. Kawanaka K, Tabata I, Katsuta S, Higuchi M. Changes in insulin-stimulated glucose transport and GLUT-4 protein in rat skeletal muscle after training. J Appl Physiol (1985) [Internet]. 1997 [cited 2025 Nov 14];83(6):2043–7. Available from: https://pubmed.ncbi.nlm.nih.gov/9390979/
28. Megeney LA, Neufer PD, Dohm GL, Tan MH, Blewett CA, Elder GCB, et al. Effects of muscle activity and fiber composition on glucose transport and GLUT-4. Am J Physiol [Internet]. 1993 [cited 2025 Nov 14];264(4 Pt 1). Available from: https://pubmed.ncbi.nlm.nih.gov/8476037/
29. Chilibeck PD, Bell G, Jeon J, Weiss CB, Murdoch G, MacLean I, et al. Functional electrical stimulation exercise increases GLUT-1 and GLUT-4 in paralyzed skeletal muscle. Metabolism [Internet]. 1999 [cited 2025 Nov 14];48(11):1409–13. Available from: https://pubmed.ncbi.nlm.nih.gov/10582549/
30. Phillips SM, Stewart BG, Mahoney DJ, Hicks AL, McCartney N, Tang JE, et al. Body-weight-support treadmill training improves blood glucose regulation in persons with incomplete spinal cord injury. J Appl Physiol (1985) [Internet]. 2004 Aug [cited 2025 Nov 14];97(2):716–24. Available from: https://pubmed.ncbi.nlm.nih.gov/15107410/
31. Blakemore J, Naftolin F. Aromatase: Contributions to physiology and disease in women and men. Physiology [Internet]. 2016 Jul 1 [cited 2025 Nov 14];31(4):258–69. Available from: https://journals.physiology.org/doi/10.1152/physiol.00054.2015
32. Dallal CM, Brinton LA, Matthews CE, Pfeiffer RM, Hartman TJ, Lissowska J, et al. Association of active and sedentary behaviors with postmenopausal estrogen metabolism. Med Sci Sports Exerc [Internet]. 2016 Mar 1 [cited 2025 Nov 14];48(3):439–48. Available from: https://pubmed.ncbi.nlm.nih.gov/26460631/
33. Simó R, Saez-Lopez C, Lecube A, Hernandez C, Fort JM, Selva DM. Adiponectin upregulates SHBG production: Molecular mechanisms and potential

implications. Endocrinology [Internet]. 2014 [cited 2025 Nov 14];155(8): 2820–30. Available from: https://pubmed.ncbi.nlm.nih.gov/24828613/
34. Helmerhorst HJF, Wijndaele K, Brage S, Wareham NJ, Ekelund U. Objectively measured sedentary time may predict insulin resistance independent of moderate- and vigorous-intensity physical activity. Diabetes [Internet]. 2009 Aug [cited 2025 Nov 14];58(8):1776–9. Available from: https://pubmed.ncbi.nlm.nih.gov/19470610/
35. Hamilton MT, Hamilton DG, Zderic TW. Sedentary behavior as a mediator of type 2 diabetes. Med Sport Sci [Internet]. 2014 Sep 15 [cited 2025 Nov 14];60:11–26. Available from: https://pubmed.ncbi.nlm.nih.gov/25226797/
36. Nead KT, Sharp SJ, Thompson DJ, Painter JN, Savage DB, Semple RK, et al. Evidence of a causal association between insulinemia and endometrial cancer: A mendelian randomization analysis. J Natl Cancer Inst [Internet]. 2015 Sep 1 [cited 2025 Nov 14];107(9). Available from: https://pubmed.ncbi.nlm.nih.gov/26134033/
37. Vrachnis N, Iavazzo C, Iliodromiti Z, Sifakis S, Alexandrou A, Siristatidis C, et al. Diabetes mellitus and gynecologic cancer: Molecular mechanisms, epidemiological, clinical and prognostic perspectives. Arch Gynecol Obstet [Internet]. 2016 Feb 1 [cited 2025 Nov 14];293(2):239–46. Available from: https://pubmed.ncbi.nlm.nih.gov/26338721/
38. Poloz Y, Stambolic V. Obesity and cancer, a case for insulin signaling. Cell Death Dis [Internet]. 2015 Dec 1 [cited 2025 Nov 14];6(12). Available from: https://pubmed.ncbi.nlm.nih.gov/26720346/
39. Pearson-Stuttard J, Papadimitriou N, Markozannes G, Cividini S, Kakourou A, Gill D, et al. Type 2 diabetes and cancer: An umbrella review of observational and mendelian randomization studies. Cancer Epidemiol Biomarkers Prev [Internet]. 2021 Jun 1 [cited 2025 Nov 14];30(6):1218–28. Available from: https://pubmed.ncbi.nlm.nih.gov/33737302/
40. Coussens LM, Werb Z. Inflammation and cancer. Nature [Internet]. 2002 Dec 26 [cited 2025 Nov 14];420(6917):860. Available from: https://pmc.ncbi.nlm.nih.gov/articles/PMC2803035/
41. Kyrgiou M, Kalliala I, Markozannes G, Gunter MJ, Paraskevaidis E, Gabra H, et al. Adiposity and cancer at major anatomical sites: Umbrella review of the literature. BMJ [Internet]. 2017 Feb 28 [cited 2025 Nov 14];356:477. Available from: https://www.bmj.com/content/356/bmj.j477
42. Avgerinos KI, Spyrou N, Mantzoros CS, Dalamaga M. Obesity and cancer risk: Emerging biological mechanisms and perspectives. Metabolism [Internet]. 2019 Mar 1 [cited 2025 Nov 14];92:121–35. Available from: https://pubmed.ncbi.nlm.nih.gov/30445141/
43. Onstad MA, Schmandt RE, Lu KH. Addressing the role of obesity in endometrial cancer risk, prevention, and treatment. J Clin Oncol [Internet]. 2016 Dec 10 [cited 2025 Nov 14];34(35):4225–30. Available from: https://pubmed.ncbi.nlm.nih.gov/27903150/
44. McTiernan A, Friedenreich CM, Katzmarzyk PT, Powell KE, Macko R, Buchner D, et al. Physical activity in cancer prevention and survival: A systematic review. Med Sci Sports Exerc [Internet]. 2019 Jun [cited 2024 Nov 8];51(6):1252–61. Available from: https://journals.lww.com/00005768-201906000-00020
45. Aicr, WCRF. Diet, nutrition, physical activity and cancer: a global perspective a summary of the third expert report. [cited 2025 Nov 14]. Available from: http://gco.iarc.fr/today
46. Moore SC, Lee IM, Weiderpass E, Campbell PT, Sampson JN, Kitahara CM, et al. Association of leisure-time physical activity with risk of 26 types of

cancer in 1.44 million adults. JAMA Intern Med [Internet]. 2016 Jun 1 [cited 2025 Nov 14];176(6):816–25. Available from: https://jamanetwork.com/journals/jamainternalmedicine/fullarticle/2521826
47. HHS. 2018 physical activity guidelines advisory committee scientific report. 2018.
48. What is prehabilitation? | Cancer Research UK [Internet]. [cited 2025 Nov 14]. Available from: https://www.cancerresearchuk.org/about-cancer/treatment/prehabilitation/what-is-prehabilitation
49. PREHABILITATION, rehabilitation, and revocation in the Army—PubMed [Internet]. [cited 2025 Nov 14]. Available from: https://pubmed.ncbi.nlm.nih.gov/20989832/
50. Stout NL, Fu J, Silver JK. Prehabilitation is the gateway to better functional outcomes for individuals with cancer. J Cancer Rehabil [Internet]. 2021 [cited 2025 Nov 14];4:283. Available from: https://pmc.ncbi.nlm.nih.gov/articles/PMC8765744/
51. Santa Mina D, Brahmbhatt P, Lopez C, Baima J, Gillis C, Trachtenberg L, et al. The case for prehabilitation prior to breast cancer treatment. PM R [Internet]. 2017 Sep 1 [cited 2025 Nov 14];9(9S2):S305–16. Available from: https://pubmed.ncbi.nlm.nih.gov/28942905/
52. Carli F, Silver JK, Feldman LS, McKee A, Gilman S, Gillis C, et al. Surgical prehabilitation in patients with cancer: State-of-the-science and recommendations for future research from a panel of subject matter experts. Phys Med Rehabil Clin N Am [Internet]. 2017 Feb 1 [cited 2025 Nov 14];28(1):49–64. Available from: https://pubmed.ncbi.nlm.nih.gov/27913000/
53. Bousquet-Dion G, Awasthi R, Loiselle SÈ, Minnella EM, Agnihotram RV, Bergdahl A, et al. Evaluation of supervised multimodal prehabilitation programme in cancer patients undergoing colorectal resection: A randomized control trial. Acta Oncol [Internet]. 2018 Jun 3 [cited 2025 Nov 14];57(6):849–59. Available from: https://pubmed.ncbi.nlm.nih.gov/29327644/
54. Brown JC, Damjanov N, Courneya KS, Troxel AB, Zemel BS, Rickels MR, et al. A randomized dose-response trial of aerobic exercise and health-related quality of life in colon cancer survivors. Psychooncology [Internet]. 2018 Apr 1 [cited 2025 Nov 14];27(4):1221–8. Available from: https://pubmed.ncbi.nlm.nih.gov/29388275/
55. Van Rooijen SJ, Molenaar CJL, Schep G, Van Lieshout RHMA, Beijer S, Dubbers R, et al. Making patients fit for surgery: Introducing a four pillar multimodal prehabilitation program in colorectal cancer. Am J Phys Med Rehabil [Internet]. 2019 Oct 1 [cited 2025 Nov 14];98(10):888–96. Available from: https://pubmed.ncbi.nlm.nih.gov/31090551/
56. Li C, Carli F, Lee L, Charlebois P, Stein B, Liberman AS, et al. Impact of a trimodal prehabilitation program on functional recovery after colorectal cancer surgery: A pilot study. Surg Endosc [Internet]. 2013 [cited 2025 Nov 14];27(4):1072–82. Available from: https://pubmed.ncbi.nlm.nih.gov/23052535/
57. Cesario A, Ferri L, Galetta D, Cardaci V, Biscione G, Pasqua F, et al. Preoperative pulmonary rehabilitation and surgery for lung cancer. Lung Cancer [Internet]. 2007 Jul [cited 2025 Nov 14];57(1):118–9. Available from: https://pubmed.ncbi.nlm.nih.gov/17475363/
58. Smith SR, Khanna A, Wisotzky EM. An evolving role for cancer rehabilitation in the era of low-dose lung computed tomography screening. PM R [Internet]. 2017 Sep 1 [cited 2025 Nov 14];9(9S2):S407–14. Available from: https://pubmed.ncbi.nlm.nih.gov/28942912/
59. van Haren IEPM, Staal JB, Potting CM, Atsma F, Hoogeboom TJ, Blijlevens NMA, et al. Physical exercise prior to hematopoietic stem cell transplantation:

A feasibility study. Physiother Theory Pract [Internet]. 2018 Oct 3 [cited 2025 Nov 14];34(10):747–56. Available from: https://pubmed.ncbi.nlm.nih.gov/29336645/

60. Liang Y, Zhou M, Wang F, Wu Z. Exercise for physical fitness, fatigue and quality of life of patients undergoing hematopoietic stem cell transplantation: A meta-analysis of randomized controlled trials. Jpn J Clin Oncol [Internet]. 2018 Dec 1 [cited 2025 Nov 14];48(12):1046–57. Available from: https://pubmed.ncbi.nlm.nih.gov/30277514/
61. Molenaar CJL, Minnella EM, Coca-Martinez M, Ten Cate DWG, Regis M, Awasthi R, et al. Effect of multimodal prehabilitation on reducing postoperative complications and enhancing functional capacity following colorectal cancer surgery: The PREHAB Randomized Clinical Trial. JAMA Surg [Internet]. 2023 Jun 14 [cited 2025 Nov 14];158(6):572. Available from: https://pmc.ncbi.nlm.nih.gov/articles/PMC10061316/
62. Maroto-Izquierdo S, Bautista IJ, Pérez-Guerrero A, Redondo-Delgado P, Jauregui-Fajardo I, Simó V, et al. Effects of prehabilitation concurrent exercise on functional capacity in colorectal cancer patients: A systematic review and meta-analysis. Healthcare (Switzerland) [Internet]. 2025 May 1 [cited 2025 Nov 14];13(10):1119. Available from: https://www.mdpi.com/2227-9032/13/10/1119/htm
63. Michael CM, Lehrer EJ, Schmitz KH, Zaorsky NG. Prehabilitation exercise therapy for cancer: A systematic review and meta-analysis. Cancer Med [Internet]. 2021 Jul [cited 2025 Jan 10];10(13):4195–205. Available from: http://www.ncbi.nlm.nih.gov/pubmed/34110101
64. Rahota RG, Salin A, Gautier JR, Almeras C, Garnault V, Tollon C, et al. A prehabilitation programme implemented before robot-assisted radical prostatectomy improves peri-operative outcomes and continence recovery. BJU Int [Internet]. 2022 Sep 1 [cited 2025 Nov 14];130(3):357–63. Available from: https://pubmed.ncbi.nlm.nih.gov/34854212/
65. Shamsesfandabadi P, Shams Esfand Abadi M, Yin Y, Carpenter DJ, Peluso C, Hilton C, et al. Resistance training and lymphedema in breast cancer survivors. JAMA Netw Open [Internet]. 2025 Jun 2 [cited 2025 Nov 14];8(6):e2514765–e2514765. Available from: https://jamanetwork.com/journals/jamanetworkopen/fullarticle/2835176
66. Toohey K, Hunter M, McKinnon K, Casey T, Turner M, Taylor S, et al. A systematic review of multimodal prehabilitation in breast cancer. Breast Cancer Res Treat [Internet]. 2023 Jan 1 [cited 2025 Nov 14];197(1):1–37. Available from: https://pubmed.ncbi.nlm.nih.gov/36269525/
67. Xu S, Yin R, Zhu H, Gong Y, Zhu J, Li C, et al. The role of exercise-based prehabilitation in enhancing surgical outcomes for patients with digestive system cancers: a meta-analysis. BMC Gastroenterol [Internet]. 2025 Dec 1 [cited 2025 Nov 14];25(1):26. Available from: https://bmcgastroenterol.biomedcentral.com/articles/10.1186/s12876-025-03626-3
68. Santa Mina D, Hilton WJ, Matthew AG, Awasthi R, Bousquet-Dion G, Alibhai SMH, et al. Prehabilitation for radical prostatectomy: A multicentre randomized controlled trial. Surg Oncol [Internet]. 2018 Jun 1 [cited 2025 Nov 14];27(2):289–98. Available from: https://pubmed.ncbi.nlm.nih.gov/29937184/
69. Paterson C, Primeau C, Pullar I, Nabi G. Development of a prehabilitation multimodal supportive care interventions for men and their partners before radical prostatectomy for localized prostate cancer. Cancer Nurs [Internet]. 2019 Jul 1 [cited 2025 Nov 14];42(4):E47–53. Available from: https://pubmed.ncbi.nlm.nih.gov/29933304/

70. Centemero A, Rigatti L, Giraudo D, Lazzeri M, Lughezzani G, Zugna D, et al. Preoperative pelvic floor muscle exercise for early continence after radical prostatectomy: A randomised controlled study. Eur Urol [Internet]. 2010 Jun [cited 2025 Nov 14];57(6):1039–44. Available from: https://pubmed.ncbi.nlm.nih.gov/20227168/
71. Singh F, Newton RU, Galvão DA, Spry N, Baker MK. A systematic review of pre-surgical exercise intervention studies with cancer patients. Surg Oncol [Internet]. 2013 Jun [cited 2025 Nov 14];22(2):92–104. Available from: https://pubmed.ncbi.nlm.nih.gov/23434347/
72. Springer BA, Levy E, McGarvey C, Pfalzer LA, Stout NL, Gerber LH, et al. Pre-operative assessment enables early diagnosis and recovery of shoulder function in patients with breast cancer. Breast Cancer Res Treat [Internet]. 2010 Feb [cited 2025 Nov 14];120(1):135–47. Available from: https://pubmed.ncbi.nlm.nih.gov/20054643/
73. Baima J, Reynolds SG, Edmiston K, Larkin A, Ward BM, O'Connor A. Teaching of independent exercises for prehabilitation in breast cancer. J Cancer Educ [Internet]. 2017 Jun 1 [cited 2025 Nov 14];32(2):252–6. Available from: https://pubmed.ncbi.nlm.nih.gov/26541465/
74. Pietrakiewicz K, Stec R, Sobocki J. Prehabilitation prior to chemotherapy in humans: A review of current evidence and future directions. Cancers (Basel) [Internet]. 2025 Aug 1 [cited 2025 Nov 14];17(16):2670. Available from: https://pmc.ncbi.nlm.nih.gov/articles/PMC12384665/
75. Harris E, Marignol L. Prehabilitation for patients with cancer undergoing radiation therapy: A scoping review. Clin Oncol. 2024 Apr 1;36(4):254–64.
76. Di Leone A, Terribile D, Magno S, Sanchez AM, Scardina L, Mason EJ, et al. Neoadjuvant chemotherapy in breast cancer: An Advanced Personalized Multidisciplinary Prehabilitation Model (APMP-M) to optimize outcomes. J Pers Med [Internet]. 2021 Apr 21 [cited 2025 Jan 10];11(5). Available from: http://www.ncbi.nlm.nih.gov/pubmed/33919061
77. Santa Mina D, van Rooijen SJ, Minnella EM, Alibhai SMH, Brahmbhatt P, Dalton SO, et al. Multiphasic prehabilitation across the cancer continuum: A narrative review and conceptual framework. Front Oncol [Internet]. 2021 Jan 11 [cited 2025 Nov 14];10:598425. Available from: https://pmc.ncbi.nlm.nih.gov/articles/PMC7831271/
78. Silver JK, Baima J. Cancer prehabilitation: An opportunity to decrease treatment-related morbidity, increase cancer treatment options, and improve physical and psychological health outcomes. Am J Phys Med Rehabil [Internet]. 2013 Aug [cited 2025 Nov 14];92(8):715–27. Available from: https://pubmed.ncbi.nlm.nih.gov/23756434/
79. Mustian KM, Sprod LK, Janelsins M, Peppone LJ, Mohile S. Exercise recommendations for cancer-related fatigue, cognitive impairment, sleep problems, depression, pain, anxiety, and physical dysfunction: A review. Oncol Hematol Rev [Internet]. 2012 [cited 2025 Jan 10];8(2):81–8. Available from: http://www.ncbi.nlm.nih.gov/pubmed/23667857
80. Courneya KS, Friedenreich CM, Quinney HA, Fields ALA, Jones LW, Fairey AS. A randomized trial of exercise and quality of life in colorectal cancer survivors. Eur J Cancer Care (Engl) [Internet]. 2003 Dec [cited 2025 Nov 14];12(4): 347–57. Available from: https://pubmed.ncbi.nlm.nih.gov/14982314/
81. Dimeo FC, Stieglitz RD, Novelli-Fischer U, Fetscher S, Keul J. Effects of physical activity on the fatigue and psychologic status of cancer patients during chemotherapy. 1999 [cited 2025 Nov 14]. Available from: https://acsjournals.onlinelibrary.wiley.com/doi/10.1002/

82. Sprod LK, Palesh OG, Janelsins MC, Peppone LJ, Heckler CE, Jacob Adams M, et al. Exercise, sleep quality, and mediators of sleep in breast and prostate cancer patients receiving radiation therapy. Community Oncol [Internet]. 2010 [cited 2025 Nov 14];7(10):463. Available from: https://pmc.ncbi.nlm.nih.gov/articles/PMC3026283/
83. The effect of aerobic exercise on self-esteem and depressive and anxiety symptoms among breast cancer survivors | Cochrane Library [Internet]. [cited 2025 Nov 14]. Available from: https://www.cochranelibrary.com/central/doi/10.1002/central/CN-00147456/full
84. Windsor PM, Nicol KF, Potter J. A randomized, controlled trial of aerobic exercise for treatment-related fatigue in men receiving radical external beam radiotherapy for localized prostate carcinoma. Cancer [Internet]. 2004 Aug 1 [cited 2025 Nov 14];101(3):550–7. Available from: https://pubmed.ncbi.nlm.nih.gov/15274068/
85. Galvão DA, Taaffe DR, Spry N, Joseph D, Newton RU. Combined resistance and aerobic exercise program reverses muscle loss in men undergoing androgen suppression therapy for prostate cancer without bone metastases: A randomized controlled trial. J Clin Oncol [Internet]. 2010 Jan 10 [cited 2025 Nov 14];28(2):340–7. Available from: https://pubmed.ncbi.nlm.nih.gov/19949016/
86. Courneya KS, Segal RJ, Mackey JR, Gelmon K, Reid RD, Friedenreich CM, et al. Effects of aerobic and resistance exercise in breast cancer patients receiving adjuvant chemotherapy: A multicenter randomized controlled trial. J Clin Oncol [Internet]. 2007 Oct 1 [cited 2025 Nov 14];25(28):4396–404. Available from: https://pubmed.ncbi.nlm.nih.gov/17785708/
87. An KY, Arthuso FZ, Kang DW, Morielli AR, Ntoukas SM, Friedenreich CM, et al. Exercise and health-related fitness predictors of chemotherapy completion in breast cancer patients: Pooled analysis of two multicenter trials. Breast Cancer Res Treat [Internet]. 2021 Jul 1 [cited 2025 Nov 14];188(2):399–407. Available from: https://pubmed.ncbi.nlm.nih.gov/33779887/
88. Groen WG, Naaktgeboren WR, van Harten WH, van Vulpen JK, Kool N, Sonke GS, et al. Physical fitness and chemotherapy tolerance in patients with early-stage breast cancer. Med Sci Sports Exerc [Internet]. 2022 Apr 1 [cited 2025 Jan 10];54(4):537–42. Available from: http://www.ncbi.nlm.nih.gov/pubmed/34961754
89. Smith SR, Zheng JY, Silver J, Haig AJ, Cheville A. Cancer rehabilitation as an essential component of quality care and survivorship from an international perspective. Disabil Rehabil [Internet]. 2020 Jan 2 [cited 2025 Nov 14];42(1):8–13. Available from: https://pubmed.ncbi.nlm.nih.gov/30574818/
90. Padgett LS, Dyk K Van, Kelly NC, Newman R, Hite S, Asher A. Addressing cancer-related cognitive impairment in cancer survivorship. Oncol Issues [Internet]. 2020 Jan 2 [cited 2025 Nov 14];35(1):52–7. Available from: https://www.tandfonline.com/doi/abs/10.1080/10463356.2020.1692601
91. Salerno EA, Rowland K, Kramer AF, McAuley E. Acute aerobic exercise effects on cognitive function in breast cancer survivors: A randomized crossover trial. BMC Cancer [Internet]. 2019 Apr 23 [cited 2025 Nov 14];19(1). Available from: https://pubmed.ncbi.nlm.nih.gov/31014267/
92. Sommer MS, Staerkind MEB, Christensen J, Vibe-Petersen J, Larsen KR, Pedersen JH, et al. Effect of postsurgical rehabilitation programmes in patients operated for lung cancer: A systematic review and meta-analysis. J Rehabil Med [Internet]. 2018 Mar 1 [cited 2025 Nov 14];50(3):236–45. Available from: https://pubmed.ncbi.nlm.nih.gov/29392334/
93. Ness KK, Leisenring WM, Huang S, Hudson MM, Gurney JG, Whelan K, et al. Predictors of inactive lifestyle among adult survivors of childhood cancer: A report from the childhood cancer survivor study. Cancer [Internet].

2009 May 1 [cited 2025 Nov 14];115(9):1984–94. Available from: https://pubmed.ncbi.nlm.nih.gov/19224548/
94. Reeves M, Eakin E, Lawler S, Demark-Wahnefried W. Health behaviours in survivors of childhood cancer. Aust Fam Physician. 36(2).
95. Robien K, Ness KK, Klesges LM, Baker KS, Gurney JG. Poor adherence to dietary guidelines among adult survivors of childhood acute lymphoblastic leukemia. J Pediatr Hematol Oncol [Internet]. 2008 Nov [cited 2025 Nov 14];30(11):815–22. Available from: https://pubmed.ncbi.nlm.nih.gov/18989158/
96. Geidl W, Schlesinger S, Mino E, Miranda L, Pfeifer K. Dose-response relationship between physical activity and mortality in adults with noncommunicable diseases: A systematic review and meta-analysis of prospective observational studies. International Journal of Behavioral Nutrition and Physical Activity [Internet]. 2020 Aug 26 [cited 2025 Nov 14];17(1):109. Available from: https://ijbnpa.biomedcentral.com/articles/10.1186/s12966-020-01007-5
97. Thraen-Borowski KM, Trentham-Dietz A, Edwards DF, Koltyn KF, Colbert LH. Dose-response relationships between physical activity, social participation, and health-related quality of life in colorectal cancer survivors. J Cancer Surviv [Internet]. 2013 Sep [cited 2025 Nov 14];7(3):369–78. Available from: https://pubmed.ncbi.nlm.nih.gov/23546822/
98. van Doorslaer de Ten Ryen S, Deldicque L. The regulation of the metastatic cascade by physical activity: A narrative review. Cancers (Basel) [Internet]. 2020 Jan 8 [cited 2025 Jan 10];12(1):153. Available from: http://www.ncbi.nlm.nih.gov/pubmed/31936342
99. Schadler KL, Thomas NJ, Galie PA, Bhang DH, Roby KC, Addai P, et al. Tumor vessel normalization after aerobic exercise enhances chemotherapeutic efficacy. Oncotarget [Internet]. 2016 [cited 2025 Nov 14];7(40):65429. Available from: https://pmc.ncbi.nlm.nih.gov/articles/PMC5323166/
100. Gustafson MP, Wheatley-Guy CM, Rosenthal AC, Gastineau DA, Katsanis E, Johnson BD, et al. Exercise and the immune system: Taking steps to improve responses to cancer immunotherapy. J Immunother Cancer [Internet]. 2021 Jul 2 [cited 2025 Nov 14];9(7):1872. Available from: https://jitc.bmj.com/content/9/7/e001872
101. Holmes MD, Chen WY, Feskanich D, Kroenke CH, Colditz GA. Physical activity and survival after breast cancer diagnosis. JAMA [Internet]. 2005 May 25 [cited 2025 Nov 14];293(20):2479–86. Available from: https://jamanetwork.com/journals/jama/fullarticle/200955
102. Meyerhardt JA, Heseltine D, Niedzwiecki D, Hollis D, Saltz LB, Mayer RJ, et al. Impact of physical activity on cancer recurrence and survival in patients with stage III colon cancer: Findings from CALGB 89803. J Clin Oncol [Internet]. 2006 Aug 1 [cited 2025 Nov 14];24(22):3535–41. Available from: https://pubmed.ncbi.nlm.nih.gov/16822843/
103. American College of Sports Medicine. ACSM's guidelines for exercise testing and prescription [Internet]. Wolters Kluwer; 2022 [cited 2025 Nov 14]. Available from: https://books.google.com/books/about/ACSM_s_Guidelines_for_Exercise_Testing_a.html?hl=sl&id=hTKvzgEACAAJ
104. Campbell KL, Winters-Stone KM, Wiskemann J, May AM, Schwartz AL, Courneya KS, et al. Exercise guidelines for cancer survivors: Consensus statement from international multidisciplinary roundtable. Med Sci Sports Exerc [Internet]. 2019 Nov 1 [cited 2025 Nov 14];51(11):2375–90. Available from: https://pubmed.ncbi.nlm.nih.gov/31626055/

3

THE CELLULAR RESPONSE TO EXERCISE IN CANCER

3.1 Mapping the cellular landscape in cancer

Tumours are more than merely aggregates of cancerous cells—they cohabit a complex, dynamic ecosystem known as the tumour microenvironment (TME). This local neighbourhood comprises not only cancer cells and a small subpopulation of cancer stem cells (CSCs) but also healthy cells from the tissue of origin and a diverse array of stromal cells, such as fibroblasts, mesenchymal stem cells (MSCs), adipocytes, endothelial cells and pericytes. These cells are embedded in a scaffold of acellular elements, including the extracellular matrix (ECM), which provides structural integrity and biochemical cues, as well as extracellular vesicles (EVs), which serve to prepare the pre-metastatic niche (1,2). Table 3.1 summarises the major cellular and structural constituents of the TME.

Together with cancer cells, these cellular and non-cellular components of the TME interact in diverse and dynamic ways to support (or sometimes suppress) the growth of the tumour, to help cancer cells evade the immune response, to enable the formation of new blood vessels (angiogenesis) in order to maintain oxygen and nutrient supplies, and to facilitate invasion and metastasis to distant sites (2). Understanding the composition and behaviour of the TME is essential to appreciate how systemic interventions such as exercise can exert anti-tumour effects. Unlike many pharmacological treatments that target a single molecule or signalling pathway, exercise interacts with the TME on multiple fronts: mechanical, metabolic, immunological and endocrine. This offers a diverse array of strategies for disrupting tumour-promoting cues, which will be explored in this chapter

DOI: 10.4324/9781003511519-4

TABLE 3.1 Key components of the TME

Component	*Function in tumourigenesis*
Cancer cells	Drive tumour growth and progression
Immune cells (e.g., T cells, NK cells, macrophages)	Mediate immune surveillance or suppression
Cancer-associated fibroblasts (CAFs)	Remodel ECM, promote invasion
MSCs	Contribute to immune modulation, repair and growth
Cancer-associated adipocytes (CAAs)	Secrete adipokines, modulate inflammation
Vasculature (endothelial cells, pericytes)	Supplies nutrients and oxygen, as well as routes for metastatic dissemination
ECM	Provides structural support and biochemical cues via integrin signalling
CSCs	Have self-renewal and differentiation capabilities that drive tumour initiation, progression and recurrence. Often exhibit chemoresistance.

Abbreviations: CAA = cancer-associated adipocyte; CAF = cancer-associated fibroblast; CSC = cancer stem cell; ECM = extracellular matrix; MSC = mesenchymal stem cell; NK = natural killer

and in Chapter 4. Figure 3.1 provides a schematic overview of the TME, illustrating the key cellular and non-cellular constituents, along with their functional interactions in promoting tumour growth, angiogenesis, immune evasion and metastasis.

3.2 Exercise and the cellular landscape of the TME

Cancer cells arise from healthy cells from the tissue of origin: e.g., breast cancer arises from mammary epithelial cells, colorectal cancer arises from epithelial cells lining the colon or rectum and so on. However, there are many different subtypes within each cancer type, arising from variations in the specific cell of origin, molecular alterations and their resulting phenotypes and differentiation states, all of which influence tumour behaviour, prognosis and response to therapy. The effects of exercise on the diverse cell types in the TME are summarised in Table 3.2 and Figure 3.2.

Exercise and physical activity interact with the TME via both direct and indirect mechanisms. Direct effects include alterations in cancer cell metabolism, growth signalling and susceptibility to apoptosis (programmed cell death). These direct effects have been demonstrated in vitro using

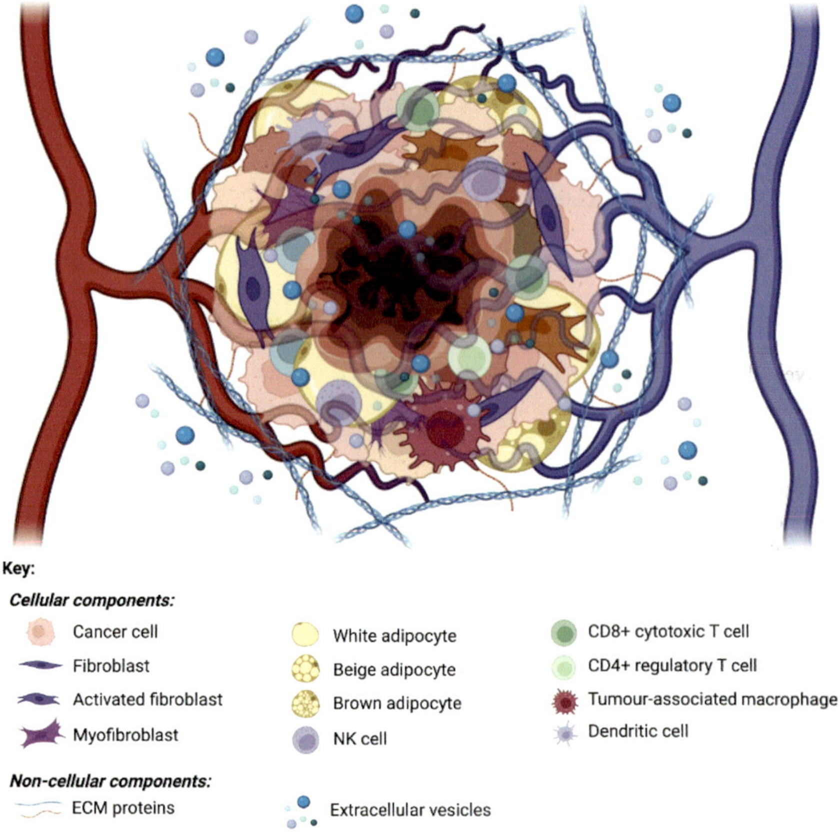

FIGURE 3.1 The cellular and structural composition of the TME. This schematic illustrates the complex and dynamic TME, comprising both cellular and non-cellular components that collectively influence tumour progression. Central to the tumour are cancer cells with a hypoxic core, surrounded by an extracellular matrix (ECM) scaffold. The ECM provides structural support and facilitates signalling interactions that enable angiogenesis and metastasis. Stromal components include cancer-associated fibroblasts (CAFs), mesenchymal stem cells (MSCs) and cancer-associated adipocytes (CAAs), all of which modulate inflammatory and mechanical cues. Immune cell populations such as CD8+ cytotoxic T cells, CD4+ regulatory T cells (Tregs), natural killer (NK) cells, dendritic cells (DCs) and tumour-associated macrophages (TAMs) interact with cancer cells to mount their anti-tumour immune response. Cancer cells often subvert these cell populations to promote immune suppression. Leaky vasculature formed by endothelial cells and pericytes facilitates nutrient delivery, oxygenation and metastatic spread. Additional layers of complexity arise from tumour-derived extracellular vesicles (EVs) and secreted cytokines (e.g., IL-6, TGFβ, CXCL12), which orchestrate local and systemic tumour-promoting signals. Created with Biorender.com.

TABLE 3.2 Summary of exercise-induced effects on cell types found in the TME

Cell type	*Exercise-induced change*	*Functional consequence*
Cytotoxic CD8+ T cells	Increased mobilisation, intratumoural infiltration and cytotoxic function (3–5)	Enhanced tumour surveillance and killing (6)
Regulatory T cells (Tregs)	Decreased frequency and suppressive function (7–9)	Reduced immunosuppression resulting in increased CD8+ T cell activity (10)
NK cells	Increased acute mobilisation, intratumoural infiltration and cytotoxicity (3,11)	Direct tumour cell lysis; improved immune priming
Myeloid-derived suppressor cells (MDSCs)	Reduced abundance in the TME and decreased immunosuppressive signalling (7,12)	Relief of immune suppression; improved anti-tumour immunity
Tumour-associated macrophages (TAMs)	Shift from M2-like (tumour-promoting) to M1-like (pro-inflammatory) phenotype (12,13)	Restoration of immune surveillance; reduced angiogenesis and matrix remodelling
Dendritic cells (DCs)	Increased numbers in circulation; increased antigen presentation potential (6,12)	Improved T cell priming and immune activation
CAFs	Limited direct evidence; potential modulation of activation state (14,15)	Possible reduction in fibrosis and barrier to immune infiltration (14)
MSCs	Increased presence in trained adipose tissue; shift towards repair-supporting phenotype (16–18)	Reduced inflammation; unclear impact on tumour-stroma signalling (19–21)
CAAs	Reduced pro-tumourigenic adipokines (e.g., leptin, FABP4); increased protective adipokines (e.g., adiponectin) (22,23)	Reduced tumour growth signalling; reduced aromatase activity in breast cancer (23–25)
Endothelial cells	Increased VEGF receptor expression; improved vascular structure and perfusion (26)	Normalised vasculature; better immune cell trafficking (26)
CSCs	Potentially reduced self-renewal signalling and increased differentiation (27)	Potentially suppressed tumour initiation and relapse
CTCs	Increased immune clearance; reduced viability (28–30)	Decreased metastatic potential

Abbreviations: CAA = cancer-associated adipocyte; CAF = cancer-associated fibroblast; CD = cluster of differentiation; CSC = cancer stem cell; DC = dendritic cell; CTC = circulating tumour cell; ECM = extracellular matrix; FABP4 = fatty acid binding protein 4; MDSC = myeloid-derived suppressor cell; MSC = mesenchymal stem cell; NK = natural killer; TAM = tumour-associated macrophage; TME = tumour microenvironment; VEGF = vascular endothelial growth factor

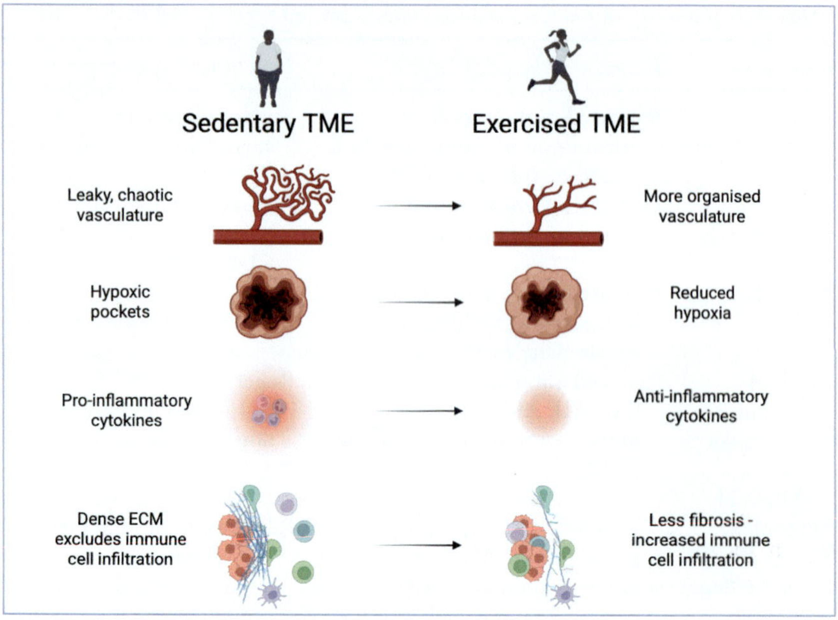

FIGURE 3.2 Exercise-mediated remodelling of the TME. This schematic illustrates the contrasting features of the TME in sedentary versus exercised states. Under sedentary conditions, the TME is characterised by disorganised and leaky tumour vasculature, pockets of hypoxia (regions of low oxygen), an excess of pro-inflammatory cytokines, and a dense extracellular matrix that precludes immune cells from infiltrating into the centre of the tumour mass. By contrast, regular exercise promotes vascular normalisation in tumours, reduces intratumoural hypoxia, shifts the cytokine profile towards an anti-inflammatory phenotype, and remodels the ECM to permit greater immune cell infiltration. Collectively, these adaptations support a more immunologically active and a microenvironment less permissive to tumour growth. Created with Biorender.com.

exercise-conditioned serum, which inhibits tumour cell proliferation and induces cell cycle arrest (31–33). Indirect effects are primarily mediated through systemic responses, particularly those initiated by skeletal muscle. On a cellular level, during exercise, repeated muscle contractions increase mechanical load and energy demand on skeletal muscle, leading to local hypoxia, changes in calcium signalling and transient oxidative stress. These physiological changes activate a variety of signalling pathways such as AMPK, SIRT1 and p38 MAPK, which promote mitochondrial biogenesis, increase oxidative capacity and enhance capillary density. Collectively, these adaptations improve systemic metabolic health, increasing insulin sensitivity, lowering circulating glucose and insulin levels and enhancing fatty acid oxidation, all of which may reduce nutrient availability to tumours (34). These molecular effects of exercise on cancer will be discussed in more detail in Chapter 4.

Importantly, skeletal muscle also functions as an endocrine organ. In response to contraction-induced stress, it releases bioactive molecules known as myokines that circulate through the blood and act on distant tissues, including tumours (35). These circulating factors can act directly on tumours or indirectly by modulating immune function. Exercise-induced immune mobilisation includes the transient recruitment of neutrophils, monocytes and lymphocytes into the bloodstream, which are subsequently redistributed to peripheral tissues, including tumours and sites of inflammation, where they may enhance anti-cancer immunity (11). This phenomenon will be discussed in more detail in Section 3.2.1. Additionally, skeletal muscle damage and regeneration following an acute bout of exercise further amplifies immune activation, facilitating the mobilisation of NK cells, T cells and monocytes into the bloodstream and potentially into the TME (3,31).

Together, these effects position skeletal muscle as a central mediator of the systemic response to exercise, helping to shape the TME in ways that may support anti-cancer immunity, reduce inflammation and disrupt tumour-supportive signalling networks (see Box-out 3.1).

BOX-OUT 3.1 SYSTEMIC MEDIATORS OF EXERCISE EFFECTS

Skeletal muscle is a powerful endocrine organ that communicates with distant organs through the release of bioactive molecules during physical activity and exercise. These molecules, collectively termed exerkines, include proteins, peptides, metabolites and EVs, many of which are specifically released from muscle and are therefore known as myokines. Well-characterised myokines, such as IL-6, SPARC, irisin and BDNF, are secreted into circulation during and after exercise, where they act systemically to modulate inflammation, metabolism, immune surveillance and tissue repair. For example, IL-6 is acutely released in response to muscle contraction and plays dual roles in promoting anti-inflammatory responses (see Chapter 4, Section 4.1.1) and enhancing immune cell recruitment (Section 4.13). SPARC is involved in ECM remodelling and has been shown to promote apoptosis in colon cancer models (Section 4.2.2). Irisin has been shown to reduce tumour cell viability and may influence the browning of adipose tissue, indirectly altering tumour metabolism (Section 4.1.2). In addition to soluble proteins, skeletal muscle also secretes EVs that contain microRNAs, lipids and proteins with the capacity to reprogramme target cells. These EVs may serve as delivery vehicles for exercise-induced signals that influence fibroblasts, immune cells, endothelial cells and even cancer cells themselves (Section 4.3.3). Importantly, not all exerkines originate from muscle: adipose tissue, the liver and even the gut microbiota contribute to this circulating pool, adding to the molecular complexity observed during and after exercise. The tissue of origin, exercise modality, intensity and duration all shape the composition of exerkines, suggesting enormous potential for personalised interventions. Together, these molecules help to rebalance the TME, pushing it away from pro-tumourigenic signalling towards a state characterised by enhanced immune surveillance, metabolic control and suppressed tumour growth. These pathways, including mechanisms and context-specific effects, are explored in more detail in Chapter 4.

3.2.1 Immune cells

The immune landscape within the TME is highly variable and dynamic but oftentimes leans towards immunosuppression rather than immunosurveillance (11). In many solid tumours, there is a mass infiltration of immunosuppressive cell types, including regulatory T cells (Tregs), myeloid-derived suppressor cells (MDSCs), bone marrow-derived dendritic cells (DCs) and tumour-associated macrophages (TAMs) (4). Bone-marrow derived DCs regulate angiogenesis and promote the formation of the pre-metastatic niche, facilitating host colonisation by the tumour cells (5). By contrast, immune cells that should be actively monitoring the local environment and eliminating cancer cells, such as cytotoxic T lymphocytes (CTLs—also known as CD8+ T cells or killer T cells) and NK cells, are unable to penetrate the tumour or are exhausted or dysfunctional (6). This functional impairment can be elicited via tumour cells themselves or by other stromal elements through the secretion of inhibitory cytokines, overexpression of immune checkpoint proteins, such as PD-L1, and competing for nutrients within the TME (7).

3.2.1.1 Exercise mobilises cytotoxic immune cells

Acute bouts of exercise promote rapid mobilisation of immune cells into the bloodstream, a phenomenon known as transient leukocytosis (8). NK cells are among the most responsive populations of immune cells, with numbers rising sharply within minutes of moderate-to-vigorous physical activity, peaking at around 30 minutes post-exercise. This mobilisation is largely driven by enhanced shear stress as the increased blood flow against the blood vessel walls stimulates the release of catecholamines, particularly adrenaline (epinephrine) and nor-adrenaline (nor-epinephrine), which bind to β-adrenergic receptors expressed on the surface of NK cells and facilitate their rapid redistribution to peripheral tissues, including tumours. Once within the TME, NK cells can exert direct cytotoxic effects on malignant cells, an effect that may be amplified by repeated bouts of exercise over time (11).

Chronic exercise training, meanwhile, improves the surveillance and cytotoxic function of these populations, increasing their infiltration into tumours and enhancing their ability to kill cancer cells. Cytotoxic T cells, which are central to the adaptive anti-tumour immune response, are also mobilised during and after exercise (8). Evidence suggests that regular physical activity enhances their activation and effector function, boosting the immune system's capacity for tumour surveillance and destruction (9). In mouse models, voluntary wheel running has been shown to increase CD8+ T cell infiltration into tumours, and this response has been demonstrated as necessary for the anti-tumour effects of exercise to occur (3). Blocking NK cell infiltration or depleting these populations using propranolol, a β-adrenergic receptor inhibitor, also blocks T cell infiltration and abrogates the tumour-suppressive benefits of exercise in these murine models (3). In preclinical models, exercise increases intratumoural infiltration of cytotoxic T cells and is associated with reduced tumour burden and improved survival (9). In women with breast cancer, 12 weeks of moderate to vigorous cycling increased the number of circulating bone marrow-derived DCs, alongside greater expression of vascular endothelial growth factor receptor 2 (VEGFR2) expression on circulating endothelial cells, suggesting enhanced vascular remodelling and immune priming within the TME that may facilitate improved tumour surveillance and perfusion (10). These observations have led to the hypothesis that exercise may serve as an immune primer, enhancing the number and function of cytotoxic immune cells prior to treatment. This concept underpins emerging interest in exercise as a form of prehabilitation, potentially improving patient readiness and response to therapies such as immunotherapy and is currently being explored in trials combining exercise with neoadjuvant therapies or immunotherapy (12,13).

3.2.1.2 Exercise reduces immunosuppression

Beyond boosting anti-tumour immunity, exercise also alleviates immunosuppressive pressures within the TME by reducing the frequency and suppressive function of regulatory T cells (Tregs) and MDSCs (14). These immunosuppressive populations are typically elevated in cancer and are associated with poor prognosis, as they inhibit CD8+ cytotoxic T cell activation and cytokine production (15). By lowering these inhibitory cells, exercise helps to rebalance the immune landscape towards a cytotoxic phenotype that favours tumour clearance. Interestingly, these effects are even seen in immunotherapy-resistant brain tumours, suggesting that exercise may serve as a sensitising agent for immune checkpoint blockade (16). Tregs, which often accumulate in tumours and suppress the anti-tumour immune response, proportionally reduce in number following regular exercise, thereby reorienting immune activity in favour of tumour rejection (17,18). Additionally, exercise influences macrophage polarisation, steering TAMs away from an M2-like, tumour-promoting towards a more inflammatory M1-like phenotype, though this remains an active area of research (19). Exercise also modulates the tumour immune environment through changes in cytokine signalling, with skeletal muscle-derived factors influencing both pro- and anti-inflammatory pathways. These dual effects of mobilising effector immune cells and suppression of immunosuppressive populations together remodel the immune landscape of the TME in favour of anti-tumour immunity (Figure 3.3). The molecular mechanisms underpinning this phenomenon will be explored further in Chapter 4.

3.2.1.3 Exercise sensitises tumours to immunotherapy

By enhancing immune surveillance and modulating immunosuppressive elements of the TME, exercise may increase tumour responsiveness to immunotherapy. In murine models, exercise prior to anti-PD-1 checkpoint blockade significantly improved therapeutic outcomes, in part by increasing the infiltration and activation of cytotoxic T cells (20,21). In support of this, combining exercise with anti-PD-1 or anti-CTLA-4 therapy has been shown to enhance therapeutic responses in preclinical models of breast and lung cancer (14,22). These findings suggest that physical activity could be a low-cost, non-toxic strategy to boost the efficacy of immune-based treatments, though translational studies in humans are still being undertaken (23).

BOX-OUT 3.2 WHAT ARE IMMUNE CHECKPOINT INHIBITORS?

Immune checkpoint inhibitors are a class of cancer immunotherapy drugs that work by releasing the "brakes" on the immune system, allowing it to recognise and destroy cancer cells more effectively. Under normal conditions, immune checkpoints like PD-1 (programmed cell death protein 1) on T cells and its respective ligand, PD-L1, on other cells, help prevent excessive immune activation that could damage healthy tissue. However, many tumours exploit these checkpoints by overexpressing PD-L1, which binds to PD-1 and shuts down cytotoxic T cell activity, effectively hiding from immune attack.

Checkpoint inhibitors are monoclonal antibodies that block PD-1, PD-L1 or CTLA-4 (another checkpoint protein), reactivating the immune system to target the tumour. Examples include Nivolumab and Pembrolizumab (anti-PD-1),

Atezolizumab and Durvalumab (anti-PD-L1) and Ipilimumab (anti-CTLA-4). While checkpoint inhibitors have revolutionised treatment for some cancers (e.g., melanoma, lung and renal cancers), their effectiveness varies, and not all patients respond (24,25). The immunosuppressive TME, poor immune cell infiltration and metabolic constraints are key barriers to their success.

Exercise is emerging as a potential adjuvant that could help prime the immune system, increasing T cell infiltration and altering the TME in ways that may enhance the efficacy of immune checkpoint inhibitors, particularly when timed before or alongside treatment (see Figure 3.4).

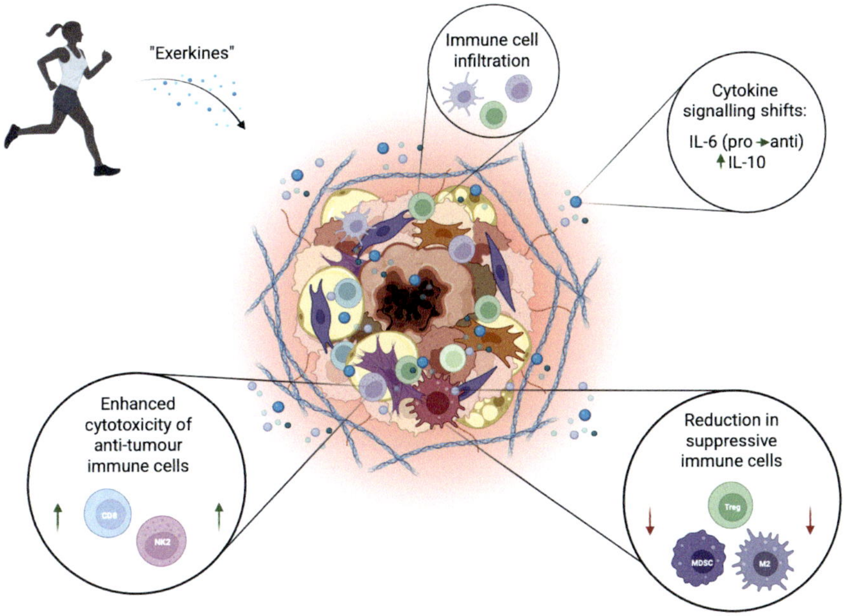

FIGURE 3.3 Immune remodelling of the (TME) in response to exercise. This schematic illustrates the dynamic impact of exercise on the immune landscape within the TME. In the sedentary state, the TME is typically characterised by low infiltration of cytotoxic immune cells (e.g., NK cells and CD8⁺ T cells), enrichment of immunosuppressive populations (e.g., Tregs and MDSCs) and a pro-inflammatory cytokine milieu that favours tumour progression and immune evasion. In contrast, regular physical activity enhances systemic immune surveillance and leads to increased infiltration of effector cells into the TME, elevated antigen presentation, and a shift towards a more anti-inflammatory, anti-tumour cytokine environment. Exercise also promotes vascular normalisation, which facilitates immune cell trafficking and may reprogramme stromal and tumour-associated immune cells towards a phenotype that supports tumour suppression. Created with Biorender.com.

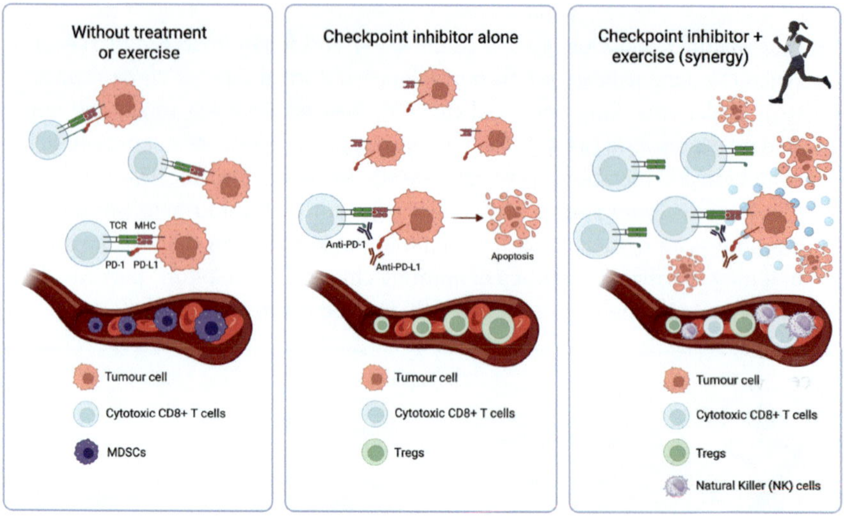

FIGURE 3.4 Synergistic potential of exercise and immune checkpoint inhibition. This schematic illustrates how exercise may enhance the efficacy of immune checkpoint inhibitors by modulating immune cell infiltration and function within the TME. Left panel: In untreated settings, tumours exploit immune checkpoints (e.g., PD-1/PD-L1) to suppress cytotoxic T cell activity, leading to immune evasion despite T cell presence. Middle panel: Checkpoint inhibitors such as anti-PD-1 or anti-PD-L1 antibodies block inhibitory signalling, restoring T cell-mediated tumour cell killing. However, in immunologically "cold" tumours, low immune infiltration and suppressive cell populations (e.g., regulatory T cells, Tregs) limit therapeutic benefit. Right panel: Exercise can act as an immunological primer, increasing intratumoural infiltration of CD8+ cytotoxic T cells and natural killer (NK) cells, enhancing antigen presentation, and reducing immunosuppressive barriers. When combined with immune checkpoint inhibitors, these adaptations may convert the TME to a more immune-responsive, "hot" state, amplifying anti-tumour responses. Created with Biorender.com.

3.2.2 Cancer-associated fibroblasts

In addition to immune cells, the TME harbours a rich population of stromal cells, among which CAFs are the most abundant and functionally versatile (26,27). Under physiological conditions, fibroblasts contribute to tissue architecture by producing ECM proteins and play key roles in the wound-healing response (28). Upon tissue injury, they become activated to myofibroblasts, secreting cytokines and growth factors that support epithelial cell proliferation and migration, ECM remodelling enzymes such as matrix metalloproteinases (MMPs) that help "clear a path" for migration, and anti-apoptotic signals that prevent anchorage-dependent cell death (anoikis) in migrating cells (29,30,36).

Tumours have been described as "wounds that do not heal" (37), and CAFs closely mimic this chronically active wound-healing phenotype. They exhibit enhanced ECM deposition, growth factor and cytokine secretion and are implicated in angiogenesis, immune modulation and invasion (38–40). CAFs can arise from multiple cellular origins, highlighting their plasticity. While they primarily derive from resident fibroblasts, other sources include epithelial cells via epithelial-to-mesenchymal transition (EMT), endothelial cells via endothelial-to-mesenchymal transition (EndMT) and bone marrow-derived MSCs; see Figure 3.5 (41–43).

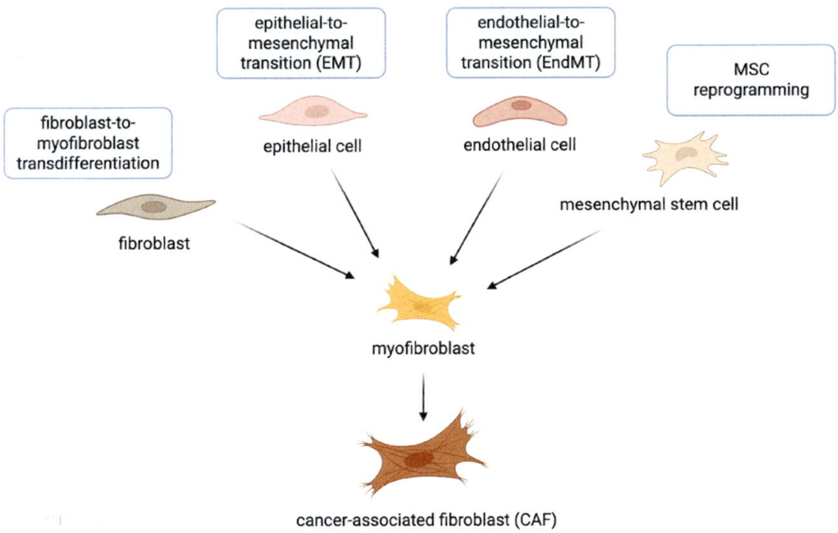

FIGURE 3.5 Cellular origins of cancer-associated fibroblasts (CAFs) within the TME. CAFs are a heterogeneous population of stromal cells that arise from multiple cellular sources in response to tumour-derived signals. This schematic illustrates the principal pathways contributing to CAF formation, including epithelial-to-mesenchymal transition (EMT), endothelial-to-mesenchymal transition (EndMT), fibroblast-to-myofibroblast transdifferentiation, and mesenchymal stem cell (MSC) reprogramming. Once activated, CAFs acquire contractile, secretory and immunomodulatory properties that support tumour progression, angiogenesis, ECM remodelling and immune evasion. Created in Biorender.com.

Activated CAFs are typically characterised by the expression of alpha-smooth muscle actin (αSMA) and fibroblast activation protein (FAP), with a loss of markers such as CD34 (44). This immunophenotypic shift from $CD34^{+/\alpha SMA-/FAP-}$ in quiescent fibroblasts to $CD34^{-/\alpha SMA+/FAP+}$ in CAFs has been well documented, although heterogeneity exists across tumour types (45). Functionally, CAFs secrete stromal cell-derived factor-1 (SDF-1/CXCL12), which promotes cancer cell proliferation and invasion through the PI3K/Akt and MAPK pathways and elevates MMP2 and MMP9 activity (46–48). This activity facilitates ECM degradation and tissue invasion, supporting metastasis. Importantly, unlike myofibroblasts in wound healing which undergo apoptosis or deactivation once repair is complete (30,36), CAFs persist and sustain the pro-tumourigenic environment.

3.2.2.1 Potential for exercise to modulate CAF activity

There is a paucity of research directly linking exercise to CAF activation or function in cancer. However, several strands of emerging evidence suggest that exercise might influence CAF biology both directly and indirectly, particularly through effects on fibrosis, inflammatory signalling and ECM remodelling. For instance, preliminary findings from Liu et al. (2023) suggest that regular aerobic training in a murine model of pancreatic cancer led to lower abundance of CAFs and CAF-activating cytokines and reduced collagen deposition, indicative of attenuated CAF-mediated fibrotic remodelling (49). These findings are consistent with other preclinical studies which demonstrated exercise suppresses fibrosis in non-cancerous tissues such as the heart (50) and reduced tumour fibrosis in pancreatic cancer models (51). In this latter study, exercise also enhanced anti-PD-1 checkpoint inhibitor delivery, indirectly implicating exercise-induced modulation of CAF activity as a driver of improved treatment access. Furthermore, interval aerobic training has been shown to reduce TGFβ expression in tumour tissue in a murine model of breast cancer (52), which is a key pathway in CAF activation and fibrotic ECM deposition. Moreover, in preclinical models of heart and liver disease, exercise has been found to downregulate the expression of fibroblast activation markers such as Col1a1 and Acta2 (53,54). In addition, exercise induces suppression of inflammatory genes including IL-6, TNF-α and IL-1β (9), all of which have been implicated in CAF activation and maintenance (55–57), supporting the idea that exercise has the potential to modulate CAF activity.

Mechanistically, exercise may alter the physical and biochemical properties of tissues in ways that influence CAF phenotype and function. For example, changes in ECM tension and stiffness associated with regular physical activity could suppress the differentiation of fibroblasts into contractile myofibroblasts. Additionally, exercise-induced modulation of MMP activity may promote ECM turnover, countering CAF-mediated ECM accumulation (58). From a cellular perspective, by recruiting and activating immune cells such as macrophages and CD8+ T cells, exercise may indirectly influence CAF function through shifts in the local cytokine milieu (59). As CAFs are known to engage in reciprocal signalling with immune cells, such changes may tip the balance away from immune suppression and towards immune surveillance.

Skeletal muscle acts as an endocrine organ, releasing systemic factors such as IL-6, irisin and SPARC during exercise (see Chapter 4), all of which have been implicated in modulating fibrotic responses (35,60–64). SPARC in particular, a matricellular protein secreted by skeletal muscle during muscle contraction, has demonstrated context-dependent anti-fibrotic and tumour-suppressive properties that could dampen CAF activity (65). Interestingly, IL-6 can exert seemingly contradictory roles in the stromal compartment: in some settings it promotes fibroblast activation, myofibroblast differentiation and ECM accumulation, thus contributing to fibrosis, while in other contexts it supports repair and resolution of the wound healing response, thereby acting in an anti-fibrotic manner (62,63,66). Whether IL-6 promotes or inhibits fibrosis appears to depend on factors like timing, the cellular context (such as acute injury versus chronic damage) and the surrounding signalling environment, including TGFβ levels. These proteins and their pleiotropic signalling roles are explored in more detail in Chapter 4. Taken together, these findings suggest a plausible, though still largely theoretical, role for exercise in reprogramming CAFs and the fibrotic stroma. By modifying fibroblast activation and ECM dynamics, exercise may help to normalise the TME, suppress tumour invasiveness and improve therapeutic delivery. Further studies are urgently needed to investigate these mechanisms directly.

3.2.3 Mesenchymal stem cells

MSCs are multipotent stromal cells capable of differentiating into various lineages including adipocytes, osteoblasts and chondrocytes (67). These cells are recruited to sites of tissue damage and inflammation, including tumours, where they are co-opted by the tumour to promote progression and immune evasion. Within the TME, MSCs can be reprogrammed into tumour-associated MSCs, exhibiting altered gene expression, cytokine secretion and cellular interactions that support tumourigenesis (68). MSCs contribute to tumour growth via several mechanisms. First, by secreting cytokines and growth factors such as TGFβ, IL-6 and VEGF, MSCs can stimulate cancer cell proliferation, angiogenesis and immune suppression (69). They are also capable of inducing EMT in cancer cells, thereby facilitating invasion and metastasis (70). Moreover, MSCs possess immunomodulatory capacity, particularly through the expansion of Tregs and concomitant suppression of NK cell and cytotoxic T cell activity (71,72), and they contribute to remodelling of the ECM within the TME, which aids tumour expansion and invasion (73). Interestingly, MSCs display a duality in their nature: while their tumour-promoting properties have been widely documented, under certain conditions they can also exhibit anti-tumourigenic effects, such as promoting immune surveillance or inducing apoptosis in cancer cells (74–77). This plasticity appears to be context-dependent, influenced by cues from the local microenvironment, including hypoxia, inflammation and cytokine gradients (78,79).

3.2.3.1 Exercise modulates MSC interactions with cancer cells

Exercise influences MSC biology both systemically and within the TME, although this remains a relatively underexplored area in exercise oncology. Emerging evidence suggests that physical activity can modulate the recruitment, differentiation and secretory profile of MSCs, potentially reprogramming them towards a more regenerative and less tumour-supportive phenotype. For instance, exercise has been shown to influence the lineage fate of MSCs (80). In the context of obesity and inflammation, MSCs are more likely to differentiate into adipocytes, contributing to a pro-tumourigenic niche (81). Exercise may counter this by promoting osteogenic over adipogenic differentiation, via activation of Wnt/β-catenin signalling and reduced PPARγ expression (80,82). By reducing systemic inflammation, exercise may suppress the tumour-promoting phenotype of MSCs. For example, regular physical activity lowers circulating levels of IL-6 and TNF-α (83), two cytokines that drive the immunosuppressive and pro-invasive behaviour of MSCs within the TME (84,85). In co-culture models, exercised serum or exercise-conditioned media appears to blunt the pro-migratory effects of MSCs on breast cancer cells, suggesting that exercise may impair the ability of MSCs to promote cancer cell invasion (86). Finally, there is growing interest in how exercise might alter the cargo of EVs secreted by MSCs. These vesicles carry miRNAs, cytokines and metabolic enzymes that can reshape the TME. Exercise-induced changes in EV content could reduce the tumour-supportive messaging transmitted by MSCs (87). Overall, while research is still evolving, these findings suggest that MSCs may represent an important and mechanistic link between systemic exercise effects and local tumour behaviour. A better understanding of how exercise reprogrammes MSC function could inform strategies to therapeutically harness or inhibit MSCs in cancer.

3.2.4 *Cancer-associated adipocytes*

Adipocytes, particularly in breast and ovarian cancers, have emerged as active modulators of the TME. Beyond their role in storing energy, they actively secrete adipokines such as leptin, IL-6, FABP4 and adiponectin, which serve a role in driving cancer cell proliferation, facilitating migration, and crucially, in metabolic reprogramming (88,89). In the context of obesity, adipocytes become hypertrophic and dysregulated, releasing more pro-inflammatory and pro-tumourigenic signals, while simultaneously lowering levels of protective factors like adiponectin (90,91). CAAs also display elevated levels of aromatase expression, an enzyme that is essential for oestrogen production, which is a key driver in hormone-responsive breast cancers (92).

3.2.4.1 *Exercise counteracts the pro-inflammatory environment in obesity*

In obesity-linked cancers such as breast cancer, exercise exerts beneficial effects in adipose tissue that extend beyond weight loss alone. Regular exercise improves adipose tissue function by reducing the secretion of pro-tumourigenic adipokines, for example the aforementioned leptin and FABP4, and increasing the release of protective adipokines such as adiponectin, further tipping the balance away from a pro-growth, inflammatory state, towards an anti-tumourigenic state (93,94). These changes help restore insulin sensitivity, which in turn lowers systemic insulin and IGF-1 levels, both of which are potent mitogens (growth stimulators) for many cancer types (95). Indeed, higher circulating levels of IGF-1 are associated with an increased risk of breast cancer (96). Further supporting this effect, a recent intervention study showed that 12 weeks of aerobic exercise led to substantial improvements in subcutaneous adipose tissue transcriptional profiles, including downregulation of inflammatory and macrophage-related genes in overweight men with dysglycaemia (abnormal blood glucose level) (97). While this study was not conducted in a cancer population, it reinforces the capacity of exercise to reprogramme adipose tissue towards a less inflammatory, more metabolically favourable phenotype.

Mechanistically, the obese adipose tissue environment is characterised by hypertrophic adipocytes, hypoxia, ECM stiffening and chronic low-grade inflammation: features that create a pro-tumourigenic TME.

Exercise appears to remodel this environment by reducing adipocyte size, enhancing mitochondrial oxidative capacity in adipose tissue, by promoting the "browning" of white adipose tissue, and by lowering pro-inflammatory immune cell infiltration (98). These adaptations lower the secretion of growth-promoting adipokines and reduce systemic levels of insulin, IGF-1 and free fatty acids, which all fuel tumour progression (Figure 3.6).

Together, these findings suggest exercise may transform the obese adipose tissue niche from one that supports tumour growth to one that is less permissive, both by modulating systemic metabolic-hormonal factors and by altering the local adipose microenvironment itself.

3.2.5 Endothelial cells and pericytes

Other key players in the TME include endothelial cells that line the blood vessels in the tumour vasculature, and pericytes embedded in the capillary walls that help regulate vascular stability. Unlike normal blood vessels, tumour vasculature is typically disorganised and leaky, contributing to poor oxygen delivery and regions of hypoxia within the tumour. This hypoxia, combined with the high metabolic activity of cancer cells, contributes to the build-up of acidic by-products like lactate, resulting in a condition known as acidosis, characterised by a drop in pH that creates a hostile, low-oxygen, low-pH environment that supports tumour progression (2). This abnormal vasculature impairs immune cell infiltration and chemotherapeutic drug delivery, driving selection pressures within the hypoxic regions for more aggressive, hypoxia-resistant cancer cell clones (99).

3.2.5.1 Exercise promotes normalisation of tumour vasculature

Another key benefit of exercise in cancer is the normalisation of tumour vasculature. Preclinical studies have demonstrated that aerobic training can remodel the chaotic and leaky vascular network typically found in tumours into more structured, functional vessels that resemble normal vasculature (100). This vascular remodelling improves tissue perfusion, thereby reducing hypoxia and enhancing the delivery of chemotherapeutic agents and enabling greater infiltration of immune cells into the core of the tumour mass. Mechanistically, exercise-induced increases in blood flow impose shear stress on endothelial cells, which triggers intracellular signalling cascades that drive these structural changes. In vitro studies using microfluidic devices to mimic flow conditions have shown that shear stress

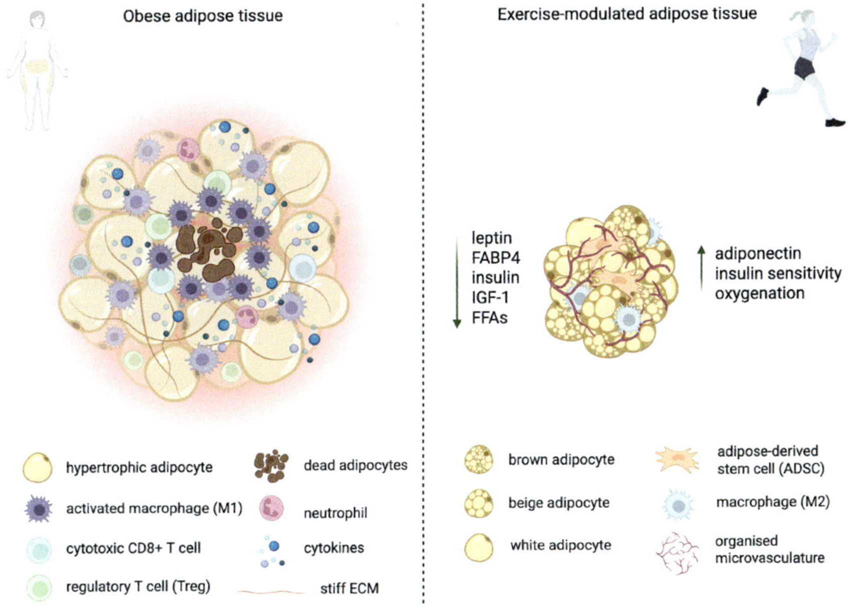

FIGURE 3.6 Exercise remodels the adipose microenvironment. This schematic compares the local stromal microenvironment in a sedentary, obese state (left) with an exercised, leaner phenotype (right). In the sedentary microenvironment, enlarged (hypertrophic) adipocytes dominate, surrounded by pro-inflammatory immune cells such as M1-like macrophages and regulatory T cells (Tregs). This environment promotes hypoxia, cell death, extracellular matrix (ECM) stiffening, and elevated secretion of adipokines (e.g., leptin, FABP4) and pro-inflammatory cytokines (e.g., IL-6, TNF-α), which supports tumour progression. In contrast, regular physical activity and exercise induces changes in adipose tissue that is anti-inflammatory and impairs tumour progression. Adipocytes become smaller and more metabolically active, with an increase in brown and beige-like adipocyte populations with enhanced mitochondrial content. The immune landscape shifts towards an anti-inflammatory profile, including greater presence of M2-like macrophages and adipose-derived stem cells (ADSCs) that support tissue repair rather than chronic inflammation, alongside improved vascularisation. These adaptations reduce systemic insulin and IGF-1 levels, improving insulin sensitivity, and are accompanied by an increase in protective adipokines, such as adiponectin. Collectively, these changes render the microenvironment less permissive to tumour growth. Created with Biorender.com.

alters the factors secreted by endothelial cells (the so-called angiogenic secretome), leading to the inhibition of aberrant endothelial sprouting and promoting vessel remodelling. Central to this process is the activation of the transcription factor NFAT (Nuclear Factor of Activated T cells), which modulates the expression of both pro- and anti-angiogenic genes. Notably, exercise-induced shear stress upregulates thrombospondin-1, a potent anti-angiogenic protein, thereby contributing to vascular normalisation in the TME (100). By improving oxygenation and reducing hypoxic stress, exercise also suppresses the hypoxia-driven signalling pathways that underpin process such as EMT, cancer stem cell (CSC) maintenance and metabolic reprogramming (101,102).

3.2.6 Cancer stem cells

Cells within the tumour mass display a wide range of genetic and phenotypic characteristics, a term known as tumour heterogeneity. CSCs are a small but highly potent subpopulation of cancer cells that have the capacity for self-renewal and initiating new tumours and are typically more resistant to chemotherapy (103). The CSC concept represents a paradigm shift in understanding tumour heterogeneity, therapeutic resistance and tumour recurrence. In many solid tumours, CSCs are enriched and closely associated with poor prognosis (104). Although their characteristics and surface marker expression profiles vary across cancer type, functionally CSCs generally exhibit increased resistance to apoptosis, enhanced DNA repair capabilities and a metabolic profile that supports quiescence and survival under stress (105,106).

The maintenance and behaviour of CSCs are highly dependent on cues from the TME. Hypoxic regions within the tumour mass promote CSC survival via HIF-1α signalling; likewise, pro-inflammatory cytokines such as IL-6, TNF-α and TGFβ can induce de-differentiation of non-stem tumour cells into a more stem-like phenotype (107). Crosstalk between CSCs and neighbouring stromal cells, particularly CAFs and CAAs, further supports the stem cell niche through the secretion of leptin, fibroblast growth factors (FGFs) and EVs carrying microRNAs and metabolites that promote stemness, such as lactate from the Warburg effect (see Chapter 4, Section 4.6) and ketone bodies secreted by CAFs (108,109).

In aggressive cancers, such as triple-negative breast cancer (TNBC), CSCs are often enriched and are thought to contribute to recurrence and metastasis (110). These CSCs are maintained in specialised micro-niches in the TME that are starved of oxygen (hypoxic), rich in inflammation and metabolically distinct from other tissues (111). Systemic influences such as obesity may further support CSC expansion. In the obesogenic microenvironment, elevated levels of leptin activate various signalling pathways, including JAK/STAT3 and PI3K/Akt, which are known to promote cancer cell proliferation and are implicated in leptin-mediated maintenance of stemness (112,113). In a similar manner, FABP4, an adipokine upregulated in hypertrophic adipocytes, can promote lipid transfer to tumour cells, enhancing their tumour-initiating capacity (114,115). These signals converge to not only sustain CSCs but also stimulate de-differentiation of tumour cells back into a stem-like state—a process known as phenotypic plasticity (116). These effects are explored in more detail in Chapter 4, which focuses on the molecular pathways underpinning signalling in cancer.

3.2.6.1 Exercise has the potential to suppress the CSC niche

Given the influential role of the systemic and microenvironmental milieu on CSC biology, it stands to reason that exercise could potentially suppress CSC function through multiple converging pathways. Although direct evidence is scarce, the theoretical rationale is compelling. Regular exercise reduces systemic inflammation, modulates adipokine profiles and alters the bioavailability of metabolic substrates, all of which can influence CSC survival. For example, exercise has been shown to reduce serum levels of leptin, IL-6 and insulin, while simultaneously increasing levels of adiponectin and anti-inflammatory cytokines such as IL-10 (117). This shift in systemic factors creates a more hostile environment that is less favourable for CSC maintenance and expansion, although research is still being undertaken in this area.

Mechanistically, exercise-induced myokines such as irisin, oncostatin M and SPARC, have demonstrated anti-tumour properties in vitro (32,118,119) (discussed in more detail in Chapter 4) and may directly influence CSC-associated pathways such as JAK/STAT3, Notch and Wnt/β-catenin. At the epigenetic level, exercise has been linked with changes in DNA methylation and microRNA expression, in both cancer and non-cancer settings. For example, in preclinical models of breast cancer, exercise (and diet) have been shown to modulate specific microRNAs, such as the upregulation of miR-873–5p, which regulates stemness and EMT, and the downregulation of miR-199a-5p, which functions as a tumour suppressor (120). These findings support the notion that exercise might suppress CSCs, not only through changes in cytokine and hormonal levels, but also by reprogramming the epigenetic landscape that sustains their identity. However, it is important to emphasise that, to date, there is a lack of robust in vivo evidence demonstrating that exercise directly reduces CSC populations, alters stem cell marker expression, or modulates microRNA expression specifically in relation to stemness, highlighting the need for further research in this emerging area.

Yet, the idea that exercise might act as a CSC-modulating strategy, through indirect rewiring of systemic and stromal cues rather than direct targeting of CSCs themselves is intriguing and given the central role of CSCs in therapy resistance and relapse, the potential for lifestyle interventions in this space is compelling but must be approached with caution until stronger empirical evidence emerges.

3.2.7 Circulating tumour cells

CTCs are cancer cells that have detached from a primary tumour and entered the bloodstream, where they serve as seeds for metastatic spread. Although CTCs are rare, often comprising only a few cells among billions of blood cells, their presence is a poor prognostic indicator and correlates with disease progression and reduced survival across multiple cancer types, including breast, lung and colorectal cancer (121). CTCs must survive a range of hostile conditions within the circulation. These include oxidative stress, anoikis (a form of cell death induced by detachment from the ECM), immune surveillance and physical forces such as shear stress from blood flow. Despite these challenges, some CTCs succeed in adhering to vascular walls, extravasating into distant tissues and establishing secondary tumours.

CTCs interact closely with other blood and stromal cells during circulation. For example, they can bind to platelets, which form a protective cloak around the tumour cells, shielding them from immune attack and enhancing their ability to adhere to the endothelium (122). Moreover, interactions with macrophages and osteoclasts have been shown to support their survival and migration, particularly to common metastatic sites such as bone. The metastatic potential of CTCs is further influenced by their molecular profile. Subsets of CTCs may exhibit stem-like characteristics, epithelial-mesenchymal plasticity, or resistance to apoptosis, enabling them to better survive in circulation and seed metastatic sites (123). Importantly, emerging data suggest that elements of the TME, including systemic factors like inflammation, cytokines and metabolic signals, can modulate CTC behaviour.

3.2.7.1 The role of exercise in modulating CTC dynamics

Although not part of the TME per se, CTCs are a critical link between the local tumour and distant sites and may be influenced by exercise through mechanical forces, immune modulation and vascular shear stress. While direct evidence linking exercise to reductions in CTC number or viability is still emerging, several mechanistic insights suggest that exercise may influence the fate of CTCs in circulation. One of the most compelling lines of evidence relates to the mechanical force of blood flow. A preclinical study using a microfluidic platform showed that increasing shear stress to levels equivalent to those seen during vigorous exercise (~45–60 dyn/cm^2) resulted in the death of up to 99% of CTCs in vitro (124). In contrast, shear levels typical of resting conditions (~15 dyn/cm^2) allowed nearly half of CTCs to remain viable, highlighting the potential for exercise-induced haemodynamic stress to compromise CTC survival. Exercise may also enhance immune-mediated clearance of CTCs. For instance, preclinical studies in mice have demonstrated that wheel running or treadmill exercise prior to tumour inoculation increases NK cell activity and macrophage cytotoxicity, both of which are critical for eliminating tumour cells in circulation (125,126). Notably, this effect appears to be timing-dependent, with greater anti-metastatic benefits observed when exercise is initiated before metastatic seeding occurs.

In addition, fluid flow has been shown to activate osteocytes (a class of cells found in bone), which in turn release factors that impair CTC migration and promote apoptosis in bone-metastatic models. This mechanosensitive signalling involves molecules such as ICAM-1 and IL-6, which reduce cancer cell extravasation into the bone matrix (127). These findings suggest that exercise-induced mechanical cues may not only affect CTC survival in circulation but also modulate the metastatic potential of target organs such as bone. Interestingly, exercise intensity may also influence these dynamics. In sedentary men with nasopharyngeal carcinoma, high-intensity cycling transiently increased platelet-tumour aggregation and pro-coagulant activity, potentially promoting metastasis. However, moderate-intensity exercise was shown to inhibit these interactions, supporting a protective effect (128).

Taken together, while clinical data remain limited, these preclinical studies highlight multiple potential mechanisms through which exercise could reduce the viability, dissemination and metastatic success of CTCs, representing an exciting and underexplored avenue for future research.

3.3 Intercellular crosstalk and the tumour ecosystem

Cancer progression is not solely driven by intrinsic changes within tumour cells but is intricately shaped by the dynamic crosstalk between various cell types within the TME. This communication occurs via soluble factors, direct cell-cell contact, and the structural cues provided by the

ECM. As a systemic physiological stimulus, exercise can disrupt or recalibrate these lines of communication in ways that restrain tumour growth and progression. A key player in this systemic influence is skeletal muscle, which functions as an endocrine organ by releasing cytokines and peptides known as myokines during contraction (see Box-out 3.1 and Chapter 4, Section 4.4). These signalling molecules exert both paracrine and endocrine effects, influencing distant tissues, including tumours. Myokines such as IL-6, SPARC and irisin have been shown to exert direct anti-tumour properties, including suppressing proliferation, promoting apoptosis and modulating immune surveillance (9,32,35,60,118,119,129,130). The effects of these and many other myokines are discussed in more detail in Chapter 4.

Importantly, the effects of myokines extend beyond cancer cells. These molecules modulate the behaviour of immune cells, fibroblasts, endothelial cells, and adipocytes, all of which play critical roles in either sustaining or constraining tumour progression (131). In doing so, exercise orchestrates a broader ecological shift within the TME, reprogramming it from a tumour-supportive to a tumour-suppressive state. While many of the underlying mechanisms remain under active investigation, including changes in gene expression, epigenetic modifications and extracellular vesicle (EV) signalling, these will be discussed in greater depth in Chapter 4. Nonetheless, current evidence clearly positions exercise as a master regulator of intercellular communication, with systemic and local ripple effects throughout the tumour ecosystem.

3.4 Chapter summary

The past few decades have transformed our understanding of the tumour as a dynamic, evolving ecosystem in which cancer cells interact with a complex microenvironment, adapt their metabolism, evade immune surveillance and respond to mechanical and systemic cues. Within this evolving landscape, exercise has emerged not merely as a supportive lifestyle factor, but as a biologically active, multi-potent intervention capable of reshaping cancer biology from the molecular to the systemic level. This chapter has mapped the cellular and structural complexity of the TME, highlighting the diverse populations of stromal, immune, vascular and CSCs that influence tumour progression. It has explored the pleiotropic effects of exercise in modulating immune cell mobilisation, altering cytokine profiles, influencing angiogenesis and ECM remodelling, and reprogramming the metabolic and inflammatory cues that underpin tumour growth. Through both direct and indirect mechanisms, physical activity can recondition the TME, potentially tipping the balance away from immune evasion, fibrosis and hypoxia towards an environment more permissive to immune surveillance and treatment response.

While many of the underlying molecular mechanisms remain under investigation, the evidence supports the view that exercise influences cancer biology at multiple levels. By treating the terrain, not just the tumour, exercise offers an opportunity to disrupt tumour-promoting networks in a coordinated way. However, despite the compelling evidence, exercise is still underutilised in standard cancer care. The challenge lies in the need for the integration of biology with behaviour: the translation of these findings into clinical practice presents both exciting opportunities and key challenges and will be addressed in greater depth in Chapter 9. Meanwhile, the next chapter will dive deeper into the molecular mechanisms underpinning these effects, exploring the intracellular pathways, metabolic shifts and transcriptional programmes activated by exercise. These insights may set the stage for more precise, biologically informed exercise prescriptions in cancer care in due course.

Chapter 3 Test your understanding question bank

1. What are the main cellular components of the tumour microenvironment (TME), and how do they influence cancer progression?
2. Describe the role of immune checkpoint proteins such as PD-1 and PD-L1 in tumour immune evasion.
3. How does exercise influence the infiltration and function of natural killer (NK) cells and CD8+ T cells within the TME?
4. What is the difference between M1-like and M2-like tumour-associated macrophages (TAMs), and how might exercise influence their polarisation?
5. Explain how regulatory T cells (Tregs) and myeloid-derived suppressor cells (MDSCs) contribute to an immunosuppressive TME.
6. In what ways does exercise alter cytokine signalling within the TME, and what are the potential implications for tumour behaviour?
7. What is the significance of cancer-associated fibroblasts (CAFs) in shaping the TME, and how might exercise modify their activity?
8. How do adipokines secreted by cancer-associated adipocytes (CAAs) impact cancer cell behaviour, particularly in obesity-associated cancers?
9. Describe how exercise affects the secretory profile of adipose tissue and the downstream consequences for tumour progression.
10. What are myokines, and which ones have been implicated in mediating anti-tumour effects of exercise?
11. Summarise how exercise-induced vascular normalisation might enhance immune cell trafficking into the tumour.

12. Explain how skeletal muscle functions as an endocrine organ. Which signalling molecules are involved, and what effects do they have on the TME?
13. How does exercise influence the viability and extravasation of circulating tumour cells (CTCs)?
14. What are the key characteristics of cancer stem cells (CSCs), and what does emerging research suggest about how exercise might affect CSC behaviour?
15. In what ways might exercise act as a primer for cancer therapies such as immune checkpoint inhibitors?
16. Discuss how obesity alters the adipose tissue microenvironment to support tumour growth. How can exercise reverse or mitigate these changes?
17. What role do extracellular vesicles (EVs) play in intracellular communication, and how might their cargo be modified by exercise?
18. Exercise exerts both systemic and local effects on the tumour ecosystem. Summarise at least three different cell types that are influenced by exercise, describing the nature and consequences of these changes.

References

1. Guo S, Huang J, Li G, Chen W, Li Z, Lei J. The role of extracellular vesicles in circulating tumor cell-mediated distant metastasis. Mol Cancer [Internet]. 2023 Dec 1 [cited 2025 Nov 16];22(1):193. Available from: https://pmc.ncbi.nlm.nih.gov/articles/PMC10688140/
2. Baghban R, Roshangar L, Jahanban-Esfahlan R, Seidi K, Ebrahimi-Kalan A, Jaymand M, et al. Tumor microenvironment complexity and therapeutic implications at a glance. Cell Communication and Signaling [Internet]. 2020 Apr 7 [cited 2025 Nov 16];18(1):59. Available from: https://biosignaling.biomedcentral.com/articles/10.1186/s12964-020-0530-4
3. Pedersen L, Idorn M, Olofsson GH, Lauenborg B, Nookaew I, Hansen RH, et al. Voluntary running suppresses tumor growth through Epinephrine- and IL-6-dependent NK cell mobilization and redistribution. Cell Metab; 2016 Mar 8;23(3):554–62.
4. Baskerville R, Castell L, Bermon S. Sports and immunity, from the recreational to the elite athlete. Infect Dis Now [Internet]. 2024 Jun 1 [cited 2025 Nov 16];54(4S). Available from: https://pubmed.ncbi.nlm.nih.gov/38531477/
5. Koelwyn GJ, Wennerberg E, Demaria S, Jones LW. Exercise in regulation of inflammation-immune axis function in cancer initiation and progression. Oncology (Williston Park) [Internet]. 2015 Dec 15 [cited 2025 Nov 16];29(12):214800. Available from: https://pmc.ncbi.nlm.nih.gov/articles/PMC4909049/
6. Jones LW, Fels DR, West M, Allen JD, Broadwater G, Barry WT, et al. Modulation of circulating angiogenic factors and tumor biology by aerobic training in breast cancer patients receiving neoadjuvant chemotherapy. Cancer Prevention Research [Internet]. 2013 Sep 1 [cited 2025 Nov 16];6(9):925–37. Available from: /cancerpreventionresearch/article/6/9/925/50183/Modulation-of-Circulating-Angiogenic-Factors-and

7. Wennerberg E, Lhuillier C, Rybstein MD, Dannenberg K, Rudqvist NP, Koelwyn GJ, et al. Exercise reduces immune suppression and breast cancer progression in a preclinical model. Oncotarget [Internet]. 2020 [cited 2025 Nov 16];11(4):452–61. Available from: www.oncotarget.com
8. Zhang X, Ashcraft KA, Warner AB, Nair SK, Dewhirst MW. Can exercise-induced modulation of the tumor physiologic microenvironment improve antitumor immunity? Cancer Res [Internet]. 2019 May 15 [cited 2025 Nov 16];79(10):2447. Available from: https://pmc.ncbi.nlm.nih.gov/articles/PMC7474542/
9. Proschinger S, Winker M, Joisten N, Bloch W, Palmowski J, Zimmer P. The effect of exercise on regulatory T cells: A systematic review of human and animal studies with future perspectives and methodological recommendations.
10. Veglia F, Sanseviero E, Gabrilovich DI. Myeloid-derived suppressor cells in the era of increasing myeloid cell diversity. Nature Reviews Immunology [Internet]. 2021 Feb 1 [cited 2025 Nov 16];21(8):485–98. Available from: https://www.nature.com/articles/s41577-020-00490-y
11. Idorn M, thor Straten P. Exercise and cancer: From "healthy" to "therapeutic"? Cancer Immunol Immunother [Internet]. 2017 May 1 [cited 2025 Nov 16];66(5):667–71. Available from: https://pubmed.ncbi.nlm.nih.gov/28324125/
12. Haist M, Stege H, Grabbe S, Bros M. The functional crosstalk between myeloid-derived suppressor cells and regulatory T cells within the immunosuppressive tumor microenvironment. Cancers [Internet]. 2021 Jan 8 [cited 2025 Nov 16];13(2):210. Available from: https://www.mdpi.com/2072-6694/13/2/210/htm
13. Lyu DW. Immunomodulatory effects of exercise in cancer prevention and adjuvant therapy: A narrative review. Front Physiol [Internet]. 2024 [cited 2025 Nov 16];14:1292580. Available from: https://pmc.ncbi.nlm.nih.gov/articles/PMC10794543/
14. Liu G, Ballarò R, Schadler K. Aerobic exercise impacts the tumor microenvironment by altering CAF abundance and CAF-activating cytokines in pancreatic cancer. Summer Experience [Internet]. 2023 Aug 9 [cited 2025 Nov 29]. Available from: https://openworks.mdanderson.org/sumexp23/81
15. Kurz E, Hirsch CA, Dalton T, Shadaloey SA, Khodadadi-Jamayran A, Miller G, et al. Exercise-induced engagement of the IL-15/IL-15Rα axis promotes anti-tumor immunity in pancreatic cancer. Cancer Cell. 2022 Jul 11;40(7):720–737.e5.
16. Case N, Xie Z, Sen B, Styner M, Zou M, O'Conor C, et al. Mechanical activation of β-catenin regulates phenotype in adult murine marrow-derived mesenchymal stem cells. J Orthop Res [Internet]. 2010 [cited 2025 Nov 16];28(11):1531. Available from: https://pmc.ncbi.nlm.nih.gov/articles/PMC3046385/
17. Xiang YY, Won JH, Lee SJ, Baek KW. The effect of exercise on mesenchymal stem cells and their application in obesity treatment. Stem Cell Rev Rep [Internet]. 2024 Oct 1 [cited 2025 Nov 16];20(7):1732–51. Available from: https://link.springer.com/article/10.1007/s12015-024-10755-x
18. Docherty S, Harley R, McAuley JJ, Crowe LAN, Pedret C, Kirwan PD, et al. The effect of exercise on cytokines: Implications for musculoskeletal health: A narrative review. BMC Sports Sci Med Rehabil [Internet]. 2022 Dec 1 [cited 2025 Nov 16];14(1):5. Available from: https://pmc.ncbi.nlm.nih.gov/articles/PMC8740100/
19. Brown MJ, Morris MA, Akam EC. Investigating the effects of indirect coculture of human mesenchymal stem cells on the migration of breast cancer cells: A systematic review and meta-analysis. Breast Cancer (Auckl) [Internet]. 2023 Jan 1 [cited 2025 Nov 16];17. Available from: https://doi.org/10.1177/11782234221145385

20. Zhang X, Hu F, Li G, Li G, Yang X, Liu L, et al. Human colorectal cancer-derived mesenchymal stem cells promote colorectal cancer progression through IL-6/JAK2/STAT3 signaling. Cell Death Dis [Internet]. 2018 Feb 1 [cited 2025 Nov 16];9(2). Available from: https://pubmed.ncbi.nlm.nih.gov/29348540/
21. Li W, Liu Q, Shi J, Xu X, Xu J. The role of TNF-α in the fate regulation and functional reprogramming of mesenchymal stem cells in an inflammatory microenvironment. Front Immunol. 2023 Feb 6;14:1074863.
22. Becic T, Studenik C, Hoffmann G. Exercise increases adiponectin and reduces leptin levels in prediabetic and diabetic individuals: Systematic review and meta-analysis of randomized controlled trials. Medical Sciences [Internet]. 2018 Oct 30 [cited 2025 Nov 16];6(4):97. Available from: https://pmc.ncbi.nlm.nih.gov/articles/PMC6318757/
23. Zhou Y, Jia N, Ding M, Yuan K. Effects of exercise on inflammatory factors and IGF system in breast cancer survivors: a meta-analysis. BMC Womens Health [Internet]. 2022 Dec 1 [cited 2025 Nov 16];22(1):507. Available from: https://bmcwomenshealth.biomedcentral.com/articles/10.1186/s12905-022-02058-5
24. Lee S, Norheim F, Langleite TM, Gulseth HL, Birkeland KI, Drevon CA. Effects of long-term exercise on plasma adipokine levels and inflammation-related gene expression in subcutaneous adipose tissue in sedentary dysglycaemic, overweight men and sedentary normoglycaemic men of healthy weight. Diabetologia [Internet]. 2019 Jun 1 [cited 2025 Nov 16];62(6):1048–64. Available from: https://link.springer.com/article/10.1007/s00125-019-4866-5
25. Garritson JD, Boudina S. The effects of exercise on white and brown adipose tissue cellularity, metabolic activity and remodeling. Front Physiol [Internet]. 2021 Nov 2 [cited 2025 Nov 16];12:772894. Available from: www.frontiersin.org
26. Schadler KL, Thomas NJ, Galie PA, Bhang DH, Roby KC, Addai P, et al. Tumor vessel normalization after aerobic exercise enhances chemotherapeutic efficacy. [cited 2025 Nov 16];7(40). Available from: www.impactjournals.com/oncotarget
27. Falzone L, Grimaldi M, Celentano E, Augustin LSA, Libra M. Identification of modulated MicroRNAs associated with breast cancer, diet, and physical activity. Cancers (Basel) [Internet]. 2020 Sep 1 [cited 2025 Nov 18];12(9):2555. Available from: https://pmc.ncbi.nlm.nih.gov/articles/PMC7564431/
28. Effect of exercise on natural cytotoxicity and pulmonary tumor metastases in mice—PubMed [Internet]. [cited 2025 Nov 18]. Available from: https://pubmed.ncbi.nlm.nih.gov/8371653/
29. Regmi S, Fu A, Luo KQ. High shear stresses under exercise condition destroy circulating tumor cells in a microfluidic system. Sci Rep [Internet]. 2017 Jan 5 [cited 2025 Nov 18];7. Available from: https://pubmed.ncbi.nlm.nih.gov/28054593/
30. Hoffman-Goetz L. Exercise, natural immunity, and tumor metastasis. Med Sci Sports Exerc [Internet]. 1994 [cited 2025 Nov 18];26(2):157–63. Available from: https://pubmed.ncbi.nlm.nih.gov/8164532/
31. Dethlefsen C, Hansen LS, Lillelund C, Andersen C, Gehl J, Christensen JF, et al. Exercise-induced catecholamines activate the Hippo tumor suppressor pathway to reduce risks of breast cancer development. Cancer Res [Internet]. 2017 Sep 15 [cited 2025 Nov 16];77(18):4894–904. Available from: https://pubmed.ncbi.nlm.nih.gov/28887324/
32. Gannon NP, Vaughan RA, Garcia-Smith R, Bisoffi M, Trujillo KA. Effects of the exercise-inducible myokine irisin on malignant and non-malignant breast

epithelial cell behavior in vitro. Int J Cancer [Internet]. 2015 Feb 15 [cited 2025 Nov 16];136(4):E197–202. Available from: https://pubmed.ncbi.nlm.nih.gov/25124080/
33. Baldelli G, De Santi M, Gervasi M, Annibalini G, Sisti D, Højman P, et al. The effects of human sera conditioned by high-intensity exercise sessions and training on the tumorigenic potential of cancer cells. Clin Transl Oncol [Internet]. 2021 Jan 1 [cited 2025 Nov 16];23(1):22–34. Available from: https://pubmed.ncbi.nlm.nih.gov/32447643/
34. Hojman P, Gehl J, Christensen JF, Pedersen BK. Molecular mechanisms linking exercise to cancer prevention and treatment. Cell Metab [Internet]. 2018 Jan 9 [cited 2025 Nov 16];27(1):10–21. Available from: https://pubmed.ncbi.nlm.nih.gov/29056514/
35. Karstoft K, Pedersen BK. Skeletal muscle as a gene regulatory endocrine organ. Curr Opin Clin Nutr Metab Care [Internet]. 2016 Jul 1 [cited 2025 Nov 16];19(4):270–5. Available from: https://pubmed.ncbi.nlm.nih.gov/27101470/
36. van Doorslaer de Ten Ryen S, Deldicque L. The regulation of the metastatic cascade by physical activity: A narrative review. Cancers (Basel) [Internet]. 2020 Jan 8 [cited 2025 Jan 10];12(1):153. Available from: http://www.ncbi.nlm.nih.gov/pubmed/31936342
37. Jiang Y, Li Y, Zhu B. T-cell exhaustion in the tumor microenvironment. Cell Death & Disease [Internet]. 2015 Jun 18 [cited 2025 Nov 16];6(6):e1792–e1792. Available from: https://www.nature.com/articles/cddis2015162
38. Zhao H, Wu L, Yan G, Chen Y, Zhou M, Wu Y, et al. Inflammation and tumor progression: Signaling pathways and targeted intervention. [cited 2025 Nov 16]. Available from: https://doi.org/10.1038/s41392-021-00658-5
39. Gustafson MP, Wheatley-Guy CM, Rosenthal AC, Gastineau DA, Katsanis E, Johnson BD, et al. Exercise and the immune system: Taking steps to improve responses to cancer immunotherapy. J Immunother Cancer [Internet]. 2021 Jul 2 [cited 2025 Nov 16];9(7):1872. Available from: https://jitc.bmj.com/content/9/7/e001872
40. Casciano F, Caruso L, Zauli E, Gonelli A, Zauli G, Vaccarezza M. Emerging mechanisms of physical exercise benefits in adjuvant and neoadjuvant cancer immunotherapy. Biomedicines [Internet]. 2024 Nov 5 [cited 2025 Nov 16];12(11):2528. Available from: https://www.mdpi.com/2227-9059/12/11/2528/htm
41. Wu G, Chen Y, Chen C, Liu J, Wu Q, Zhang Y, et al. Role and mechanisms of exercise therapy in enhancing drug treatment for glioma: A review. 2025.
42. Gomes-Santos IL, Amoozgar Z, Kumar AS, Ho WW, Roh K, Talele NP, et al. Exercise training improves tumor control by increasing CD8+ T-cell infiltration via CXCR3 signaling and sensitizes breast cancer to immune checkpoint blockade. Cancer Immunol Res [Internet]. 2021 Jul 1 [cited 2025 Nov 16];9(7):765. Available from: https://pmc.ncbi.nlm.nih.gov/articles/PMC8295193/
43. Yan H, Jiang A, Huang Y, Zhang J, Yang W, Zhang W, et al. Exercise sensitizes PD-1/PD-L1 immunotherapy as a hypoxia modulator in the tumor microenvironment of melanoma. Front Immunol. 2023 Oct 9;14:1265914.
44. Exercise and Immunotherapy 101.
45. Brummer C, Pukrop T, Wiskemann J, Bruss C, Ugele I, Renner K. Can exercise enhance the efficacy of checkpoint inhibition by modulating anti-tumor immunity? Cancers (Basel) [Internet]. 2023 Sep 1 [cited 2025 Nov 29];15(18):4668. Available from: https://pmc.ncbi.nlm.nih.gov/articles/PMC10526963/

46. Marei HE, Hasan A, Pozzoli G, Cenciarelli C. Cancer immunotherapy with immune checkpoint inhibitors (ICIs): Potential, mechanisms of resistance, and strategies for reinvigorating T cell responsiveness when resistance is acquired. Cancer Cell International 2023 23:1 [Internet]. 2023 Apr 10 [cited 2025 Nov 16];23(1):64. Available from: https://cancerci.biomedcentral.com/articles/10.1186/s12935-023-02902-0
47. Darvin P, Toor SM, Sasidharan Nair V, Elkord E. Immune checkpoint inhibitors: Recent progress and potential biomarkers. Experimental & Molecular Medicine [Internet]. 2018 Dec 13 [cited 2025 Nov 16];50(12):1–11. Available from: https://www.nature.com/articles/s12276-018-0191-1
48. Liu T, Han C, Wang S, Fang P, Ma Z, Xu L, et al. Cancer-associated fibroblasts: An emerging target of anti-cancer immunotherapy. J Hematol Oncol [Internet]. 2019 Aug 28 [cited 2025 Nov 16];12(1). Available from: https://pubmed.ncbi.nlm.nih.gov/31462327/
49. Bhowmick NA, Neilson EG, Moses HL. Stromal fibroblasts in cancer initiation and progression. Nature [Internet]. 2004 Nov 18 [cited 2025 Nov 16];432(7015):332–7. Available from: https://pubmed.ncbi.nlm.nih.gov/15549095/
50. Li B, Wang JHC. Fibroblasts and myofibroblasts in wound healing: Force generation and measurement. J Tissue Viability [Internet]. 2011 Nov [cited 2025 Nov 16];20(4):108–20. Available from: https://pubmed.ncbi.nlm.nih.gov/19995679/
51. Miles FL, Sikes RA. Insidious changes in stromal matrix fuel cancer progression. Mol Cancer Res [Internet]. 2014 [cited 2025 Nov 16];12(3):297–312. Available from: https://pubmed.ncbi.nlm.nih.gov/24452359/
52. Desmoulière A. Factors influencing myofibroblast differentiation during wound healing and fibrosis. Cell Biol Int [Internet]. 1995 May [cited 2025 Nov 16];19(5):471. Available from: https://pubmed.ncbi.nlm.nih.gov/7640660/
53. Darby IA, Laverdet B, Bonté F, Desmoulière A. Fibroblasts and myofibroblasts in wound healing. Clin Cosmet Investig Dermatol [Internet]. 2014 Nov 6 [cited 2025 Nov 16];7:301–11. Available from: https://pubmed.ncbi.nlm.nih.gov/25395868/
54. Dvorak HF. Tumors: Wounds that do not heal-redux. Cancer Immunol Res. 2015 Jan 1;3(1):1–11.
55. Taguchi A, Kawana K, Tomio K, Yamashita A, Isobe Y, Nagasaka K, et al. Matrix Metalloproteinase (MMP)-9 in Cancer-Associated Fibroblasts (CAFs) is suppressed by Omega-3 polyunsaturated fatty acids in vitro and in vivo. PLoS One [Internet]. 2014 Feb 27 [cited 2025 Nov 16];9(2):e89605. Available from: https://journals.plos.org/plosone/article?id=10.1371/journal.pone.0089605
56. Coussens LM, Werb Z. Inflammation and cancer. Nature 2002 420:6917 [Internet]. 2002 Dec 26 [cited 2025 Nov 16];420(6917):860–7. Available from: https://www.nature.com/articles/nature01322
57. Morris MA. Cancer-associated fibroblasts in undifferentiated nasopharyngeal carcinoma: A putative role for the EBV-encoded oncoprotein, LMP1. Pathogens [Internet]. 2019 Jan 1 [cited 2025 Nov 16];9(1). Available from: https://pubmed.ncbi.nlm.nih.gov/31861782/
58. Fukino K, Shen L, Matsumoto S, Morrison CD, Mutter GL, Eng C. Combined total genome loss of heterozygosity scan of breast cancer stroma and epithelium reveals multiplicity of stromal targets. Cancer Res [Internet]. 2004 Oct 15 [cited 2025 Nov 16];64(20):7231–6. Available from: https://pubmed.ncbi.nlm.nih.gov/15492239/

59. Petersen OW, Nielsen HL, Gudjonsson T, Villadsen R, Rønnov-Jessen L, Bissell MJ. The plasticity of human breast carcinoma cells is more than epithelial to mesenchymal conversion. Breast Cancer Res [Internet]. 2001 [cited 2025 Nov 16];3(4):213. Available from: https://pmc.ncbi.nlm.nih.gov/articles/PMC138684/
60. Quante M, Tu SP, Tomita H, Gonda T, Wang SSW, Takashi S, et al. Bone marrow-derived myofibroblasts contribute to the mesenchymal stem cell niche and promote tumor growth. Cancer Cell [Internet]. 2011 Feb 15 [cited 2025 Nov 16];19(2):257–72. Available from: https://pubmed.ncbi.nlm.nih.gov/21316604/
61. [Changes of fibroblast immunophenotype and their clinical significance in stromal remodeling of breast tumors]—PubMed [Internet]. [cited 2025 Nov 16]. Available from: https://pubmed.ncbi.nlm.nih.gov/25620480/
62. Öhlund D, Handly-Santana A, Biffi G, Elyada E, Almeida AS, Ponz-Sarvise M, et al. Distinct populations of inflammatory fibroblasts and myofibroblasts in pancreatic cancer. J Exp Med [Internet]. 2017 Mar 6 [cited 2025 Nov 16];214(3):579–96. Available from: https://pubmed.ncbi.nlm.nih.gov/28232471/
63. Wei L, Ye H, Li G, Lu Y, Zhou Q, Zheng S, et al. Cancer-associated fibroblasts promote progression and gemcitabine resistance via the SDF-1/SATB-1 pathway in pancreatic cancer. Cell Death Dis [Internet]. 2018 Nov 1 [cited 2025 Nov 16];9(11). Available from: https://pubmed.ncbi.nlm.nih.gov/30337520/
64. Teng F, Tian WY, Wang YM, Zhang YF, Guo F, Zhao J, et al. Cancer-associated fibroblasts promote the progression of endometrial cancer via the SDF-1/CXCR4 axis. J Hematol Oncol [Internet]. 2016 Feb 6 [cited 2025 Nov 16];9(1):8. Available from: https://pmc.ncbi.nlm.nih.gov/articles/PMC4744391/
65. Orimo A, Gupta PB, Sgroi DC, Arenzana-Seisdedos F, Delaunay T, Naeem R, et al. Stromal fibroblasts present in invasive human breast carcinomas promote tumor growth and angiogenesis through elevated SDF-1/CXCL12 secretion. Cell [Internet]. 2005 May 6 [cited 2025 Nov 16];121(3):335–48. Available from: https://pubmed.ncbi.nlm.nih.gov/15882617/
66. Kwak H, Kim J, Joshi K, Yeh A, Martinez DA, Lawler JM. Exercise training reduces fibrosis and matrix metalloproteinase dysregulation in the aging rat heart. The FASEB Journal [Internet]. 2011 Mar [cited 2025 Nov 16];25(3):1106. Available from: https://pmc.ncbi.nlm.nih.gov/articles/PMC3042845/
67. Gholamian S, Hosseini SRA, Rashidlamir A, Aghaalinejad H. The effects of interval aerobic training on mesenchymal biomarker gene expression, the rate of tumor volume, and cachexia in mice with breast cancer. Iran J Basic Med Sci [Internet]. 2020 [cited 2025 Nov 16];23(2):244. Available from: https://pmc.ncbi.nlm.nih.gov/articles/PMC7211355/
68. Lighthouse JK, Burke RM, Velasquez LS, Dirkx RA, Aiezza A, Moravec CS, et al. Exercise promotes a cardioprotective gene program in resident cardiac fibroblasts. JCI Insight [Internet]. 2019 Jan 10 [cited 2025 Nov 16];4(1):e92098. Available from: https://pmc.ncbi.nlm.nih.gov/articles/PMC6485363/
69. Zou YY, Tang X Bin, Chen ZL, Liu B, Zheng L, Song MY, et al. Exercise intervention improves mitochondrial quality in non-alcoholic fatty liver disease zebrafish. Front Endocrinol (Lausanne). 2023 May 22;14:1162485.
70. Koncina E, Nurmik M, Pozdeev VI, Gilson C, Tsenkova M, Begaj R, et al. IL1R1+ cancer-associated fibroblasts drive tumor development and immunosuppression in colorectal cancer. Nat Commun [Internet]. 2023 Dec 1 [cited 2025 Nov 16];14(1):4251. Available from: https://pmc.ncbi.nlm.nih.gov/articles/PMC10352362/

71. Wu X, Tao P, Zhou Q, Li J, Yu Z, Wang X, et al. IL-6 secreted by cancer-associated fibroblasts promotes epithelial-mesenchymal transition and metastasis of gastric cancer via JAK2/STAT3 signaling pathway. Oncotarget [Internet]. 2017 [cited 2025 Nov 16];8(13):20741. Available from: https://pmc.ncbi.nlm.nih.gov/articles/PMC5400541/
72. Chaudhry SI, Hooper S, Nye E, Williamson P, Harrington K, Sahai E. Autocrine IL-1β-TRAF6 signalling promotes squamous cell carcinoma invasion through paracrine TNFα signalling to carcinoma-associated fibroblasts.
73. Suhr F. Extracellular matrix, proteases and physical exercise. Dtsch Z Sportmed. 2019 Apr 1;70(4):97–103.
74. Xie Q, Ding J, Chen Y. Role of CD8+ T lymphocyte cells: Interplay with stromal cells in tumor microenvironment. Acta Pharm Sin B. 2021 Jun 1;11(6):1365–78.
75. Aoi W, Naito Y, Takagi T, Tanimura Y, Takanami Y, Kawai Y, et al. A novel myokine, secreted protein acidic and rich in cysteine (SPARC), suppresses colon tumorigenesis via regular exercise. Gut [Internet]. 2013 Jun 1 [cited 2025 Nov 16];62(6):882–9. Available from: https://gut.bmj.com/content/62/6/882
76. Fiuza-Luces C, Garatachea N, Berger NA, Lucia A. Exercise is the real polypill. Physiology [Internet]. 2013 Sep 1 [cited 2025 Nov 16];28(5):330–58. Available from: www.physiologyonline.org
77. Li F, Liu X, Bai N, Li Y, Hou M, Hou Y, et al. Irisin attenuates liver fibrosis by regulating energy metabolism and HMGB1/β-catenin signaling in hepatic stellate cells. Eur J Pharmacol. 2025 Jul 5;998:177519.
78. Kobayashi T, Tanaka K, Fujita T, Umezawa H, Amano H, Yoshioka K, et al. Bidirectional role of IL-6 signal in pathogenesis of lung fibrosis. Respir Res [Internet]. 2015 Aug 20 [cited 2025 Nov 16];16(1):99. Available from: https://respiratory-research.biomedcentral.com/articles/10.1186/s12931-015-0261-z
79. Sangaletti S, Tripodo C, Cappetti B, Casalini P, Chiodoni C, Piconese S, et al. SPARC oppositely regulates inflammation and fibrosis in bleomycin-induced lung damage. Am J Pathol. 2011 Dec 1;179(6):3000–10.
80. Sangaletti S, Tripodo C, Cappetti B, Casalini P, Chiodoni C, Piconese S, et al. SPARC oppositely regulates inflammation and fibrosis in bleomycin-induced lung damage. Am J Pathol. 2011 Dec 1;179(6):3000–10.
81. Johnson BZ, Stevenson AW, Prêle CM, Fear MW, Wood FM. The role of IL-6 in skin fibrosis and cutaneous wound healing. Biomedicines [Internet]. 2020 May 1 [cited 2025 Nov 16];8(5). Available from: https://pubmed.ncbi.nlm.nih.gov/32365896/
82. Ullah I, Subbarao RB, Rho GJ. Human mesenchymal stem cells—current trends and future prospective. Biosci Rep [Internet]. 2015 [cited 2025 Nov 16];35(2):e00191. Available from: https://pmc.ncbi.nlm.nih.gov/articles/PMC4413017/
83. Li X, Fan Q, Peng X, Yang S, Wei S, Liu J, et al. Mesenchymal/stromal stem cells: Necessary factors in tumour progression. Cell Death Discov [Internet]. 2022 Dec 1 [cited 2025 Nov 16];8(1):333. Available from: https://pmc.ncbi.nlm.nih.gov/articles/PMC9307857/
84. Xuan X, Tian C, Zhao M, Sun Y, Huang C. Mesenchymal stem cells in cancer progression and anticancer therapeutic resistance. Cancer Cell Int [Internet]. 2021 Dec 1 [cited 2025 Nov 16];21(1):595. Available from: https://pmc.ncbi.nlm.nih.gov/articles/PMC8570012/
85. Martin FT, Dwyer RM, Kelly J, Khan S, Murphy JM, Curran C, et al. Potential role of mesenchymal stem cells (MSCs) in the breast tumour microenvironment:

Stimulation of epithelial to mesenchymal transition (EMT). Breast Cancer Res Treat [Internet]. 2010 Nov [cited 2025 Nov 16];124(2):317–26. Available from: https://pubmed.ncbi.nlm.nih.gov/20087650/
86. Spaggiari GM, Capobianco A, Becchetti S, Mingari MC, Moretta L. Mesenchymal stem cell-natural killer cell interactions: Evidence that activated NK cells are capable of killing MSCs, whereas MSCs can inhibit IL-2-induced NK-cell proliferation. Blood [Internet]. 2006 Feb 15 [cited 2025 Nov 16];107(4):1484–90. Available from: https://pubmed.ncbi.nlm.nih.gov/16239427/
87. Mittal SK, Cho WK, Elbasiony E, Guan Y, Foulsham W, Chauhan SK. Mesenchymal stem cells augment regulatory T cell function via CD80-mediated interactions and promote allograft survival. Am J Transplant [Internet]. 2022 Jun 1 [cited 2025 Nov 16];22(6):1564. Available from: https://pmc.ncbi.nlm.nih.gov/articles/PMC11261724/
88. Kundu AK, Khatiwala CB, Putnam AJ. Extracellular matrix remodeling, integrin expression, and downstream signaling pathways influence the osteogenic differentiation of mesenchymal stem cells on poly(Lactide-Co-Glycolide) substrates. Tissue Eng Part A [Internet]. 2008 Feb 1 [cited 2025 Nov 16];15(2):273. Available from: https://pmc.ncbi.nlm.nih.gov/articles/PMC2810215/
89. Rhee KJ, Lee JI, Eom YW. Mesenchymal stem cell-mediated effects of tumor support or suppression. Int J Mol Sci [Internet]. 2015 Dec 16 [cited 2025 Nov 16];16(12):30015–33. Available from: https://pubmed.ncbi.nlm.nih.gov/26694366/
90. Klopp AH, Gupta A, Spaeth E, Andreeff M, Marini F. Concise review: Dissecting a discrepancy in the literature: Do mesenchymal stem cells support or suppress tumor growth? Stem Cells [Internet]. 2011 Jan [cited 2025 Nov 16];29(1):11–9. Available from: https://pubmed.ncbi.nlm.nih.gov/21280155/
91. Ridge SM, Sullivan FJ, Glynn SA. Mesenchymal stem cells: Key players in cancer progression. Mol Cancer [Internet]. 2017 Feb 1 [cited 2025 Nov 16];16(1). Available from: https://pubmed.ncbi.nlm.nih.gov/28148268/
92. Atiya H, Frisbie L, Pressimone C, Coffman L. Mesenchymal stem cells in the tumor microenvironment. Adv Exp Med Biol [Internet]. 2020 [cited 2025 Nov 16];1234:31–42. Available from: https://pubmed.ncbi.nlm.nih.gov/32040853/
93. Ramdasi S, Sarang S, Viswanathan C. Potential of mesenchymal stem cell based application in cancer. Int J Hematol Oncol Stem Cell Res [Internet]. 2015 [cited 2025 Nov 16];9(2):95. Available from: https://pmc.ncbi.nlm.nih.gov/articles/PMC4410295/
94. Ritter A, Kreis NN, Hoock SC, Solbach C, Louwen F, Yuan J. Adipose tissue-derived mesenchymal stromal/stem cells, obesity and the tumor microenvironment of breast cancer. Cancers [Internet]. 2022 Aug 12 [cited 2025 Nov 16];14(16):3908. Available from: https://www.mdpi.com/2072-6694/14/16/3908/htm
95. Brown MJ, Nickels M, Akam EC, Morris MA. The protective effect of endurance running against the pro-invasive effects of ageing in breast cancer cells and mesenchymal stem cells in vitro. In Vitro Models [Internet]. 2023 Aug 2 [cited 2025 Nov 16];2(6):263–80. Available from: https://pubmed.ncbi.nlm.nih.gov/39872498/
96. Li H, Liu G, Wang B, Momeni MR. Exosomes and microRNAs as mediators of the exercise. European Journal of Medical Research [Internet]. 2025 Jan 19 [cited 2025 Nov 16];30(1):38. Available from: https://eurjmedres.biomedcentral.com/articles/10.1186/s40001-025-02273-4

97. Kounatidis D, Vallianou NG, Karampela I, Grivakou E, Dalamaga M. The intricate role of adipokines in cancer-related signaling and the tumor microenvironment: Insights for future research. Semin Cancer Biol. 2025 Aug 1;113:130–50.
98. Gyamfi J, Eom M, Koo JS, Choi J. Multifaceted roles of interleukin-6 in adipocyte-breast cancer cell interaction. Transl Oncol [Internet]. 2018 [cited 2025 Nov 16];11:275–85. Available from: https://doi.org/10.1016/j.tranon.2017.12.009
99. Divella R, De Luca R, Abbate I, Naglieri E, Daniele A. Obesity and cancer: The role of adipose tissue and adipo-cytokines-induced chronic inflammation. J Cancer [Internet]. 2016 [cited 2025 Nov 16];7(15):2346–59. Available from: http://www.jcancer.org
100. Hildebrandt X, Ibrahim M, Peltzer N. Cell death and inflammation during obesity: "Know my methods, WAT(son)." Cell Death & Differentiation [Internet]. 2022 Sep 29 [cited 2025 Nov 16];30(2):279–92. Available from: https://www.nature.com/articles/s41418-022-01062-4
101. Wu C, Dong S, Huang R, Chen X. Cancer-associated adipocytes and breast cancer: Intertwining in the tumor microenvironment and challenges for cancer therapy. 2023 [cited 2025 Nov 16]. Available from: https://doi.org/10.3390/cancers15030726
102. Coughlin SS, Smith SA. The insulin-like growth factor axis, adipokines, physical activity, and obesity in relation to breast cancer incidence and recurrence. Cancer Clin Oncol [Internet]. 2015 Jul 20 [cited 2025 Nov 16];4(2):24. Available from: https://pmc.ncbi.nlm.nih.gov/articles/PMC4524449/
103. Tan L, Mei J, Tang R, Huang D, Qi K, Ossowski Z, et al. Can exercise as a complementary technique manage inflammatory markers in women with breast cancer who are overweight and obese? A systematic review and meta-analysis. Complement Ther Med. 2025 Mar 1;88:103119.
104. Villa C, Chaplain MAJ, Lorenzi T. Evolutionary dynamics in vascularised tumours under chemotherapy.
105. Ashcraft KA, Betof Warner A, Jones LW, Dewhirst MW. Exercise as adjunct therapy in cancer.
106. Chen Z, Han F, Du Y, Shi H, Zhou W. Hypoxic microenvironment in cancer: molecular mechanisms and therapeutic interventions. Signal Transduction and Targeted Therapy [Internet]. 2023 Feb 17 [cited 2025 Nov 16];8(1):70. Available from: https://www.nature.com/articles/s41392-023-01332-8
107. Naz F, Shi M, Sajid S, Yang Z, Yu C. Cancer stem cells: A major culprit of intra-tumor heterogeneity. Am J Cancer Res [Internet]. 2021 [cited 2025 Nov 16];11(12):5782–811. Available from: www.ajcr.us/
108. Saygin C, Matei D, Majeti R, Reizes O, Lathia JD. Cell stem cell perspective targeting cancer stemness in the clinic: From hype to hope. Stem Cell [Internet]. 2019 [cited 2025 Nov 16];24:25–40. Available from: https://doi.org/10.1016/j.stem.2018.11.017
109. Milella M, Rutigliano M, Pandolfo SD, Aveta A, Crocetto F, Ferro M, et al. The metabolic landscape of cancer stem cells: Insights and implications for therapy. Cells [Internet]. 2025 May 1 [cited 2025 Nov 16];14(10):717. Available from: https://pmc.ncbi.nlm.nih.gov/articles/PMC12109792/
110. Rich JN. Cancer stem cells: Understanding tumor hierarchy and heterogeneity. Medicine (United States) [Internet]. 2016 [cited 2025 Nov 16];95(1):S2–7. Available from: https://journals.lww.com/md-journal/fulltext/2016/09081/cancer_stem_cells__understanding_tumor_hierarchy.3.aspx
111. Liu Q, Guo Z, Li G, Zhang Y, Liu X, Li B, et al. Cancer stem cells and their niche in cancer progression and therapy. Cancer Cell Int [Internet]. 2023 Dec

1 [cited 2025 Nov 16];23(1):305. Available from: https://pmc.ncbi.nlm.nih.gov/articles/PMC10693166/
112. Martinez-Outschoorn UE, Lin Z, Whitaker-Menezes D, Howell A, Sotgia F, Lisanti MP. Ketone body utilization drives tumor growth and metastasis. Cell Cycle [Internet]. 2012 Nov 1 [cited 2025 Nov 16];11(21):3964–71. Available from: https://pubmed.ncbi.nlm.nih.gov/23082722/
113. Pan Y, Yuan C, Zeng C, Sun C, Xia L, Wang G, et al. Cancer stem cells and niches: Challenges in immunotherapy resistance. Molecular Cancer [Internet]. 2025 Feb 25 [cited 2025 Nov 16];24(1):52. Available from: https://molecular-cancer.biomedcentral.com/articles/10.1186/s12943-025-02265-2
114. Fultang N, Chakraborty M, Peethambaran B. Regulation of cancer stem cells in triple negative breast cancer. Cancer Drug Resist [Internet]. 2021 [cited 2025 Nov 18];4(2):321–42. Available from: https://pubmed.ncbi.nlm.nih.gov/35582030/
115. Liu Q, Guo Z, Li G, Zhang Y, Liu X, Li B, et al. Cancer stem cells and their niche in cancer progression and therapy. Cancer Cell Int [Internet]. 2023 Dec 1 [cited 2025 Nov 18];23(1):305. Available from: https://pmc.ncbi.nlm.nih.gov/articles/PMC10693166/
116. Park J, Morley TS, Kim M, Clegg DJ, Scherer PE. Obesity and cancer—mechanisms underlying tumour progression and recurrence. Nat Rev Endocrinol [Internet]. 2014 [cited 2025 Nov 18];10(8):455. Available from: https://pmc.ncbi.nlm.nih.gov/articles/PMC4374431/
117. Zheng Q, Banaszak L, Fracci S, Basali D, Dunlap SM, Hursting SD, et al. Leptin receptor maintains cancer stem-like properties in triple negative breast cancer cells. Endocr Relat Cancer [Internet]. 2013 Dec 1 [cited 2025 Nov 18];20(6):797–808. Available from: https://erc.bioscientifica.com/view/journals/erc/20/6/797.xml
118. Zeng J, Sauter ER, Li B. FABP4: A new player in obesity-associated breast cancer. Trends Mol Med [Internet]. 2020 May 1 [cited 2025 Nov 18];26(5):437. Available from: https://pmc.ncbi.nlm.nih.gov/articles/PMC7646254/
119. Yu L, Wei W, Lv J, Lu Y, Wang Z, Cai C. FABP4-mediated lipid metabolism promotes TNBC progression and breast cancer stem cell activity. Cancer Lett. 2024 Nov 1;604:217271.
120. Gupta PB, Pastushenko I, Skibinski A, Blanpain C, Kuperwasser C. Phenotypic plasticity as a driver of cancer formation, progression and resistance to therapy. Cell Stem Cell [Internet]. 2018 Jan 3 [cited 2025 Nov 18];24(1):65. Available from: https://pmc.ncbi.nlm.nih.gov/articles/PMC7297507/
121. Golbidi S, Laher I. Exercise induced adipokine changes and the metabolic syndrome. J Diabetes Res [Internet]. 2014 [cited 2025 Nov 18];2014. Available from: https://pubmed.ncbi.nlm.nih.gov/24563869/
122. Ma J, Gao S, Xie X, Sun E, Zhang M, Zhou Q, et al. SPARC inhibits breast cancer bone metastasis and may be a clinical therapeutic target. Oncol Lett [Internet]. 2017 Nov 1 [cited 2025 Nov 18];14(5):5876. Available from: https://pmc.ncbi.nlm.nih.gov/articles/PMC5661402/
123. Ghanemi A, Yoshioka M, St-Amand J. Therapeutic potential of exercise-induced SPARC in bone health? Biomedicines [Internet]. 2025 Apr 1 [cited 2025 Nov 18];13(4):945. Available from: https://pmc.ncbi.nlm.nih.gov/articles/PMC12024751/
124. Alix-Panabières C, Pantel K. Challenges in circulating tumour cell research. Nat Rev Cancer [Internet]. 2014 [cited 2025 Nov 18];14(9):623–31. Available from: https://pubmed.ncbi.nlm.nih.gov/25154812/
125. Labelle M, Begum S, Hynes RO. Direct signaling between platelets and cancer cells induces an epithelial-mesenchymal-like transition and promotes

metastasis. Cancer Cell [Internet]. 2011 [cited 2025 Nov 18];20(5):576–90. Available from: https://pubmed.ncbi.nlm.nih.gov/22094253/
126. Plaks V, Koopman CD, Werb Z. Circulating tumor cells. Science [Internet]. 2013 [cited 2025 Nov 18];341(6151):10.1126/science.1235226. Available from: https://pmc.ncbi.nlm.nih.gov/articles/PMC3842225/
127. Ma YHV., Lam C, Dalmia S, Gao P, Young J, Middleton K, et al. Mechanical regulation of breast cancer migration and apoptosis via direct and indirect osteocyte signaling. J Cell Biochem [Internet]. 2018 Jul 1 [cited 2025 Nov 18];119(7):5665–75. Available from: https://pubmed.ncbi.nlm.nih.gov/29384215/
128. Wang JS, Chang CY, Chow SE, Chen YW, Yang CM. Exercise modulates platelet-nasopharyngeal carcinoma cell aggregation and subsequent tissue factor and matrix metalloproteinase activities. J Appl Physiol [Internet]. 2007 Sep [cited 2025 Nov 18];103(3):763–70. Available from: https://journals.physiology.org/doi/10.1152/japplphysiol.00165.2007
129. Li Y, Zhao J, Yin Y, Li K, Zhang C, Zheng Y. The role of IL-6 in fibrotic diseases: Molecular and cellular mechanisms. Int J Biol Sci [Internet]. 2022 [cited 2025 Nov 18];18(14):5405. Available from: https://pmc.ncbi.nlm.nih.gov/articles/PMC9461670/
130. Yoshida S, Asanoma K, Yagi H, Onoyama I, Hori E, Matsumura Y, et al. Fibronectin mediates activation of stromal fibroblasts by SPARC in endometrial cancer cells. BMC Cancer [Internet]. 2021 Dec 1 [cited 2025 Nov 18];21(1):156. Available from: https://pmc.ncbi.nlm.nih.gov/articles/PMC7881467/
131. Leal LG, Lopes MA, Batista ML. Physical exercise-induced myokines and muscle-adipose tissue crosstalk: A review of current knowledge and the implications for health and metabolic diseases. Front Physiol [Internet]. 2018 Sep 24 [cited 2025 Nov 18];9(SEP):1307. Available from: https://pmc.ncbi.nlm.nih.gov/articles/PMC6166321/

4

THE MOLECULAR BASIS OF EXERCISE IN CANCER

4.1 Introduction

Building on the systemic and cellular effects of exercise described in Chapter 3, this chapter shifts the focus to the molecular mechanisms that underpin these exercise-induced adaptations in cancer. Exercise is not only a physiological stressor but also an active regulator of intracellular signalling, gene expression and the TME. These molecular changes translate into wide-ranging effects on tumour biology, influencing metabolic pathways, immune activity, vascular function, mechanical forces and systemic hormonal balance. Understanding these molecular pathways is critical for two main reasons. First, it enables the identification of key molecular pathways where exercise might disrupt cancer progression, such as reprogramming tumour metabolism, suppressing angiogenesis, enhancing immune surveillance or altering the mechanical properties of the TME. Second, this knowledge lays the foundation for precision exercise prescriptions, where training modality, dose and intensity are tailored to individual tumour phenotypes and patient physiology. This chapter therefore explores the intracellular cascades, molecular messengers and systemic signals mobilised by exercise and how these converge to remodel the tumour ecosystem.

4.2 Gene expression and epigenetic regulation

Exercise induces dynamic changes in gene expression and epigenetic regulation, influencing both tumour cells and the surrounding host tissues (1). These molecular alterations underpin many of the protective effects of

DOI: 10.4324/9781003511519-5

exercise against cancer and are an area of growing research interest, especially for designing precision oncology interventions. These molecular adaptations often align with several of the recognised hallmarks of cancer, including sustained proliferative signalling, evasion of growth suppression and resistance to cell death (2), offering mechanistic insights into how exercise may interfere with tumour-promoting pathways.

4.2.1 Exercise-induced transcriptional changes

Regular exercise, particularly at moderate to high intensity, induces widespread transcriptional remodelling in skeletal muscle, immune cells and even tumour tissue. Preclinical transcriptomic analyses reveal that exercise modulates the expression of genes involved in apoptosis, cell cycle control, immune surveillance and metabolism. In a mouse model of colorectal cancer, high-intensity aerobic exercise significantly altered the expression of over 23,000 genes in skeletal muscle, including the upregulation of Col1a1, closely linked to EMT, and Six2, a gene associated with cancer stemness and metastatic potential. Conversely, expression of the proto-oncogene Fos and the colorectal cancer marker Trim63 was downregulated. Functional studies demonstrated that manipulating these genes in vitro led to a 20% reduction in cancer cell viability, suggesting that exercise-induced transcriptional changes may exert direct anti-tumour effects (3). Notably, many of these differentially expressed genes regulate immune evasion and metabolic reprogramming, two key traits of tumour adaptation, indicating that transcriptional changes in peripheral tissues, such as muscle, can indirectly influence tumour phenotype via systemic signalling. Additional studies have reported systemic transcriptomic shifts in exercised animals, impacting inflammatory mediators and immune regulation (4,5), supporting the view that exercise modulates the TME not only locally but through broader host tissue gene regulation.

4.2.2 Impact on tumour suppressors and oncogenes

Exercise modulates the expression and activity of several key tumour suppressors and oncogenes. *TP53*, a central regulator of cell cycle arrest, DNA damage repair and apoptosis, is frequently upregulated following exercise, contributing to the tumour-suppressive effects of exercise (see Section 4.2.3.3.; (5). Conversely, oncogenes such as *MYC* and anti-apoptotic regulators like *BCL2* are often suppressed in exercised models, contributing to reduced tumour proliferation and enhanced cell death (6). These transcriptional changes are tissue-specific and influenced by the type, intensity and duration of exercise. Their variability underscores the potential for using such molecular responses as biomarkers for patient responsiveness to exercise oncology interventions.

4.2.3 Epigenetic modifications

Epigenetic changes are heritable but reversible post-transcriptional modifications to chromatin structure that regulate gene expression without altering the underlying DNA sequence. Exercise acts as a potent modulator of the epigenome in skeletal muscle, inducing changes in DNA methylation, histone modifications and microRNAs (miRNAs)—small non-coding RNAs that fine-tune gene expression (7). Increasing evidence now also highlights its role in shaping the cancer-related epigenetic network, with implications for tumour suppression and disease progression (8–10). Importantly, some epigenetic changes appear to be reversible and sensitive to environmental inputs such as diet, stress and exercise, suggesting that the epigenome serves as a flexible interface between lifestyle and cancer risk (11).

4.2.3.1 DNA methylation

Exercise appears to promote global DNA methylation stability while also targeting specific gene loci involved in tumour suppression and oncogenesis (10). Aberrant methylation patterns, particularly promoter hypermethylation of tumour suppressor genes and global hypomethylation of repetitive elements, are characteristic traits of tumourigenesis (12). Physical activity and exercise have been linked with the partial reversal of these changes. For instance, individuals with higher levels of physical activity display reduced methylation of tumour suppressor genes such as *CACNA2D3*, a calcium channel gene whose silencing is linked to gastric cancer progression (13). Similar effects have been reported in breast cancer, where long-term exercise training over 6 months was associated with reduced leukocyte promoter methylation of the tumour suppressor gene L3MBTL1. In a separate tumour sample cohort, high L3MBTL1 expression correlated with low-grade, hormone receptor-positive tumours and reduced recurrence and mortality risk (14). Other genes frequently implicated in breast cancer, such as *APC* and *RASSF1A*, also show reduced promoter hypermethylation in response to regular physical activity, suggesting that exercise-linked epigenetic modulation of tumour suppressor genes may contribute to cancer risk reduction (15). Furthermore, physical activity and exercise are also associated with reduced promoter hypermethylation of tumour suppressor gene promoters in breast tissue. While lower oestrogen levels are one potential mechanism linking exercise to epigenetic regulation, direct evidence that exercise-mediated reductions in circulating oestrogen drive hypermethylation reversal remains limited (15,16). Longitudinal studies are now beginning to assess how persistent these demethylation effects are post-intervention, with preliminary findings suggesting some epigenetic benefits may be maintained with consistent exercise but fade upon cessation (17).

4.2.3.2 Histone modifications

Exercise also alters the activity of histone-modifying enzymes, such as histone acetyltransferases (HATs) and histone deacetylases (HDACs), thereby modifying chromatin accessibility and gene transcription. Acetylation of histone tails typically correlates with gene activation, and exercise has been shown to enhance this process at key gene loci involved in metabolism, apoptosis and immune regulation. One well-characterised mechanism involves the regulation of *GLUT4*, the insulin-responsive glucose transporter. At rest, *GLUT4* expression is suppressed by the interaction of HDAC5 with the transcription factor MEF2, which maintains chromatin in a deacetylated, repressive state. Following acute exercise, AMP-activated protein kinase (AMPK) phosphorylates HDAC5, promoting its dissociation from MEF2. This allows MEF2 to recruit co-activators such as PPARγ, PGC-1α, and HATs, leading to increased histone acetylation and GLUT4 transcription (18–20). This mechanism also underlies improved systemic glucose handling, linking epigenetics to metabolic reprogramming (see Figure 4.1 and Section 4.6). Similar regulatory mechanisms underlie the effects of exercise on tumour cells, enhancing expression of genes involved in apoptotic signalling and immune surveillance through increased histone acetylation (9,21).

4.2.3.3 MicroRNAs and inflammatory modulation

Physical activity and exercise also influence the expression of microRNAs (miRNAs), which act as post-transcriptional regulators of gene expression. Exercise-induced miRNAs have been linked to reduced expression of inflammatory mediators and restoration of tumour suppressor gene activity. For example, miR-630 and miR-5703 were shown to be upregulated by a low-intensity resistance training programme in a cohort of participants with no exercise habits. Moreover, these miRNAs were found to be enriched in numerous signalling pathways, including TGFβ, Wnt and PI3K/Akt, suggestive of their tumour-suppressive effects and immune-activating properties (22). Similarly, regular moderate-intensity exercise has been shown to reduce the expression of *ASC* (apoptosis-associated speck-like protein containing a caspase recruitment domain), a pro-inflammatory mediator

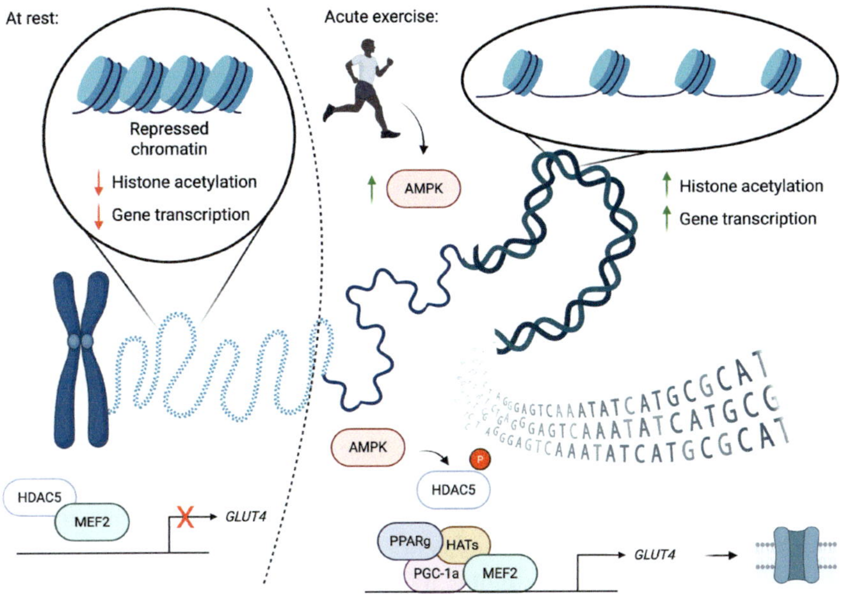

FIGURE 4.1 Exercise-induced histone acetylation and gene activation via AMPK-HDAC5-MEF2 signalling. Acute exercise activates AMP-activated protein kinase (AMPK), which phosphorylates and inhibits histone deacetylase 5 (HDAC5). At rest (left panel), HDAC5 interacts with the transcription factor MEF2, maintaining chromatin in a deacetylated, transcriptionally repressed state. Upon exercise (right panel), AMPK activation leads to HDAC5 dissociation, allowing MEF2 to recruit transcriptional co-activators including PGC-1α, PPARγ, and histone acetyltransferases (HATs). This results in increased histone acetylation, relaxed chromatin structure, and enhanced transcription of target genes such as GLUT4, and their subsequent translation to a fully functional protein. This mechanism not only improves glucose handling but may also contribute to broader gene activation in tumour and immune cells, linking epigenetic reprogramming to exercise-induced modulation of the TME. Created with Biorender.com.

implicated in carcinogenesis, resulting in reduced activity of the gene in human monocytic cells, thereby preventing activation of pro-inflammatory cytokines (23,24). Circulating exosomal miRNAs are also emerging as key mediators of systemic anti-cancer effects. Exercise increases the secretion of exosomes enriched in muscle-derived miRNAs, such as miR-1, miR133a/b and miR-206, and some miRNAs such as miR0233–3p and miR-486–5p have been implicated in tumour-suppressive pathways (25). However, definitive identification of specific exosomal miRNAs with anti-cancer effects remains an active area of research.

The tumour suppressor gene, *TP53*, which is frequently downregulated or silenced in many cancers, is also regulated at the epigenetic level via miRNAs. For instance, miR-125b has been shown to directly target the 3' untranslated region (UTR) of *TP53* mRNA, leading to its downregulation. Similarly, miR-504 and miR-25 can inhibit *TP53* translation, thereby lowering the tumour-suppressive activities of the p53 protein (26). While a direct link between exercise-induced miRNA modulation and p53 upregulation in cancer has yet to be established, exercise does appear to modulate relevant miRNAs, such as miR-16, which may indirectly influence p53 signalling (27). Moreover, acute bouts of exercise have been shown to activate p53 function in the liver (28), supporting a potential pathway through which physical activity influences this key tumour suppressor. Taken together, these findings suggest that regular exercise remodels the cancer epigenome through multiple coordinated mechanisms: Reversing promoter hypermethylation of tumour suppressors, enhancing histone acetylation, and modulating miRNA expression. These epigenetic effects may collectively contribute to a less inflammatory, more tumour-suppressive environment, with the potential to slow disease progression.

BOX-OUT 4.1 HOW DOES EXERCISE AFFECT CANCER AT THE EPIGENETIC LEVEL?

Exercise can "switch on" protective genes and "switch off" harmful ones without changing the actual DNA code. It does this by:

1. Removing chemical tags (methyl groups) from tumour suppressor genes, so they can be expressed.
2. Loosening the packaging around DNA (via histone acetylation), making genes more accessible for activation (see Figure 4.1).
3. Disrupting proteins (like HDAC5) that keep protective genes turned off.
4. Producing small regulatory RNAs (miRNAs) that fine-tune inflammation and cancer cell behaviour.

This means exercise can help reprogramme cancer cells and their environment, making them less aggressive and more vulnerable to treatments.

4.3 Key signalling pathways

Exercise modulates several intracellular signalling cascades that collectively suppress tumourigenesis and remodel the TME. These include canonical energy-sensing and stress-activated pathways, as well as mechanotransduction signalling pathways that convert biomechanical stress into biochemical signals. This section explores three key signalling systems affected by exercise: AMPK, mitogen-activated protein kinases (MAPKs) and the Hippo-YAP pathway.

4.3.1 AMPK pathway

AMPK is a serine-threonine kinase that functions as a central cellular energy sensor, becoming activated by increases in AMP:ATP ratios observed under conditions of energy stress, such as during exercise. Often described as the master regulator of energy homeostasis, AMPK plays a pivotal role in shifting cellular metabolism from anabolic to catabolic states, restoring ATP levels. It is strongly activated by exercise in metabolically active tissues, including skeletal muscle, liver and adipose tissue (29). In cancer, AMPK plays tumour-suppressive functions via three primary mechanisms: mTOR inhibition, autophagy induction; and apoptosis and cell cycle arrest. These effects are particularly relevant in metabolically dysregulated or hypoxic TMEs, where energy stress is frequent and may be exacerbated by exercise-induced metabolic demand. Perhaps unsurprisingly, AMPK is also induced in tumours during exercise, indicating its potential as a mediator of anti-cancer effects (30,31).

4.3.1.1 mTOR inhibition

AMPK inhibits the mechanistic target of rapamycin (mTOR), a key regulator of protein synthesis, cell growth and proliferation that is frequently hyperactivated in cancer. It does so by phosphorylating tuberous sclerosis complex 2 (TSC2) protein and Raptor, a component of the mTORC1 complex, thereby suppressing mTOR activity and halting proliferative signalling (32). Exercise-induced AMPK activation inhibits mTOR in both skeletal muscle and tumour tissue, suggesting that systemic energetic stress may constrain tumour growth via this pathway. This is consistent with preclinical observations of reduced tumour proliferation following exercise (3,33). It is plausible that AMPK activation is mediating this effect, however a direct causal link between exercise-induced AMPK activation, mTOR inhibition and tumour suppression remains to be conclusively demonstrated (34).

4.3.1.2 Autophagy induction

AMPK also promotes autophagy, a catabolic process that recycles intracellular components and removes damaged organelles and proteins. Autophagy has dual roles in cancer, but under energetic stress it may prevent tumour progression by reducing genomic instability and oxidative stress, as well as supporting immune surveillance. Mechanistically, AMPK activates autophagy via phosphorylation of unc-51 like autophagy activating kinase 1 (ULK1) and inhibition of mTORC1 (35,36). However, more recent evidence suggests a more nuanced relationship whereby AMPK-mediated ULK1 phosphorylation may inhibit autophagy under certain conditions, highlighting the context-dependent nature of this pathway (37). Further research is needed to delineate how these dynamics play out in tumours during exercise, however it appears that exercise-induced autophagy in tumours may contribute to the maintenance of cellular homeostasis and prevent the accumulation of DNA damage (38).

4.3.1.3 Apoptosis and cell cycle arrest

AMPK can also enhance pro-apoptotic signalling and enforce cell cycle arrest, particularly in the G1 phase. This involves regulation of p53, p21 and BCL-2 family proteins that govern mitochondrial integrity and apoptosis. Exercise-induced AMPK activation upregulates the expression of tumour suppressors such as Trim63 and downregulates oncogenes, reducing tumour viability (3). Additionally, AMPK may increase sensitivity to pro-apoptotic signals in metabolically stressed tumour cells, making them more vulnerable to immune attack or chemotherapeutic agents (39).

4.3.2 MAPK pathways

MAPK family includes ERK1/2, JNK/SAPK and p38 MAPK pathways and are key mediators of cellular responses to extracellular stress, growth factors and cytokines that are often deregulated in cancer. Sustained ERK signalling in cancer supports ongoing proliferation and survival, whereas stress-activated JNK and p38 drive cell cycle arrest, differentiation or apoptosis. Critically, however, their activity is highly context-dependent, shaped by both the pattern and duration of activation. Acute exercise imposes transient physiological stressors in the form of catecholamines, myokines (e.g., IL-6), ROS, as well as haemodynamic and mechanical changes. These cellular stresses briefly engage MAPK signalling systemically, while chronic training remodels the TME, improving perfusion and lowering hypoxia, thereby shifting baseline stress signalling, enhancing therapy delivery and boosting anti-tumour immunity (see Chapter 3, Section 3.2). Together, these effects offer multiple, complementary routes by which exercise can diminish tumour growth while improving host anti-tumour responses (34,40,41).

4.3.2.1 ERK1/2

The Ras-Raf-MEK1/2-ERK1/2 cascade promotes proliferation and survival in cancers, driven by either oncogenic mutations in the Ras or Raf kinases, or constitutive receptor tyrosine kinase activation, resulting in increased cyclin D expression and c-Myc activity, forcing cells through the cell cycle (42). By contrast, transient ERK activation, such as that induced by exercise, may favour differentiation or quiescence in some contexts (43,44). This dual nature, or "double-edged sword" effect of ERK-MAPK adds complexity to the field but also provides novel and exciting potential therapeutic strategies that target ERK-mediated apoptosis in cancer cells (45).

In skeletal muscle, intermittent physiological stress induced by exercise promotes transient ERK activation through integrins, catecholamines and growth factors, supporting adaptation and growth (46), while in tumour cells, the same transient activation can induce the expression of tumour suppressor genes and promotion of differentiation pathways (43). Moreover, exercise improves vascular maturity and blood flow, which helps reduce intratumoural hypoxia. Since hypoxia impairs NK cell cytotoxicity in an ERK-dependent manner (47), this supports a role for inhibition of ERK signalling in the anti-tumour effects of exercise. Meanwhile, other studies have demonstrated that exercise can reduce ERK activation, for example in rodent colon cancer (48) and prostate cancer models (49). ERK1/2 also interacts with p53 and other checkpoint proteins to limit uncontrolled cell division in the context of intermittent stress, potentially sensitising cancer cells to apoptosis or growth arrest (45).

4.3.2.2 JNK/SAPK

The c-Jun N-terminal kinase/stress-activated protein kinase (JNK/SAPK) pathway is primarily activated by stress stimuli such as ROS, DNA damage and pro-inflammatory cytokines—conditions that are still transiently elevated during exercise. In normal tissues, JNK activation can mediate adaptive responses to stress, including repair and remodelling. In cancer cells, JNK activation is often pro-apoptotic, acting via phosphorylation of transcription factors such as c-Jun and p53, and through modulation of Bcl-2 family proteins to promote mitochondrial outer membrane permeabilisation. Additionally, JNK signalling contributes to immune modulation within the TME by influencing cytokine production and promoting the recruitment and activation of cytotoxic lymphocytes (50).

The relationship between exercise and JNK signalling is complex and its role in the tumour context remains underexplored. In skeletal muscle, high-intensity exercise, particularly when inducing muscular damage, stimulates JNK activation, with phosphorylation levels increasing proportionally to contraction intensity (46). Adding to the complexity, while many studies report increased JNK activation following exercise, others have shown suppression of JNK activity in different contexts. For example, in a mouse model of metabolic dysfunction-associated steatotic liver disease (MASLD—formerly NAFLD) (51). These divergent findings highlight the need for targeted research to clarify the conditions under which exercise-induced JNK signalling may exert tumour-suppressive effects.

4.3.2.3 p38 MAPK

The p38 MAPK pathway is another stress-activated kinase cascade that is activated in response to inflammatory cytokines, UV radiation and ROS. Downstream, p38 phosphorylates transcription factors, such as ATF2 and MEF2, various kinases and RNA-binding proteins to coordinate inflammation, cell cycle arrest, cellular senescence, differentiation and apoptosis. In non-malignant cells, p38 activation regulates cell cycle checkpoints, DNA repair and senescence. In many models, p38 can act as a tumour suppressor by inducing growth arrest, promoting differentiation and triggering apoptosis, particularly in response to genotoxic or metabolic stress (52). However, in chronic inflammatory or hypoxic contexts, p38 can support tumour invasion, angiogenesis and chemotherapy tolerance (53,54).

Exercise transiently activates p38 MAPK in both muscle and tumour tissue, likely through mechanical stress, ROS generation and cytokine signalling (e.g., IL-6, TNF-α) (55,56). In skeletal muscle, exercise-induced p38 activation promotes skeletal muscle mitochondrial biogenesis (57). In tumour cells, p38 activation can phosphorylate p53 and other checkpoint regulators, leading to cell cycle arrest and apoptosis (58). However, p38 also regulates mRNA stability and translation of cytokines and other stress-response genes, potentially contributing to the inflammatory TME (59). Blockade of p38 signalling in a model of triple-negative breast cancer inhibited tumour angiogenesis and reduced recruitment and expansion of pro-tumourigenic TAMs and MDSCs (60). Moreover, p38 links oxidative stress to autophagy-related gene expression, offering a route whereby acute exercise-associated redox signalling could tip malignant cells towards self-damage rather than proliferation (61). These contrasting findings suggest that p38 MAPK may have both tumour-suppressive and tumour-promoting roles, depending on the cellular context, tumour type, and composition of the TME, underscoring the need for studies that specifically dissect the effects of exercise-induced p38 activation in cancer.

Collectively, the ERK, JNK and p38 MAPK pathways illustrate how the pattern, duration and cellular context of activation determine biological outcomes (see Figure 4.2). By inducing brief pulses of MAPK activation while concurrently remodelling the TME, exercise may redirect these

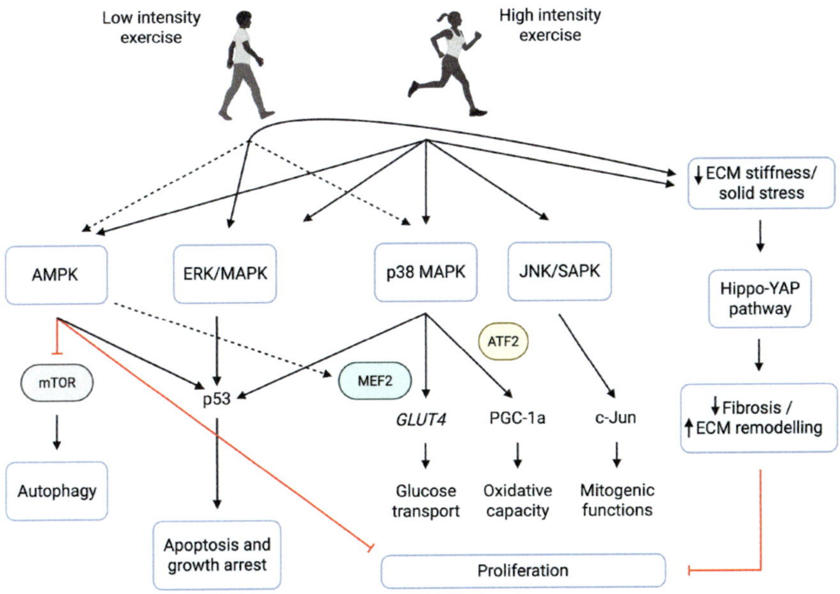

FIGURE 4.2 Exercise-modulated signalling pathways that remodel the TME. Exercise activates a range of signalling pathways that converge to suppress tumour progression and remodel the TME. Energy stress induced by exercise activates AMP-activated protein kinase (AMPK), which inhibits mTOR, promotes autophagy and contributes to apoptosis and growth arrest. AMPK also indirectly suppresses proliferation. Parallel activation of MAPK pathways occurs in response to mechanical cues and oxidative stress, with intensity-dependent effects: Low-intensity exercise predominantly activates ERK/MAPK to support metabolism, while high-intensity exercise activates p38 MAPK and JNK/SAPK, promoting transcriptional reprogramming via MEF2 and ATF2, influencing apoptosis or proliferation, depending on context. Exercise also reduces extracellular (ECM) stiffness and solid stress, leading to Hippo pathway activation. This sequesters YAP/TAZ in the cytoplasm, limiting oncogenic transcription and reducing proliferation. Collectively, these signalling cascades coordinate a multilevel anti-tumour response that integrates mechanical, metabolic and transcriptional cues. Solid black arrows = activation or promotion; red blunt arrows = inhibition; dashed arrows = indirect effects. Created in Biorender.com.

signalling cascades away from pro-tumour functions and towards differentiation, apoptosis, immune activation and vascular normalisation, offering multiple avenues to restrain tumour progression.

4.3.3 Hippo-YAP pathway

The Hippo pathway regulates organ size, tissue regeneration and tumour suppression. Its terminal effectors, Yes-associated protein (YAP) and transcriptional co-activator with PDZ-binding motif (TAZ) shuttle between cytoplasm and nucleus, where unphosphorylated YAP/TAZ bind TEA domain (TEAD) transcription factors and drive the expression of genes involved in proliferation, survival, EMT and maintenance of stem cell traits (62,63). Activation of upstream kinases, MST1/2 and LATS1/2, leads to YAP/TAZ phosphorylation, causing their cytoplasmic retention and subsequent ubiquitin-mediated degradation. This suppresses TEAD-driven transcription and thus limits oncogenic signalling (62).

Exercise modulates Hippo-YAP signalling systemically via catecholamine release during high-intensity exercise. Adrenaline (epinephrine) and noradrenaline (norepinephrine) bind to and activate β-adrenergic receptors, which in turn stimulate LATS1/2 phosphorylation and nuclear exclusion of YAP/TAZ. Blockade of β-adrenergic receptors with propranolol abrogates these effects (63,64). In preclinical breast cancer models, this mechanism has been shown to reduce proliferation in both hormone-sensitive and triple-negative cell lines, as well as lowering tumour initiation rates in vivo (64,65).

Beyond systemic effects, exercise also influences YAP/TAZ activity via mechanical and metabolic stress pathways. Different exercise modalities engage distinct upstream regulators of YAP/TAZ. For instance, endurance exercise is linked to glucose depletion, AMPK activation, IL-6 signalling and hypoxia, whereas resistance training triggers mechanotransduction cascades, PI3K/Akt signalling and SMAD pathways (66). These upstream pathways all converge on LATS1/2 and the YAP/TAZ-TEAD transcriptional axis, modulating tumour cell behaviour in response to exercise-induced cellular stress. Similarly, the duration and intensity of exercise have differential effects on YAP/TAZ activity. Serum collected after an initial bout of high-intensity endurance exercise (pre-training) increases YAP phosphorylation in both triple-negative breast and prostate cancer cells. Following a 9-week structured training period, exercise-conditioned serum was shown to modulate Wnt/β-catenin signalling and reduce GSK3β phosphorylation, suggesting that acute bouts of exercise preferentially suppress YAP activity, while longer-term training introduces further pathway adaptations downstream that influence the growth of tumour cells (65).

YAP/TAZ are increasingly recognised as key regulators of CSC biology, promoting self-renewal, EMT, drug resistance and metastatic potential (67). CD44 is a key CSC marker in many cancers, including breast and bladder cancer, that can activate YAP through cytoskeletal remodelling and Rho GTPase signalling, creating a feed-forward loop that sustains stemness and promotes chemoresistance (68,69). In breast cancer, TAZ is enriched in CSC fractions and is required for self-renewal and tumour initiation. YAP/TAZ signalling is also implicated in resistance to taxanes, anthracyclines and other chemotherapeutic agents (70). Thus, suppression of YAP, whether by pharmacological inhibitors or by upstream physiological inputs such as exercise-induced β-adrenergic activation, may represent a mechanism for targeting CSC populations, potentially reducing CSC frequency, sensitising tumours to therapy, and potentially lowering the risk of disease recurrence.

The direct anti-tumour effects of exercise-induced YAP suppression include the reduction of proliferation and viability in cancer cells (64). Alternatively, exercise-induced YAP suppression may arise as a result of alterations in the TME, for instance, via inhibition of cancer-associated fibroblast (CAF) activation and ECM remodelling, leading to reduced mechanical cues that otherwise drive YAP activation (71). Moreover, YAP/TAZ activity is highly sensitive to substrate stiffness, cell shape and cytoskeletal tension, which may mediate autophagy responses, although it remains unclear whether exercise-induced mechanical remodelling of the ECM can modulate YAP/TAZ-driven transcriptional activity (66).

Mechanical signals transmitted via integrins, FAK and Rho/ROCK are central to the cellular interpretation of mechanical stress, and they directly converge on Hippo-YAP signalling. Integrin clustering and FAK activation promote cytoskeletal rearrangement and Rho-GTPase activity, increasing actomyosin tension. This mechanical force can inhibit LATS1/2 activity, resulting in nuclear translocation and activation of YAP/TAZ (72,73). Conversely, exercise-induced changes in ECM composition and stiffness, along with systemic catecholamine release, may downregulate these mechanotransductive signals, leading to increased YAP phosphorylation and cytoplasmic retention (66,74). Indeed, activation of AMPK during exercise has been shown to reduce FAK phosphorylation in skeletal muscle (75), and therefore it is plausible that similar AMPK-dependent mechanisms could reduce FAK-driven mechanotransductive signalling within tumours, indirectly promoting YAP phosphorylation and cytoplasmic retention.

Emerging research suggests integration between Hippo-YAP and other metabolic and inflammatory signals. For example, circulating miRNAs clustered around indicators of exercise stress showed Hippo pathway enrichment in KEGG analyses (76). It is likely that there is extensive integration with other signalling pathways, including crosstalk with AMPK, p38-MAPK, ERK-MAPK and PI3K-Akt signalling, which may converge on Hippo-YAP regulation (77,78) (see Figure 4.2). Together, these findings position Hippo-YAP as a plausible mediator of the anti-tumour and CSC-targeting effects of exercise, although direct clinical evidence of the latter is currently limited. Mechanistic studies in patient-derived models, particularly tracking CSC populations and YAP activity over time with exercise interventions, are required to confirm this link.

4.4 Myokines and exerkines

Skeletal muscle is now recognised as a dynamic endocrine organ that communicates with distant tissues through the secretion of a particular class of signalling molecules, known as myokines, released into the circulation during contraction (79). Alongside these, adipose tissue secretes adipokines and other organs contribute a range of exercise-induced bioactive factors, including metabolites and EVs (80). Collectively, these diverse molecules are termed exerkines: Exercise-responsive messengers that exert autocrine effects within muscle, paracrine effects on neighbouring tissues, and systemic effects that reach distant sites including tumours (81). The composition of exerkines varies depending on the type, intensity and duration of exercise, as well as the individual's metabolic status, age and disease state. These molecules play key roles in mediating the systemic benefits of exercise, from modulating immune surveillance and inflammation to influencing tumour metabolism and microenvironmental structure and are summarised in Table 4.1.

4.4.1 Interleukin-6

Interleukin-6 (IL-6) is one of the most extensively studied myokines. Circulating IL-6 levels rise sharply during acute exercise and can increase up to 100-fold following prolonged endurance exercise bouts (82,83). Although chronically elevated IL-6 from tumour and stromal cells drives inflammation and tumour progression, exercise-derived IL-6 exerts distinctly anti-inflammatory actions, mediated via induction of IL-10, IL-1 receptor antagonist (IL-1Ra) and suppression of TNF-α (84–86). These opposing effects are partly explained by differential IL-6 receptor engagement: Pro-inflammatory signalling occurs primarily through the soluble IL-6R, whereas the membrane-bound receptor mediates its anti-inflammatory effects (87).

In cancer, acute surges of IL-6 elicited by exercise can directly inhibit proliferation, and in some contexts, promote apoptosis (88). Exercise-conditioned serum from colorectal and breast cancer survivors reduces tumour cell growth in vitro, partly attributable to IL-6 (89–91). Recombinant IL-6 at physiological concentrations reduces proliferation and DNA

TABLE 4.1 Summary of exercise-induced myokine function and regulation

Myokine	*Action*	*Change with exercise*
IL-6	Anti-inflammatory (via IL-10, IL-1Ra); metabolic regulation; immune modulation; context-dependent tumour effects	Up (acute)
IL-15	Promotes NK and CD8+ T cell proliferation; muscle anabolism; adipose tissue reduction; glucose uptake	Up
SPARC	Direct anti-proliferative; ECM remodelling; adipogenesis inhibition; promotes apoptosis	Up (high intensity)
Irisin	Promotes browning of adipose tissue; inhibits proliferation; enhances immune cell function; apoptosis and autophagy	Up (acute, more in fit individuals)
Oncostatin M	Pro-apoptotic; induces senescence; fibroblast reprogramming (context-dependent)	Up (acute)
Musclin	Enhances endurance; reduces glucose uptake; influences adipose browning; suppresses FOXO1	Up
FGF21	Glucose and fatty acid uptake; improves energy homeostasis; browning of adipose tissue	Up
Decorin	Antagonises myostatin; preserves muscle mass; inhibits EGFR/PI3K/AR; induces apoptosis	Up (resistance)
Myostatin	Inhibits muscle growth via Smad2/3; activates FOXO1; suppresses PI3K/Akt/mTOR	Down
Fractalkine (CX3CL1)	Recruits immune cells (CD8+, NK); context-dependent tumour effects; adhesion and chemoattraction	Up (low intensity)

Abbreviations: AR = androgen receptor; CD = cluster of differentiation; CXC3L1 = chemokine (C-X3-C motif) ligand 1; ECM = extracellular matrix; EGFR = epidermal growth factor receptor; FOXO1 = forkhead box O1; FGF21 = fibroblast growth factor 21; IL = interleukin; IL-1Ra = interleukin 1 receptor antagonist; NK = natural killer; PI3K = phosphatidylinositol 3-kinase; SPARC = secreted protein acidic and rich in cysteine.

damage markers in colorectal (89) and breast cancer cells (92), and lowers prostate cancer cell growth at slightly higher doses (93). However, IL-6 is not universally anti-tumourigenic. In some tumour models, IL-6 stimulates tumour cell proliferation and survival via the Ras/Raf/MEK/ERK-MAPK, PI3K/Akt, JAK/STAT (94–96) or NF-κB/IL-6/STAT3 pathways (97). Moreover, in prostate cancer cells, IL-6 exposure enhanced cell viability in a dose-dependent manner, both in the presence and absence of doxorubicin (98). These discrepancies likely reflect differences in IL-6 concentration, exposure duration and tumour cell type, as well as whether IL-6 originates from muscle, immune cells or tumour tissue.

Within the TME, chronically elevated IL-6, such as that observed in obesity or advanced cancer, is generally pro-tumourigenic (99). In this context, cellular sources of IL-6 include tumour cells, TAMs, CAAs and CAFs, all serving to drive cancer-supportive inflammation and dysregulated IL-6/IL-6 receptor signalling (100–103). The source, duration and concentration of IL-6 release therefore shape its divergent biological effects.

Beyond inflammation, IL-6 contributes to metabolic regulation. Muscle-derived IL-6 enhances insulin sensitivity and stimulates glucose uptake and fatty acid oxidation via AMPK (104,105), potentially reducing systemic nutrient availability to metabolically demanding tumours. Much less is known about the role of IL-6 in regulating immune cell function, but recent work has shown that it contributes to exercise-induced intratumoural immune cell infiltration (106). In mouse models, blockade of IL-6 during voluntary wheel running reduced the tumour-suppressive effects of exercise. Notably, however, this effect could not be reproduced by direct administration of IL-6, indicating that prior exercise-driven mobilisation and priming of immune cells are required for IL-6 to exert these effects (106).

Overall, the balance of evidence suggests a dichotomy: Acute, exercise-induced IL-6 promotes anti-inflammatory, metabolic and potentially tumour-suppressive effects, whereas chronically elevated IL-6, as observed in obesity and advanced cancer, supports tumour progression. Understanding IL-6 kinetics in relation to exercise modality and intensity is therefore critical in determining its diverse roles in cancer biology.

4.4.2 Interleukin-15

Interleukin-15 (IL-15) is constitutively expressed in skeletal muscle and has potent anabolic and immunomodulatory properties. Its expression is upregulated during and after exercise, particularly in response to resistance training, where it promotes muscle growth through enhanced myosin production (107). In direct contrast to its role in skeletal muscle anabolism, IL-15 has been shown to reduce adipose tissue mass, contributing to a shift in body composition favouring lean mass over fat (108,109). These effects are supported by experimental models showing that IL-15 reduces lipid accumulation in adipocytes and decreases white adipose tissue in rats in vivo (110,111). By modulating muscle-to-fat crosstalk, exercise-induced IL-15 may help generate a metabolically unfavourable environment for tumour growth, thereby indirectly reducing cancer risk.

IL-15 also plays a critical role in immune surveillance. Exercise-induced IL-15 promotes proliferation and activation of NK cells and CD8+ cytotoxic T cells, particularly IL-15Ra+ effector memory populations. In murine models of pancreatic ductal adenocarcinoma, these effects translate into increased tumour infiltration of cytotoxic T lymphocytes and improved response to immune checkpoint inhibitors (107). Clinically, IL-15 super-agonists such as NIZ985 have shown promise in early-phase trials for treating refractory solid tumours, offering a pharmacological mimic of the immune-stimulating effects of exercise (112–115).

Skeletal muscle is responsible for the majority of glucose metabolism that occurs in the body and IL-15 promotes skeletal muscle glucose uptake by increasing GLUT4 expression via JAK3/STAT3 signalling, further improving mitochondrial oxidative functions via AMPK (see also Section 4.3.1.) (116,117). These effects may further restrict nutrient availability to tumours while supporting muscle health.

4.4.3 Secreted protein acidic and rich in cysteine

SPARC, also known as osteonectin or BM-40, is an ECM-associated matricellular protein secreted by contracting skeletal muscle during exercise. Among the many exercise-induced myokines, SPARC is one of the most extensively studied and has shown direct anti-proliferative effects in preclinical models of colorectal and prostate cancer (118). Its effects in cancer are context dependent. In rectal, prostate, ovarian and pancreatic ductal carcinomas, SPARC often acts as a tumour suppressor (119,120), whereas in melanoma, glioblastoma and non-small cell lung cancer, it can instead promote tumour progression (121,122). These divergent effects are thought to reflect cell-type-specific expression patterns and differential regulation within the TME (122).

SPARC also regulates adipose tissue dynamics by modulating cell-ECM interactions essential for adipogenesis, including ECM remodelling and cytoskeletal reorganisation (119). Through inhibition of adipocyte progenitor proliferation and hypertrophy, SPARC elicits anti-obesity effects, which may indirectly influence cancer risk (119,123). Additionally, SPARC modulates key cellular behaviours, including adhesion, invasion, angiogenesis and apoptosis, linking it to both metabolic and oncogenic pathways (124–129). Within the TME, SPARC interacts with MMPs and growth factors such as TGFβ and FGF to remodel the ECM, reducing stiffness and diminishing integrin-mediated signalling in a manner that may suppress tumour progression (130). However, when overexpressed in stromal cells, SPARC may instead support tumour growth (131), for example, as observed in glioma, where it is highly expressed in tumour cells and promotes their invasion (132,133).

Both preclinical and clinical studies support a role for exercise-induced SPARC in suppressing tumour growth. High-intensity exercise increases circulating SPARC, which promotes apoptosis in colorectal cancer models by targeting aberrant crypt foci and upregulating caspase-3 and -9 (134,135). Similar tumour-suppressive effects have been observed in prostate cancer models, where serum from exercised individuals inhibited tumour cell growth in vitro (136). Clinically, elevated SPARC levels have been associated with improved recurrence-free survival in digestive tract cancers, suggesting its potential as both a therapeutic target and prognostic biomarker (137).

Several mechanisms underlie SPARC's anti-cancer effects. In colorectal cancer cells, SPARC induces endoplasmic reticulum (ER) stress and downregulates the anti-apoptotic protein, Bcl-2, triggering autophagy and apoptosis (138). In medulloblastoma, SPARC induces G2/M cell cycle arrest by inhibiting cyclin B and reducing STAT3 phosphorylation (139). In prostate cancer, exogenous SPARC suppresses proliferation by inactivating Akt via integrin β1 binding (140). Additionally, in pancreatic ductal adenocarcinoma, SPARC disrupts angiogenesis by interfering with VEGF-VEGFR signalling and sequestering PDGF and bFGF, thereby limiting their pro-angiogenic activity (141).

Overall, SPARC represents a compelling example of how exercise-induced myokines can influence tumour biology both directly and indirectly. Its dual roles in metabolic regulation and tumour suppression highlight it as a candidate for future therapeutic exploration in both oncology and metabolic disease.

4.4.4 Irisin

Irisin is a myokine derived from the cleavage of the transmembrane protein fibronectin type III domain-containing protein 5 (FNDC5), whose expression in skeletal muscle is upregulated by peroxisome proliferator-activated receptor gamma coactivator 1-alpha (PGC-1α) during exercise (142). Circulating irisin levels rise following acute physical activity and correlate positively with lean body mass and can also be elevated by cold exposure (143,144). Initially characterised for its metabolic role, irisin promotes the "browning" of white adipose tissue via upregulation of uncoupling protein 1 (UCP1), thereby increasing thermogenesis and supporting energy balance (145,146). However, growing evidence reveals its broader roles in tumour suppression and immune modulation and regulation of the TME (147). A 2017 meta-analysis confirmed a consistent rise in circulating irisin post-exercise, with greater responses observed in fitter individuals and those with lower BMI (148).

In cancer, irisin demonstrates a highly context-dependent effect. Anti-tumourigenic properties have been reported in multiple cancers. In pancreatic and glioblastoma models, irisin suppresses proliferation through inhibition of AMPK-mTOR and PI3K/Akt signalling, and upregulation of p21, resulting in G1/S cell cycle arrest (149–151). Similar anti-proliferative and pro-apoptotic effects are observed in lung, osteosarcoma and prostate cancer models (152–155), and irisin has also been shown to enhance chemotherapy sensitivity in pancreatic and breast cancer by suppressing PI3K/Akt and NF-κB signalling (142,156). Despite this, the effects of irisin are not universally tumour suppressive. In hepatocellular carcinoma, it has been shown to promote proliferation via PI3K/Akt activation (157), while in thyroid, oesophageal and colorectal cancers, no significant effects on proliferation were reported (158). These discrepancies likely reflect cell type differences, receptor expression and intracellular context.

Nonetheless, most data support the prevailing sentiment that irisin is tumour suppressive. It inhibits EMT and reduces invasion in lung and osteosarcoma models (159,160), and has been shown to protect against breast cancer metastasis to the spine (161). Higher resting irisin levels are associated with a reduced risk of invasive breast cancer, with one study reporting up to 90% reduction in risk per unit increase in irisin (162). Moreover, in glioblastoma, irisin reduces cell invasion by upregulating the ECM-remodelling protein tissue factor pathway inhibitor-2 (TFPI-2), and reverses the aggressive phenotype induced by CAAs (151).

Irisin also remodels the TME. In a high-intensity interval training (HIIT) intervention for breast cancer prevention, increases in circulating irisin correlated with greater NK cell cytotoxic activity (163). Additionally, both FNDC5 and irisin modulate macrophage polarisation, shifting adipose-resident macrophages from pro-inflammatory M1 to anti-inflammatory M2 phenotype, diminishing cytokine production and supporting phagocytic function (164–166). Furthermore, irisin improves tumour vascular architecture, reducing hypoxia and enhancing perfusion, which may enhance chemotherapeutic drug delivery and limit metastasis (167).

Mechanistically, irisin promotes apoptosis by upregulating pro-apoptotic proteins such as Bad, downregulating anti-apoptotic Bcl-2 and inhibiting survival pathways including PI3K/Akt and elevating ROS levels to trigger oxidative damage and cell death (168–170). Irisin can also trigger ferroptosis in pancreatic cells by enhancing erastin-induced iron accumulation and glutathione depletion (171). Irisin has also been linked to autophagy regulation, a process with paradoxical roles in cancer progression, treatment and drug resistance. While excessive or sustained autophagy can support tumour survival under stress, its controlled activation can suppress growth and metastasis, making it a promising therapeutic target. Irisin appears to promote protective autophagy in cardiomyocytes via AMPK-ULK1 signalling (172), suggesting a possible mechanism for tumour suppression that warrants further investigation. Therefore, as an endogenous, exercise-inducible molecule with multiple tumour inhibitory effects, irisin is an attractive candidate for adjunct cancer therapies. However, its tissue-specific and sometimes contradictory effects highlight the need for rigorous mechanistic and translational research before clinical application (173).

4.4.5 Oncostatin M

Oncostatin M (OSM) is a multifunctional cytokine belonging to the IL-6 family, produced by a range of immune cells including macrophages, monocytes, T cells and neutrophils (174). Much like IL-6 and irisin, OSM exhibits highly context-dependent effects in cancer, acting as either a tumour suppressor or promoter depending on the cellular and microenvironmental setting (175–178). In some cancers, OSM exerts potent anti-proliferative and pro-apoptotic effects. Early studies in melanoma and breast cancer showed OSM-mediated inhibition of cell growth (175,179), while in glioblastoma, it drives G1 cell cycle arrest through upregulation of p21 and p27, and suppression of cyclin A (180). In breast epithelial cells, OSM promotes senescence via persistent STAT3 activation and suppression of c-Myc, independent of p16 and p53 (181). OSM also activates the STAT3-Smad3 axis, linking transcriptional reprogramming to cell cycle arrest and survival inhibition (182). However, in other contexts, particularly in fibroblast-rich or chronically inflamed microenvironments, OSM can drive tumour progression. In breast cancer, for example, OSM is predominantly secreted by myeloid cells, while its receptor (OSMR) is largely expressed on fibroblasts. In this context, OSM reprogrammes fibroblasts into CAFs, stimulating VEGF, CXCL1 and CXCL16 secretion, promoting a pro-tumourigenic niche (183). Similar pro-tumourigenic roles have been observed in ovarian, prostate and cervical cancers, where stromal overexpression of OSM correlates with increased invasiveness (177,178,184). This duality likely reflects the complexity of TME signalling networks and highlights the importance of cellular source, receptor expression and the balance of downstream pathways engaged.

Evidence from both in vitro and in vivo studies suggests that OSM may be a key mediator of exercise-induced tumour suppression (88). Acute exercise elevates circulating OSM levels in cancer patients, including those with advanced disease or undergoing androgen deprivation therapy (ADT) for prostate cancer (185,186). Serum collected immediately post-exercise suppresses tumour cell proliferation in vitro. These effects are attenuated when OSM is neutralised (187). Furthermore, exercise-conditioned serum induces caspase activity in breast cancer cells, with OSM required for this effect (187). Notably, skeletal muscle itself can produce OSM during contraction. In vitro, electrically stimulated myotubes upregulate OSM expression, and their conditioned medium mimics the anti-proliferative effects of post-exercise serum (187). Together, OSM is emerging as a candidate myokine with significant context-dependent effects on tumour biology. In the exercise setting, transient surges of muscle- and immune-derived OSM contribute to the anti-proliferative and pro-apoptotic effects across a range of tumour types. While its dual roles in cancer warrant careful interpretation, the accumulating evidence supports a predominantly tumour suppressive role for OSM in response to exercise, making it a compelling target for further mechanistic and translational investigation.

4.4.6 Musclin

Musclin, also known as osteocrin, is a myokine encoded by the *Ostn* gene. It was initially identified for its role in enhancing exercise performance, with studies showing that it supports physical endurance by promoting mitochondrial biogenesis and mitogenesis, contributing to improved aerobic capacity (188). Mechanistically, musclin activates calcium-dependent signalling pathways, particularly via Akt1, while concurrently suppressing the transcription factor FOXO1, a key regulator of muscle atrophy and energy homeostasis. Beyond its role in endurance, musclin also influences metabolic processes. It has been proposed as a novel factor in the browning of white adipose tissue (189), and in rodent models, it has been shown to reduce glucose uptake in skeletal muscle by inhibiting the Akt/PKB pathway, a central player in insulin signalling and glucose transport. This inhibitory effect may be regulated through upstream interactions with PPARγ/LXRα, suggesting a broader role for musclin in metabolic regulation through nuclear receptor signalling pathways (190).

4.4.7 FGF21

Fibroblast growth factor 21 (FGF21) is a polypeptide hormone secreted by multiple tissues, including skeletal muscle, where it functions as a stress-responsive myokine (191). Its expression is induced by fasting, endoplasmic reticulum stress, mitochondrial dysfunction and metabolic disorders, often via PPARα signalling pathways (192,193). FGF21 binds fibroblast growth factor receptors (FGFRs) in complex with the co-receptor β-klotho to exert its biological effects (194). It plays a key role in regulating systemic energy homeostasis, promoting glucose uptake in skeletal muscle through GLUT4 and PKCζ-dependent mechanisms independent of insulin-Akt signalling (195,196), and via GLUT1 in other tissues (197,198). It also enhances fatty acid oxidation and induces the browning of white adipose tissue, contributing to hypoglycaemic and weight-reducing effects. These properties have made FGF21 an attractive candidate for treating metabolic diseases such as obesity and type 2 diabetes (191). Together, these findings highlight the pleiotropic roles of FGF21 in energy metabolism, with potential relevance to tumour energetics and systemic metabolic regulation in cancer. Further studies are needed to clarify its specific roles in tumour-bearing hosts and the effects of exercise-induced modulation of FGF21 in this context.

4.4.8 Decorin

Decorin is a small leucine-rich repeat proteoglycan (SLRP) that is widely expressed in connective tissues such as skin, bone, cartilage, and the mammary stroma (199). More recently, it has been recognised as a myokine, with skeletal muscle capable of producing and secreting decorin in response to exercise (200). In humans, acute resistance exercise has been shown to elevate circulating decorin levels (201).

Functionally, decorin antagonises myostatin, a member of the TGFβ superfamily and a potent negative regulator of muscle growth (201). Through this interaction, decorin helps preserve muscle mass by counteracting myostatin-mediated atrophy (202). This role may be clinically relevant, as reduced decorin expression has been observed in multiple tumour types, spanning urogenital (bladder, prostate, testis), gastrointestinal (colon, rectum, stomach, pancreas) and other sites, including breast, cervix, kidney, ovary, skin and lung cancers (203).

Evidence also suggests that decorin may exert direct anti-tumour effects. In prostate cancer patients undertaking long-term exercise training, serum decorin levels were increased; when these sera were applied to prostate cancer cells in vitro, cancer cell proliferation was suppressed (185). Although the precise mechanisms underlying these anti-tumour effects are not fully defined, several tumour-suppressive activities have been described for recombinant or exogenous decorin. In multiple cancer models, decorin reduces DNA synthesis, inhibits epidermal growth factor receptor (EGFR) activity, and suppresses downstream androgen receptor (AR)-PI3K-Akt signalling (204). In vivo, recombinant decorin administration significantly impairs tumour growth and activates caspase-3-mediated apoptosis (205). Decorin can also modulate pro-tumour signalling pathways: In TNBC, it downregulates TGFβ1 and oncogenic miR-21, thereby reducing metastatic potential (206,207). In lung cancer cells, decorin decreases TGFβ1 and cyclin D1 expression, inhibits EGFR phosphorylation and increases p53 and p21 levels (208). In hepatoma cells, it induces p21 WAF1/CIP1, inactivates c-Myc and β-catenin, and reduces phosphorylation of EGFR, GSK3β and ERK1/2 (209). Taken together, these findings indicate that exercise can increase circulating decorin levels in both healthy individuals and cancer patients, with potential benefits extending beyond muscle maintenance to direct suppression of tumour growth and progression. However, the precise role of muscle-derived decorin in mediating the anti-cancer effects of exercise is still not fully understood.

4.4.9 Myostatin

Myostatin is one of the earliest identified myokines that belongs to the TGFβ superfamily and is predominantly expressed in skeletal muscle (210). Unlike many other myokines, its levels in both muscle and plasma decrease following exercise, with significant reductions reported in healthy young men within 24 hours post-exercise (211). Functionally, myostatin acts as a negative regulator of muscle mass: High levels promote atrophy, whereas inhibition or deletion, for example in knockout mice, induces hypertrophy (212). However, clinical findings are less straightforward. For instance, lung cancer patients with cachexia exhibited lower circulating myostatin than non-cachectic patients, raising questions about its role in cancer-associated muscle loss (213).

Mechanistically, myostatin is secreted by skeletal muscle and binds to activin receptor IIB (ActRIIB), which activates ALK4/5 and phosphorylates Smad2/3 (210,214). Inhibition of ActRIIB signalling, or myostatin knockout, increases muscle mass in mice (215,216). Downstream, myostatin suppresses the PI3K/Akt/mTOR axis while activating FOXO1, thereby upregulating genes associated with muscle atrophy (217–219). Myostatin also inhibits protein synthesis by inactivating IGF-1/PI3K/Akt signalling (220). Together, these findings position myostatin as a key negative regulator of muscle mass and a central player in the muscle wasting observed in cancer cachexia. While exercise-induced reductions in myostatin are well established, their precise implications in cancer settings remain complex. Nonetheless, the ability of exercise to downregulate myostatin, alongside efforts to therapeutically inhibit its signalling, highlights this pathway as a promising target for preserving muscle integrity and improving outcomes in cancer patients.

BOX-OUT 4.2 EMERGING TARGET: FRACTALKINE (CX3CL1)

Fractalkine (CX3CL1) is a unique chemokine that exists in both membrane-bound and soluble forms, capable of mediating leukocyte adhesion and chemoattraction (221). It signals primarily through its receptor, CX3CR1, which is expressed on various immune cells, including CD8+ T lymphocytes and NK cells (222). Recent studies suggest that fractalkine may function as an exercise-responsive exerkine. Low-intensity resistance exercise has been shown to increase circulating levels of fractalkine (223). Its elevation post-exercise may enhance immune surveillance by recruiting CX3CR1+ effector cells to peripheral tissues. In cancer, the role of fractalkine is highly context-dependent. On one hand, fractalkine expression within tumours has been associated with improved prognosis in colorectal, gastric and breast cancers, presumably due to enhanced cytotoxic immune infiltration (224–226). On the other hand, some tumours may exploit fractalkine signalling to promote metastasis via CX3CR1-expressing tumour cells (227). This dual role complicates its therapeutic targeting. To date, no studies have directly demonstrated a causal link between exercise-induced fractalkine and tumour control; however, its known functions in immune cell trafficking and emerging links with exercise highlight it as a promising target for future research. Understanding how exercise modulates fractalkine expression and how this influences tumour-immune interactions, could unlock new insights into personalised exercise oncology strategies.

4.4.10 Extracellular vesicles and exosome-mediated signalling

EVs, including exosomes released via multivesicular bodies and microvesicles shed from the plasma membrane, serve as intercellular couriers of bioactive cargo such as proteins, lipids, messenger RNAs and microRNAs (228). Contracting skeletal muscle, activated adipose tissue, endothelial and immune cells release EVs in response to mechanical, metabolic and redox stressors induced by exercise. Several studies have shown increased EV counts and altered cargo profiles immediately following acute exercise bouts (228–230). The secretory profile is influenced by exercise modality, intensity, duration and the individual's baseline metabolic state (229,231). The molecular cargo of exercise-induced EVs includes muscle-derived myokines, metabolites, microRNAs (miRNAs) and signalling proteins. For example, skeletal muscle-specific miRNAs in EVs (myomiRs) have been documented post-exercise (229,231). Muscle-derived EVs constitute a relatively small proportion of circulating EVs (~5%), but the functional impact may be disproportionately large given their enriched cargo (230,231).

Emerging preclinical data suggest that exercise-conditioned EVs can modulate tumour biology, either by delivering anti-proliferative cargo to tumour cells, by altering tumour metabolism, or by modulating the TME. For instance, animal models show that EVs collected after exercise reduce tumour growth and incidence (229). While direct human tumour data are limited, these findings raise important mechanistic possibilities for exercise oncology. Beyond direct tumour-cell effects, exercise-released EVs may alter immune cell behaviour. They can enhance NK cell and CD8+ T cell activation or trafficking, improve antigen presentation and modulate metabolic pathways in circulating immune cells or tumour-infiltrating lymphocytes. These immune-mediated pathways present another route through which exercise-derived EVs might impact cancer outcomes.

Since EVs are stable in circulation and carry a unique molecular "fingerprint" of their tissue of origin and stimulation history, they hold promise as minimally invasive biomarkers of exercise response, tumour biology or even patient responsiveness to exercise-based therapies. Moreover, they could potentially serve as therapeutic vectors, either harnessed from exercise itself or engineered to mimic exercise-EV cargo in patients unable to engage in physical activity. Nevertheless, substantial mechanistic, standardisation and safety work remains before clinical application is feasible (230).

4.4.11 *Section summary*

Collectively, myokines and exerkines act as systemic messengers of physical activity and exercise, translating the mechanical and metabolic demands of exercise into biochemical signals that influence tumour growth, immunity and metabolism. By mobilising anti-inflammatory and anti-proliferative factors (IL-6, SPARC, irisin, OSM), stimulating cytotoxic immunity (IL-15), and suppressing cachexia drivers (myostatin, FGF21), exercise exerts a myriad of molecular effects that complement the vascular, metabolic and mechanical remodelling described in later sections (see Figure 4.3).

4.5 Myokines, exerkines and cancer cachexia

Cancer cachexia is a multifactorial syndrome affecting 50–80% of patients with advanced disease, characterised by progressive skeletal muscle loss, adipose tissue depletion and significant metabolic dysregulation (232). Chronic inflammation, particularly elevated levels of cytokines, such as IL-6, plays a central role in muscle wasting. In cachectic patients with gastric, lung and

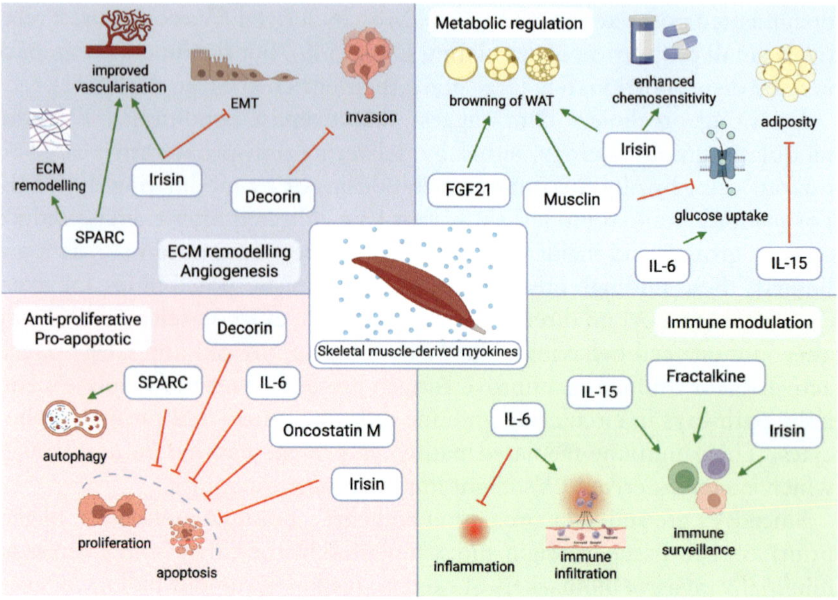

FIGURE 4.3 Exercise-induced myokines exert diverse anti-cancer effects via metabolic, immune and tumour-intrinsic mechanisms. Skeletal muscle releases a wide array of bioactive myokines in response to exercise, many of which influence cancer biology through multiple, overlapping mechanisms. This schematic illustrates the varied effects of key myokines across four domains: Metabolic regulation, immune modulation, anti-proliferative/pro-apoptotic signalling and ECM remodelling/angiogenesis. Myokines such as IL-6, IL-15, irisin, SPARC and decorin have been shown to promote tumour-suppressive outcomes including apoptosis, immune cell recruitment, ECM remodelling and reduced adiposity, while inhibiting tumour-promoting features such as proliferation, invasion, inflammation and EMT. Arrows indicate stimulatory effects (green) or inhibitory actions (red) based on current evidence. This network highlights the potential of exercise-induced myokines to shape both systemic and local TMEs in a manner that limits cancer progression and enhances therapy responses. Created in Biorender.com.

breast cancer, tumour-derived IL-6 is significantly upregulated at the mRNA level compared with non-cachectic counterparts (233,234). These persistently elevated IL-6 levels contrast sharply with the short-lived, exercise-induced IL-6 surges that are associated with anti-inflammatory responses and improved metabolic regulation rather than muscle degradation (235). Understanding this distinction is critical for interpreting how exercise training may help mitigate cachexia while simultaneously influencing tumour biology.

Several other myokines and exerkines have been implicated in the regulation of muscle mass and function in cancer cachexia. IL-15 is a promising anti-catabolic factor that inhibits the secretion of pro-inflammatory cytokines such as TNF-α, potentially limiting inflammation-driven muscle atrophy (236). In preclinical models, IL-15 suppresses protein degradation by modulating the ATP-dependent ubiquitin-proteasome pathway, a central driver of muscle wasting (237), an effect that appears to occur independently of IGF-1 signalling (238), highlighting IL-15 as a distinct therapeutic target for muscle preservation in cancer. Musclin also shows promise: In mouse models of colorectal cancer, whereby musclin-deficient animals exhibit more severe muscle wasting, whereas elevated musclin levels following exercise correlate with skeletal muscle preservation (190). Although the mechanisms remain to be fully elucidated, these findings suggest that musclin may help counteract tumour-induced catabolic signals. FGF21 adds further complexity. While it is known to enhance glucose uptake and promote metabolic balance in certain contexts, chronically elevated levels, such as those observed in older cancer patients with cachexia, have been linked to muscle atrophy and sarcopenia (239,240). Mechanistically, this involves upregulation of mitophagy via BNIP3, leading to loss of muscle mass, highlighting the context-dependent effects of FGF21 and the importance of tightly regulated expression (241).

Decorin has been shown to antagonise myostatin, a potent negative regulator of muscle growth. By inhibiting myostatin signalling, decorin can attenuate muscle atrophy and may therefore play a protective role against cachexia (202,203). Notably, decorin expression is often reduced in a wide range of tumour types, which could further contribute to the muscle-wasting phenotype observed in cancer (203). Conversely, the role of myostatin in cancer cachexia remains debated. While preclinical studies confirm its atrophic effects and show that its inhibition leads to muscle hypertrophy, clinical findings are less consistent. For instance, some studies report lower circulating myostatin levels in cachectic versus non-cachectic patients, suggesting a complex relationship that may vary with tumour type, disease stage or compensatory mechanisms (213). Activin A, which shares downstream Smad2/3 signalling with myostatin, has been more consistently linked with cachexia and poor survival outcomes (213,242). Elevated circulating activin A levels have been observed in cancer patients and are associated with muscle wasting in preclinical models. Importantly, blockade of the activin A/ActRIIB and myostatin/ActRIIB pathways has been shown to mitigate muscle loss, with several early-phase clinical trials now investigating these strategies in patients with cancer (213,243–245).

Overall, these findings underscore the importance of myokines and exerkines as modulators of muscle metabolism in cancer cachexia (246). Exercise may help counteract tumour-driven muscle loss by redirecting these molecular signals towards muscle preservation and repair, offering a promising non-pharmacological strategy to support physical function and treatment tolerance in patients with advanced cancer (247).

4.6 Metabolic reprogramming

Exercise exerts substantial effects on tumour metabolism, both systemically and within the TME. Most cancer cells display altered metabolic pathways to support rapid proliferation, immune evasion and treatment resistance. Chief among these adaptations is the Warburg effect whereby cancer cells exhibit a preference for aerobic glycolysis even in the presence of sufficient oxygen (248). This phenomenon drives excessive glucose consumption, allowing for rapid ATP generation and biomass accumulation, but at the cost of efficiency. It also results in lactate accumulation, which acidifies the TME, driving invasion, angiogenesis and contributing to immune evasion.

Skeletal muscle accounts for ~80% of whole-body glucose metabolism (88,249,250) and becomes a highly active metabolic organ during exercise. Contracting muscle competes with tumours for glucose, thereby reducing its systemic availability and diminishing the metabolic advantage of cancer cells (Figure 4.4). Additionally, regular aerobic and resistance exercise improves insulin sensitivity, enhances glucose uptake and clearance by skeletal muscle, and lowers circulating glucose and insulin levels, thereby limiting growth signals mediated by insulin/IGF-1 (249,250). Exercise also promotes mitochondrial biogenesis and oxidative phosphorylation, helping to restore metabolic flexibility and reduce lactate build-up, thus neutralising the acidified, immunosuppressive TME (251).

4.6.1 Intrinsic metabolic shifts in tumours

Emerging evidence demonstrates that exercise can disrupt the metabolic adaptations observed in cancer. One of the most consistently reported findings is a reduction in glucose uptake by cancer cells following exposure to exercise-conditioned serum or in exercised animal models (252), largely due to the competition for glucose consumption by contracting skeletal muscle. This is mediated in part by the upregulation of GLUT4 transporters and activation of AMPK. In vitro studies have shown that exercise-conditioned serum can inhibit glycolysis and increase mitochondrial respiration in cancer cells, reversing the Warburg phenotype (253,254). Exercise has also been shown to increase mitochondrial biogenesis and activity in various cell types, including cancer cells. This mitochondrial shift may restore normal metabolic checkpoints, sensitise cells to oxidative stress and tip the balance towards apoptosis (253), and is often accompanied by an increase in ROS production within tumour cells, which can lead to oxidative damage and activation of programmed cell death pathways when left unresolved (255).

In addition, exercise has been implicated in inducing G1/S cell cycle arrest through upregulation of cyclin-dependent kinase inhibitors such as p21 and p27, or through stabilisation of tumour suppressor proteins

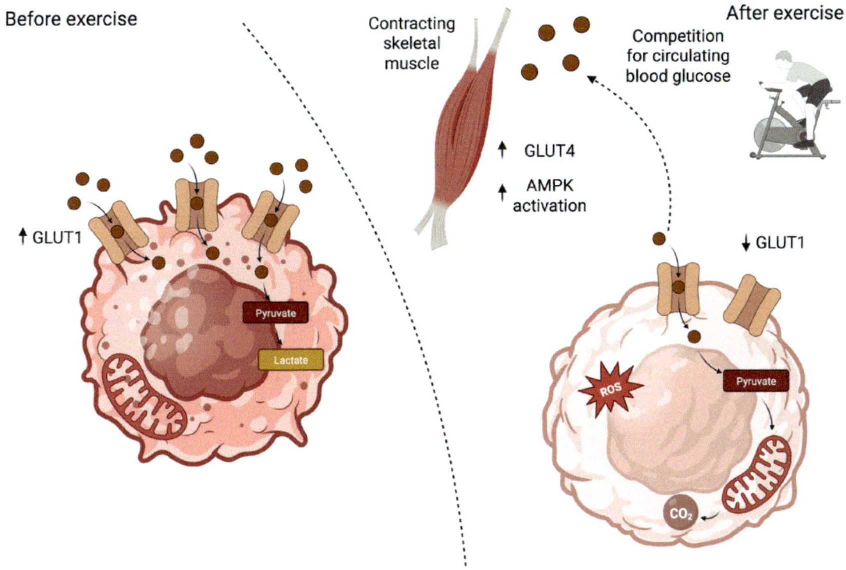

FIGURE 4.4 Exercise-induced glucose competition between skeletal muscle and tumour cells. Exercise stimulates skeletal muscle glucose uptake via upregulation of GLUT4 transporters and activation of AMPK, increasing metabolic demand. This reduces systemic glucose availability to tumour cells, which typically overexpress GLUT1 and rely heavily on aerobic glycolysis (the Warburg effect) for energy. In sedentary states, tumours outcompete inactive muscle, taking up more glucose, which is converted to lactate and supports tumour progression. During exercise (right panel), active muscle competes more effectively for glucose, decreasing tumour access and thereby limiting proliferation. Enhanced mitochondrial metabolism in tumour cells following exercise leads to increased pyruvate oxidation and ROS generation, contributing to metabolic stress in tumours. Created in Biorender.com.

like p53 (256). Importantly, many of these cellular responses are downstream of metabolic sensors and stress pathways activated by exercise, such as the AMPK and MAPK signalling cascades discussed earlier, including ERK1/2, p38 MAPK and JNK/SAPK (257). By targeting metabolic checkpoints, exercise disrupts tumour cell survival and proliferation. Within the TME, improved oxygenation via vascular normalisation suppresses hypoxia-driven stabilisation of HIF-1α, reducing pro-metastatic and glycolytic programming (258). Preclinical studies show that exercise-conditioned environments decrease expression of key nutrient transporters such as GLUT1, CD36, CPT1A and FABP4 in cancer and stromal cells (259,260). This impairs the tumour's metabolic flexibility, especially in stem-like cells, and reduces access to fuels that support resistance and recurrence.

4.6.2 Obesity and the metabolic TME

Obesity radically reshapes both the systemic metabolism and rewires metabolic pathways within the TME, creating a nutrient-rich and inflammatory microenvironment that favours tumour growth. Hypertrophic adipocytes secrete elevated levels of leptin, IL-6, TNF-α and FABP4, which collectively promote cancer cell proliferation, invasion and survival (261,262). Importantly, adipocytes also act as a direct fuel source for tumour cells, supplying free fatty acids (FFAs) and ketone bodies, particularly in breast and ovarian cancers (263). These fuels are delivered to cancer cells via lipid droplet transfer and EVs, where they are oxidised to support energy production and anabolic biosynthesis. At the same time, obesity promotes systemic metabolic dysfunction, characterised by insulin resistance, elevated blood glucose (hyperglycaemia) and high circulating insulin levels (hyperinsulinaemia). These changes stimulate tumour growth through IGF-1/PI3K/Akt/mTOR signalling, rendering tumours highly metabolically adaptable, enabling them to thrive under nutrient-limited conditions by outcompeting surrounding stromal and immune cells (264).

4.6.3 Exercise remodels adipose tissue

Epidemiological studies show that higher levels of physical activity are associated with lower risks of obesity-related cancers (e.g., post-menopausal breast, endometrial and colorectal cancers), even after adjusting for BMI, suggesting direct effects beyond weight reduction (265). Exercise and physical activity can influence many aspects of obesity-driven cancer risk and progression, including the remodelling of adipose tissue, particularly in the context of obesity. Regular exercise reduces adipose tissue mass, particularly visceral fat, curtailing the systemic supply of endocrine signals that drive tumour growth (266,267). In addition, exercise enhances fatty acid oxidation and promotes the "beiging" of white adipose tissue, whereby white adipocytes adopt thermogenic properties resembling brown adipose tissue. Beiging increases mitochondrial density and fatty acid oxidation within adipose depots, therefore reducing the availability of FFAs and ketone bodies that tumour cells would otherwise use as fuel (268). Interestingly, a preclinical study found that browning of white adipose tissue via a β3-adrenergic receptor agonist, Mirabegron, markedly suppressed tumour growth in multiple cancer models, supporting the idea that reducing white adipose tissue and the adipocyte-derived fuel supply can significantly hinder tumour growth (269). Given that exercise-induced catecholamine release also stimulates β-adrenergic receptors, not only in promoting adipose tissue beiging but also in mobilising NK cells, enhancing their cytotoxicity (270) (see Chapter 3, Section 3.2.1.1), it is plausible that β-adrenergic signalling represents a shared regulatory pathway linking metabolic and immune-mediated anti-tumour effects of exercise, and warrants further investigation.

Exercise also improves the inflammatory and secretory profile of adipose tissue, which redirects signalling from pro-tumourigenic adipokines such as leptin, IL-6 and TNF-α, towards anti-inflammatory factors such as adiponectin and omentin-1, resulting in a reduction in tumour-supporting inflammation (271,272). Moreover, exercise improves insulin sensitivity and lowers circulating levels of insulin (273,274). These changes may activate AMPK signalling and promote fatty oxidation in metabolic tissues, which in turn could reduce the endocrine and paracrine support adipocytes provide to tumours (275,276). From a stromal perspective, exercise reduces aromatase activity in adipocytes, lowering oestrogen production, which is particularly relevant in hormone-sensitive cancers such as breast and ovarian cancer (277). Exercise also improves adipose vascularisation and perfusion, reversing the hypoxia that otherwise drives fibrosis, inflammation and the de-differentiation of adipocyte progenitors into CAFs or CAAs; see Chapter 3, Section 3.2.4 (278–281).

In the context of obesity, exercise therefore acts on multiple fronts: It limits fuel supply, modulates inflammatory and endocrine signalling, and alters the microenvironment to a hostile state less favourable to tumour growth. This metabolic reprogramming strengthens the case for structured exercise as an integral component of cancer prevention and adjunctive therapy in obesity-related cancers.

BOX-OUT 4.3 ADIPOSE REMODELLING IN RESPONSE TO EXERCISE

Adipose tissue was once considered a passive energy store but is increasingly recognised as an active player in tumour progression, particularly in obesity-associated cancers. However, exercise has the power to reprogramme adipose tissue, transforming it from a tumour-promoting environment into one that is less permissive to tumour growth.

Adipokine rebalancing

Regular exercise reduces the levels of tumour-promoting adipokines such as leptin, IL-6 and TNF-α, while increasing the levels of protective adipokines such as adiponectin and omentin–1. This shift promotes a more anti-inflammatory adipose profile, diminishing pro-tumourigenic signalling.

Hormonal regulation

Exercise downregulates aromatase activity in adipose stromal cells, reducing local oestrogen production. This is particularly relevant in hormone-sensitive cancers like breast and ovarian cancer, where oestrogen fuels tumour growth.

Improved vascularisation

Physical activity enhances blood flow and perfusion within adipose tissue, alleviating hypoxia. This helps prevent fibrosis and blocks the de-differentiation of adipocyte progenitor cells into CAFs, key drivers of tumour progression.

Beiging of white adipose tissue

Exercise promotes the "browning" of WAT, increasing mitochondrial content and fatty acid oxidation. This metabolic shift limits lipid availability for tumour cells and boosts systemic energy expenditure.

Systemic impact

Together, these changes reduce nutrient supply, lower inflammatory and hormonal support for tumour growth, rewiring adipose tissue from supporting tumour metabolism to actively resisting it.

4.7 Tumour angiogenesis and vascular function

When tumours exceed a few millimetres in size, they must establish new blood vessels to sustain their growth. This process, known as angiogenesis, is frequently disordered in cancers. Tumour blood vessels are typically leaky, tortuous and poorly organised, leading to impaired perfusion, chronic hypoxia and acidosis. Such a dysfunctional vasculature not only fuels tumour progression but also fosters immune evasion and creates selection pressures that favour aggressive, therapy-resistant clones. In addition to molecular drivers, angiogenesis is shaped by mechanical forces within the TME. Abnormal interstitial pressure, vascular compression, fluid shear stress and matrix tension can all alter endothelial cell behaviour, vessel permeability and immune cell trafficking, reinforcing a vicious cycle of vascular dysfunction (282).

4.7.1 Exercise-induced vascular normalisation

Exercise has emerged as a key regulator of tumour vascular structure and function. Preclinical studies demonstrate that endurance exercise promotes vascular normalisation, characterised by increased pericyte recruitment, reduced endothelial permeability, and improved perfusion (283). These effects are largely mediated by temporally and spatially regulated vascular endothelial growth factor (VEGF) expression, together with suppression of pro-angiogenic inflammatory mediators such as TNF-α and IL-1β (284,285). This contrasts with tumour-driven angiogenesis, which is excessive and inefficient, perpetuating hypoxia and instability within the tumour vasculature. Exercise-induced mechanical stimuli, such as fluid shear stress and cyclic vascular strain, further promote endothelial quiescence, stabilise cell-cell junctions and enhance nitric oxide (NO) bioavailability, improving vascular tone and function (286).

4.7.2 Impact on hypoxia and intravasation

Hypoxia-inducible factor 1 alpha (HIF-1α) is a key transcriptional regulator linking hypoxia to angiogenesis and metastatic spread. Elevated HIF-1α expression correlates with increased invasiveness and motility of tumour cells, promoting intravasation into the vasculature (287,288). While pathological HIF-1α activation under resting tumour hypoxia drives aberrant angiogenesis, exercise-induced vascularisation is physiological and restorative, reducing hypoxia and thereby limiting EMT and intravasation (288). Importantly, voluntary wheel running in murine models of breast and prostate cancer led to reduced metastasis despite elevated HIF-1α, indicating that the context and downstream consequences of HIF-1α activation differ depending on the initiating signal (e.g., hypoxia versus exercise) (288–290). Circulating endothelial progenitor cells (EPCs) may also contribute to exercise-induced angiogenesis by incorporating into new vessels (291). Although EPCs have been implicated in pre-metastatic niche formation (292), the balance of evidence suggests that exercise-driven angiogenesis improves vascular quality and limits malignant potential.

4.7.3 *Dual roles of VEGF and nitric oxide*

The relationship between angiogenic mediators and metastasis is complex. Chronic physical activity elevates VEGF expression, enhancing endothelial-pericyte interactions and vessel stability, reducing leakiness (293). In female rats inoculated with breast cancer, treadmill running for 35 weeks increased VEGF-A expression and enhanced tumour vascularisation, which actually increased tumour growth. However, the tumours were less aggressive than those inoculated into their sedentary control counterparts and the time to onset of tumour development was also delayed in the exercising rats (293). Interestingly, in mice inoculated with lung tumours, 4 weeks of wheel running did not alter tumour volume nor metastasis when compared with the sedentary control group (294). However, VEGF also induces MCP-1, a chemokine which can support lymph node metastases. In a study using mouse Lewis lung carcinoma models, exercise did not prevent VEGF-induced MCP-1 elevation, raising questions about threshold and timing effects (295).

Similarly, NO exhibits context-dependent effects whereby it may promote proliferation and invasion under some conditions, but its cytotoxic actions on damaged DNA can inhibit tumour growth (296). A mouse study found that 4 weeks of wheel running led to lower NO production but greater pulmonary metastasis, suggesting that under specific conditions, reduced NO may impair cytotoxic defences (297). These paradoxes emphasise the importance of context, intensity, and timing in the effects of exercise-induced angiogenesis, shaped not only by molecular factors but also by the mechanical and inflammatory milieu of the tumour (288).

4.7.4 *Therapeutic implications*

Improved vascular function has two major clinical consequences. First, enhanced oxygenation reduces HIF-1α stabilisation, suppressing hypoxia-driven transcriptional programmes linked to EMT and metastasis. Second, normalised vessels improve intratumoural drug delivery, facilitating the penetration of chemotherapy, immunotherapy and effector immune cells. In preclinical models of breast and prostate cancer, exercise-induced vascular normalisation has been shown to synergise with anti-PD-1 therapy, enhancing T cell infiltration and therapeutic efficacy (298). Together, these findings position exercise as a physiological regulator of angiogenesis, capable of offsetting tumour-induced vascular dysfunction and enhancing the efficacy of systemic therapies (Figure 4.5).

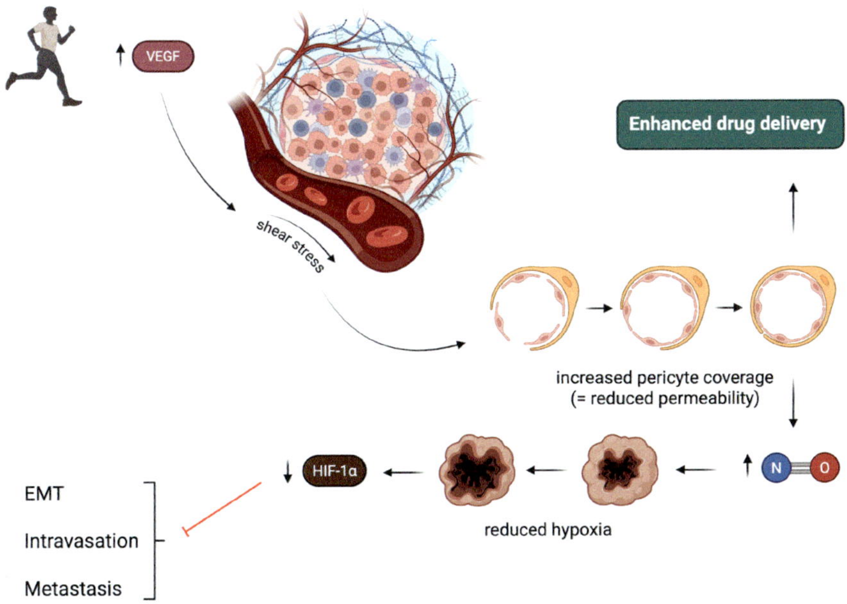

FIGURE 4.5 Exercise-induced vascular normalisation enhances tumour perfusion and therapy delivery. Regular exercise promotes physiological angiogenesis, leading to vascular normalisation within the TME. Exercise induces VEGF expression in a controlled, spatially restricted manner, enhancing pericyte recruitment and stabilising endothelial junctions. These changes improve vascular integrity, reduce leakiness and restore blood flow to the centre of the tumour, enabling deeper penetration of chemotherapeutic agents. Mechanical forces such as shear stress and cyclic strain further upregulate nitric oxide (NO) production, promoting endothelial quiescence and vascular tone. Together, these adaptations lower hypoxia, suppress HIF-1α, reducing EMT and metastatic potential. In addition to enhanced drug delivery, improved perfusion also increases immune cell infiltration, which may support chemotherapeutic efficacy. Created in Biorender.com.

4.8 Non-cellular components of the TME: ECM and mechanical properties

The TME is not only defined by its cellular composition but also by its ECM and the physical forces that shape cell behaviour. Structural remodelling of the ECM and the dysregulation of mechanical cues such as stiffness, solid stress and interstitial flow are increasingly recognised as key drivers of tumour progression, therapeutic resistance and immune exclusion (299). Exercise influences these non-cellular aspects of the TME, restoring mechanical homeostasis and thereby enhancing perfusion, drug delivery and immune infiltration (300).

4.8.1 Extracellular matrix remodelling

In healthy tissue, the ECM provides architectural support, regulates adhesion and migration and stores signalling molecules. In cancer, however, the ECM becomes desmoplastic, enriched in fibrillar collagens (types I and III), fibronectin and laminin (301). These components are frequently hyper-crosslinked by lysyl oxidase (LOX), leading to increased stiffness that promotes proliferation, migration, EMT and stemness through integrin and YAP/TAZ signalling (302,303). CAFs are central to this process, depositing ECM components while secreting pro-fibrotic cytokines such as TGFβ (304).

Emerging evidence suggests that exercise counteracts ECM stiffening (305). Myokines such as irisin and SPARC have been implicated in ECM turnover: Irisin has been shown to inhibit oxidative stress and fibrosis in a mouse model of chronic pancreatitis (306), and SPARC can regulate ECM-integrin interactions and inhibit fibrotic signalling (307). Through these mechanisms, exercise may serve to remodel the ECM into a structure more permissive to drug penetration and immune cell infiltration.

4.8.2 Mechanical properties and physical forces

The ECM surrounding a tumour generates physical forces that shape its growth. As a tumour expands, it distorts its surroundings, causing the tissue to become stiffer. This builds a compressive stress known as "solid stress" that presses on blood vessels and affects fluid flow through the tissue. These forces cut off oxygen and nutrients to the tumour, impeding drug delivery and creating a physical barrier that prevents immune cell infiltration (308). Exercise helps to rebalance tumour mechanics by reducing ECM stiffness and collagen density, which in turn alleviates the compressive solid stress on blood vessels, allowing them to open up again

(305,309). Increased vascular shear stress during exercise also promotes endothelial stability and vessel normalisation (283). These biomechanical changes reduce the physical barriers to immune surveillance, creating a microenvironment less hospitable to tumour growth and more responsive to treatment. Exercise may also enhance matrix degradation via the upregulation of MMPs, further helping to reduce mechanical compression (305).

BOX-OUT 4.4 STIFFNESS VERSUS SOLID STRESS

Stiffness

Stiffness refers to the intrinsic material property of a tissue, i.e., how resistant it is to deformation. In tumours, stiffness primarily arises from excessive deposition and crosslinking of ECM components, such as collagen, laminin and fibronectin. Enzymes like LOX catalyse collagen crosslinking, increasing matrix rigidity. As a consequence, the increase in stiffness activates mechanosensitive signalling pathways, such as the Hippo-YAP/TAZ pathway discussed earlier (Section 4.3.3.). This promotes cancer cell proliferation, EMT and the maintenance of CSC properties.

Solid stress

Unlike stiffness, solid stress is a mechanical force exerted by expanding tumour cells and their surrounding ECM. As the tumour grows, these forces compress intratumoural blood and lymphatic vessels, leading to elevated interstitial pressure. This vessel compression reduces perfusion, impairs drug delivery and aggravates hypoxia, which in turn promotes therapy resistance, tumour invasion and immunosuppression.

The effect of exercise

Regular aerobic or resistance exercise can remodel the TME by targeting both stiffness and solid stress. Exercise can reduce stiffness by decreasing ECM deposition, lowering LOX activity and improving collagen organisation through remodelling the ECM. Moreover, it can relieve solid stress by normalising stromal architecture, which in turn decompresses the vasculature. As a result, these changes enhance vascular perfusion, tumour oxygenation and immune infiltration, making the TME more permissive to treatment and less favourable for tumour progression.

4.8.3 Mechanotransduction pathways

Cells sense and respond to mechanical cues via mechanotransduction pathways, including integrins, focal adhesion kinase (FAK), Rho/ROCK signalling and the Hippo-YAP/TAZ axis (310,311). In tumours, stiff ECM and abnormal mechanical pressures chronically activate these pathways, driving proliferation, invasion and resistance to apoptosis (312,313). Mechanotransduction, particularly ECM stiffness, drives nuclear localisation of YAP/TAZ, which triggers oncogenic and pro-fibrotic transcriptional programmes (314–316). Exercise may reset some of these mechanosignals, for example, by modulating tissue deformation, ECM remodelling and interstitial pressure dynamics.

At the vascular level, exercise-induced shear stress enhances endothelial function and barrier integrity via shear stress-mediated signalling, enhanced NO availability, and mobilisation of endothelial progenitor cells for vascular repair (317–319). In muscle and cardiac tissues, exercise also modulates matrix metalloproteinases (MMP2 and MMP9), indicating controlled ECM turnover and capillary remodelling in response to physiological stress (320–322). While MMP-mediated matrix remodelling is often linked to tumour invasion in pathological contexts, it is plausible that exercise-induced ECM remodelling might improve stromal flexibility and vascular function, although as yet this remains unexplored.

Overall, exercise influences both the structural components and biophysical forces within the TME. By modulating ECM composition, reducing stiffness, relieving solid stress and restoring mechanical homeostasis, exercise may reduce aberrant mechanotransduction pathways, such as YAP/TAZ activation. These biomechanical adaptations enhance vascular perfusion, improve immune cell infiltration and may suppress oncogenic and pro-fibrotic signalling. In doing so, exercise may act as a physiological regulator of tumour mechanics, targeting a dimension of cancer biology that is otherwise difficult to address with conventional treatments.

4.9 Epithelial-to-mesenchymal transition

The EMT is a cellular programme in which epithelial cells lose polarity and adhesion, while acquiring mesenchymal traits such as motility and invasiveness. EMT contributes to tumour progression by enabling invasion, intravasation, dissemination and resistance to therapy. It is tightly regulated by transcription factors including Snail, Twist, ZEB1/2 and by signalling pathways such as TGFβ, Wnt/β-catenin and NF-κB, all of which are influenced by hypoxia, inflammation, metabolic stress and ECM stiffness (323–325).

4.9.1 Exercise, EMT markers and invasion

Preclinical evidence suggests that exercise can modulate EMT marker expression in tumours. In a murine prostate cancer model, 8 weeks of voluntary wheel running altered pro-metastatic gene expression, with downregulation of COX2, hepatocyte growth factor receptor (HGFR) and IGF-1 receptor (IGF1R), although increases in CXCR4 and MMP-9 were also observed (290). In mouse models of liver cancer, voluntary swimming (8 minutes per day for 9 weeks) suppressed TGFβ1-induced EMT, reducing expression of TGFβ1, vimentin and N-cadherin, while increasing E-cadherin expression. By contrast, the group of mice forced to undergo prolonged swimming (16–32 minutes per day) exhibited a markedly increased number of lung metastases, underscoring the importance of dose and context (326). These findings suggest that moderate, voluntary exercise exerts effects that oppose EMT, whereas prolonged or excessive stress may paradoxically promote invasion.

4.9.2 Matrix metalloproteinases and ECM degradation

EMT is closely linked with ECM degradation, particularly through MMPs that facilitate invasion. In nasopharyngeal carcinoma cells incubated with platelet-enriched plasma from a group of sedentary men recruited onto an exercise intervention, high-intensity exercise reduced MMP-2 and MMP-9 activities, while moderate exercise reduced platelet-tumour cell aggregation without affecting MMP activity (327). These findings highlight the dual role of exercise in modulating both proteolytic activity and platelet-tumour interactions that facilitate metastatic spread.

4.9.3 Tight junction integrity and vascular escape

EMT also weakens tight junctions between epithelial cells and endothelial barriers, promoting dissemination. Voluntary wheel running in mice increased expression of the tight junction protein claudin-5, thereby enhancing blood-brain barrier integrity and reducing metastasis following intracardiac tumour cell injection (328). These data suggest that exercise not only suppresses EMT within tumours but also strengthens vascular barriers, limiting the escape and colonisation of CTCs.

In summary, while preclinical evidence suggests that exercise can influence EMT-related processes in tumours, for example by downregulating pro-metastatic genes (COX2, HGFR, IGF1R) in some models and suppressing mesenchymal markers (vimentin, N-cadherin) while restoring epithelial markers (E-cadherin) in others, the effects are mixed and likely highly context-dependent. Some studies report exercise-associated reductions in invasion and markers of EMT, whereas others find increased expression of migratory or proteolytic factors (e.g., CXCR4, MMP9) or even enhanced metastatic outgrowth under certain exercise regimens (288). This suggests that the impact of exercise on EMT, invasion and metastasis depends critically on the nature, intensity and duration of exercise, the tumour type and stage, and the surrounding microenvironment. Therefore, while exercise has potential as a modulator of tumour invasiveness and metastatic potential via EMT and ECM-dependent mechanisms, more rigorous and systematic in vivo and in vitro mechanistic studies are needed before definitive conclusions can be drawn.

4.10 Systemic modulation of the TME (endocrine and hormonal factors)

While much of this chapter has focused on local effects within the TME, exercise also exerts widespread systemic influences. These endocrine and hormonal changes shape the physiological "terrain" in which tumours exist, providing another layer of regulation that complements the mechanisms described above. Historically, most cancer research has targeted mutations within tumour cells themselves. Increasingly, however, it is recognised that the systemic milieu, comprising circulating hormones, cytokines and metabolic substrates, plays an equally important role in determining tumour behaviour and therapeutic response. Unlike targeted therapies, which focus on single molecular targets and risk driving resistance, exercise exerts a myriad of systemic effects that are difficult for a tumour to escape.

4.10.1 Insulin and IGF-1

One of the best characterised systemic effects of exercise is its ability to reduce circulating levels of insulin and insulin-like growth factor-1 (IGF-1). Chronic hyperinsulinaemia, a hallmark of obesity and metabolic syndrome, promotes tumour growth via the PI3K/Akt/mTOR and MAPK pathways. IGF-1 similarly enhances proliferation, survival and angiogenesis across multiple cancer types (329). Regular exercise improves insulin sensitivity and lowers fasting insulin and glucose. These changes reduce growth-promoting signals and may lessen the selective pressures within the TME that promote plasticity and resistance. Moreover, in breast cancer survivors, structured exercise has been linked with reductions in inflammatory factors and IGF-1 (330,331).

4.10.2 Sex hormones

Exercise also modifies sex hormone profiles, particularly oestrogens and androgens. In adipose tissue, the enzyme aromatase converts androgens to oestrogens. In women, particularly post-menopausal, increased adiposity is associated with elevated aromatase expression, driving higher circulating and local oestrogen levels, which contribute to hormone-sensitive cancers such as breast cancer (277,332,333). Exercise has been shown to reduce adiposity in breast cancer survivors and at-risk women (334–337). By reducing the source tissue for aromatase activity, such reductions in adiposity may lead to lower oestrogen biosynthesis, thereby diminishing a key endocrine driver of hormone-sensitive tumour growth. In men, regular exercise is associated with reduced risk and progression of prostate cancer. Modulation or stabilisation of androgen levels may contribute, at least in part, to this effect but RCTs have shown no consistent effect of exercise on serum testosterone in prostate cancer patients, arguing against a dominant hormonal-mediated mechanism (338,339). Therefore, non-hormonal mechanisms, such as metabolic, immunologic or vascular, may play a larger role. By reshaping these endocrine networks, exercise helps reduce hormonal growth signals that cancers exploit.

4.10.3 Cortisol and stress hormones

The acute rise in cortisol and catecholamines during exercise helps mobilise glucose and immune cells, but chronic dysregulation of stress hormones can promote tumour progression. Exercise training appears to "reset" the hypothalamic-pituitary-adrenal (HPA) axis, lowering basal cortisol and restoring physiological cortisol rhythms in many individuals (340,341). This "resetting" of stress hormone dynamics may help attenuate chronic stress signalling, reduce systemic inflammation and mitigate immune suppression. These factors could render the TME less permissive to cancer progression, however direct evidence linking exercise-induced HPA regulation to long-term tumour suppression remains limited and further research is needed.

4.10.4 Adipokines and inflammatory mediators

As described in Section 4.6, obesity and adipose dysfunction are major systemic drivers of cancer. Exercise remodels adipose tissue, reducing secretion of pro-tumourigenic adipokines such as leptin, IL-6 and TNF-α, while increasing protective adipokines such as adiponectin and omentin-1 (271,272). These shifts improve metabolic homeostasis and reduce inflammatory signalling within the TME.

Taken together, these endocrine and hormonal adaptations highlight how exercise functions as a systemic intervention that reshapes the physiological terrain in which tumours arise and evolve. By lowering insulin and

IGF-1 signalling, improving insulin sensitivity, modulating sex hormones, rebalancing stress hormone dynamics and influencing adipokine and inflammatory mediator profiles, exercise reduces several systemic growth and survival cues that tumours commonly exploit (Figure 4.6). While direct evidence linking some of these systemic changes to reduced tumour progression or improved therapeutic response remains limited, the consistency of these hormonal changes across diverse human cohorts, including cancer survivors, supports the concept of exercise acting as a whole-body modulator of tumour permissiveness. As such, exercise may complement local tumour-targeted therapies by altering the "soil" (systemic environment) rather than the "seed" (tumour cells), an approach less prone to resistance than targeting single molecular targets (288,342).

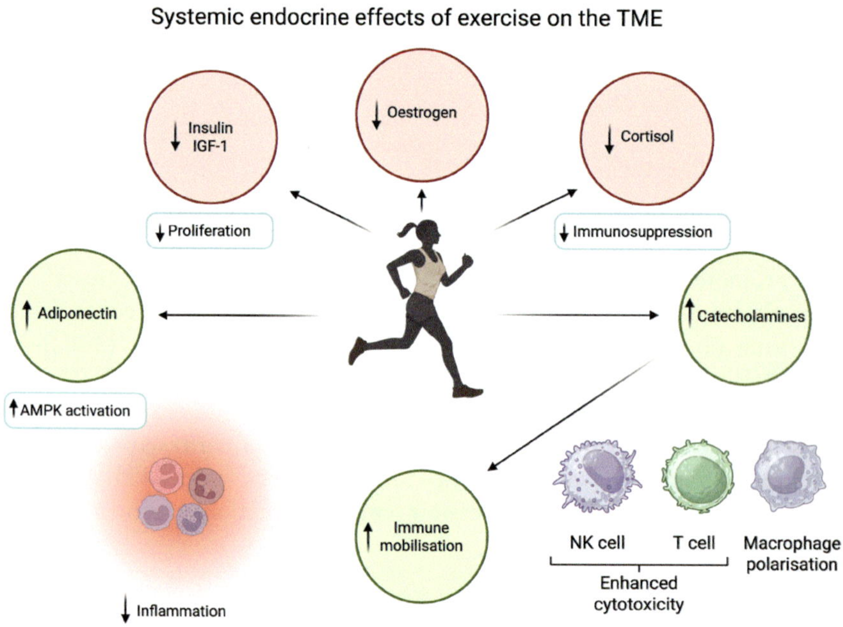

FIGURE 4.6 Systemic endocrine and immune responses to exercise. Exercise triggers a coordinated set of systemic changes that modulate tumour biology. Acute and chronic exercise lower circulating levels of insulin, IGF-1, oestrogen and cortisol, all of which can support tumour proliferation and immune evasion. In addition, exercise also increases adiponectin and catecholamine release (adrenaline, noradrenaline), which enhance AMPK activation, suppress inflammation and mobilise immune cells. These endocrine shifts create a less permissive environment for tumour growth and development. Created in Biorender.com.

4.11 Future directions and therapeutic potential

The evidence presented in this chapter highlights how exercise engages multiple molecular pathways to reprogramme the TME. Yet, while the biological rationale is strong, translating these insights into clinical benefit requires careful attention to the detailed understanding of underlying mechanisms, biomarker development and a move towards precision exercise prescription.

4.11.1 Towards biomarker-informed exercise prescriptions

One of the major future challenges is developing biomarker-informed exercise interventions. Just as cancer therapy is moving towards personalised medicine, exercise prescriptions may need to be tailored to the molecular and metabolic profile of individual patients. Biomarkers such as circulating cytokines, myokines, lactate, adipokine profiles or tumour hypoxia signatures could help stratify patients and guide exercise dose, intensity and modality. For example, patients with highly hypoxic tumours may benefit from interventions prioritising vascular normalisation, while those with obesity-driven cancers may respond best to adipose remodelling strategies. However, to date, there are no clinical studies to have successfully accomplished this. While the concept of "precision exercise oncology" is attractive, there is still a lack of validated biomarkers, standardised exercise protocols, and evidence that tailored exercise interventions produce better outcomes than general recommendations.

4.11.2 Exercise as a potential adjuvant therapy

Exercise holds promise as an adjuvant that can enhance the efficacy of established treatments. Preclinical evidence suggests that exercise synergises with chemotherapy, radiotherapy and immunotherapy, by improving perfusion, reducing hypoxia, mobilising anti-tumour cytotoxic lymphocytes and reducing immunosuppressive cells (343,344). Importantly, these benefits arise without the systemic toxicity associated with pharmacological adjuvants, making exercise an attractive, low-cost and accessible addition to cancer care. However, robust clinical trials designed to test exercise in combination with specific therapies, powered for cancer-specific endpoints (e.g., recurrence, survival), are still lacking (345,346).

4.11.3 Translational gaps

Despite compelling preclinical data, clinical evidence remains limited. Exercise oncology trials are often small, heterogeneous and focused on feasibility or QoL outcomes, rather than mechanistic endpoints. Moreover, murine exercise models fail to fully capture the complexity of human physiology or treatment regimens. Bridging this bench-to-bedside gap will require larger RCTs powered for biological endpoints, integration of imaging with circulating biomarkers (e.g., perfusion imaging, immunophenotyping, metabolic profiles), and standardisation of exercise protocols across studies (type, intensity, duration). Given the complexity of both human physiology and cancer heterogeneity, this will require coordinated, multi-disciplinary efforts.

4.11.4 Mechanistic clarity and model innovation

The field still faces challenges in defining how exercise interacts with specific molecular pathways. Many findings are context-dependent, influenced by tumour type, stage, exercise modality and host physiology. To advance the field further, more mechanistic clarity is needed with studies designed to dissect the pathways by which exercise modulates cellular signalling and mechanotransduction cascades across different tumour contexts. Model innovations, including patient-derived organoids, 3D bioreactors and in vivo imaging to capture dynamic TME responses, will be needed to drive these studies forward. Moreover, the development of precision interventions will require aligning exercise prescriptions with tumour biology and patient comorbidities. The therapeutic potential of exercise lies in its ability to reprogramme the host-tumour ecosystem rather than targeting a single molecular node. By simultaneously modulating metabolism, immunity, vasculature, mechanics and systemic hormones, exercise offers a unique, holistic approach that complements conventional therapies. If the challenges ahead can be overcome, exercise could become not merely supportive care but a recognised component of precision oncology, used to optimise treatment responses, prevent recurrence and improve long-term survival.

4.12 Chapter summary

This chapter has explored how exercise remodels the TME through diverse molecular pathways and systemic adaptations. Far beyond its role in supportive care, exercise has been shown to modify the biology of cancer: From transcriptional regulation and epigenetic remodelling, activation of metabolic and stress signalling pathways, to the release of myokines and exerkines, the molecular consequences of exercise extend across virtually every aspect of cancer. It reduces proliferative signalling, enhances immune surveillance, normalises vasculature, remodels the ECM and rebalances endocrine and metabolic inputs. Rather than acting through a single molecular target, exercise coordinates the reconditioning of the host-tumour ecosystem. These diverse effects make exercise uniquely difficult for tumours to evade, offering a complementary strategy to conventional targeted therapies, to which tumours often develop resistance. Looking forward, translating these insights into the clinic will depend on advancing mechanistic understanding, biomarker development and designing trials that move beyond feasibility to assess biological impact.

Chapter 4 Test your understanding question bank

A. *Epigenetic regulation*

1. How does exercise influence DNA methylation patterns in tumour suppressor genes, and why is this important for cancer control?
2. Describe how AMPK activation affects histone acetylation and transcriptional regulation in both muscle and tumour cells.
3. Which exercise-responsive miRNAs are implicated in anti-tumour pathways, and what cellular processes do they regulate?
4. Explain how exercise-induced activation of p53 may occur, despite the lack of direct evidence linking exercise-modulated miRNAs to p53 in cancer.

B. *AMPK and metabolic stress pathways*

5. What triggers AMPK activation during exercise, and why is this relevant to the tumour microenvironment?
6. Explain how AMPK inhibits mTOR signalling and how this may contribute to tumour suppression.
7. Describe the dual role of AMPK in regulating autophagy in cancer cells.
8. How might AMPK activation increase tumour cell vulnerability to apoptosis or therapy?

C. *MAPK signalling*

9. Why does the duration and pattern of ERK activation lead to different biological outcomes in cancer versus exercise?
10. How might exercise-induced JNK activation contribute to anti-tumour immunity?
11. Explain the context-dependent, dual roles of p38 MAPK in tumour suppression and progression.
12. How does improved vascular perfusion alter MAPK signalling within tumours?

D. *Hippo-YAP/TAZ mechanotransduction*

13. What systemic signals during exercise lead to YAP/TAZ inhibition, and how is this mediated?
14. How do mechanical cues from ECM stiffness support YAP/TAZ-driven oncogenic transcription?
15. Explain how exercise-induced ECM remodelling could reduce nuclear YAP/TAZ localisation.
16. Why is YAP/TAZ signalling considered important for cancer stem cell maintenance and therapeutic resistance?

E. *Myokines and exerkines*

17. Contrast tumour-derived IL-6 with exercise-induced IL-6 in terms of signalling and biological outcomes.
18. How does IL-15 support anti-tumour immune responses during exercise?
19. Describe how SPARC exerts anti-proliferative effects in colorectal and prostate cancer models.
20. Summarise the context-dependent effects of irisin on tumour proliferation and metastasis.
21. How might OSM contribute to the anti-tumour effects of exercise-conditioned serum?
22. What roles do musclin and FGF21 play in cancer cachexia, and how is exercise involved?
23. Explain how decorin may suppress tumour growth and modulate cachexia-related signalling.
24. What is the role of myostatin and activin A in cancer cachexia, and how might exercise counteract these pathways?
25. How do exercise-induced extracellular vesicles (EVs) influence tumour metabolism or immune evasion?

F. *Cachexia and muscle-tumour crosstalk*

26. Why is chronic IL-6 elevation associated with muscle wasting, and how does this differ from exercise-induced IL-6 dynamics?
27. Which exercise-responsive myokines show the strongest evidence for attenuating muscle loss in cancer?
28. How do myostatin/ActRIIB inhibitors reduce cachexia, and what is the link to exercise?

G. *Metabolic reprogramming of tumour cells*

29. How does exercise-conditioned serum shift cancer cell metabolism away from the Warburg phenotype?
30. What features of the obesogenic metabolic microenvironment promote tumour initiation and progression?

31. Describe how exercise remodels adipose tissue to decrease tumour fuel availability.
32. How does improved tumour perfusion alter hypoxia-driven metabolic signalling?

H. Angiogenesis and vascular function

33. What features of tumour vasculature distinguish pathological angiogenesis from physiological vascularisation?
34. How does exercise promote vascular normalisation in tumour tissue?
35. Explain how vascular normalisation improves drug delivery and immune infiltration.
36. Why can VEGF and NO have both tumour-promoting and tumour-suppressive roles depending on context?

I. ECM mechanics and interstitial pressure

37. How do the ECM and interstitial pressure activate oncogenic mechanotransduction pathways?
38. In what ways might exercise reduce ECM stiffness or solid stress in tumours?
39. How could reduced mechanical barriers improve immune infiltration into tumour tissue?

J. Systemic endocrine and hormonal modulation

40. How does exercise reduce insulin and IGF-1 signalling, and why is this important for cancer progression?
41. Explain how exercise affects oestrogen biosynthesis via adipose tissue and its implications for hormone-sensitive cancers.
42. Describe how chronic stress hormone signalling contributes to tumour progression and how exercise may reset these dynamics.
43. What changes occur in adipokine secretion with exercise, and how do these shape the TME?

References

1. Liu Q. Role of exercise on the reduction of cancer development: A mechanistic review from the lncRNA point of view. Clin Exp Med [Internet]. 2025 Dec 1 [cited 2025 Nov 29];25(1):77. Available from: https://pmc.ncbi.nlm.nih.gov/articles/PMC11893680/
2. Hanahan D. Hallmarks of cancer: New dimensions. Cancer Discov [Internet]. 2022 Jan 1 [cited 2025 Nov 29];12(1):31–46. Available from: https://pubmed.ncbi.nlm.nih.gov/35022204/
3. Jee H, Park E, Hur K, Kang M, Kim Y. High-intensity aerobic exercise suppresses cancer growth by regulating skeletal muscle-derived oncogenes and

tumor suppressors. Front Mol Biosci [Internet]. 2022 Jun 21 [cited 2025 Nov 29];9:818470. Available from: www.frontiersin.org

4. Liu L, Kim S, Buckley MT, Reyes JM, Kang J, Tian L, et al. Exercise reprograms the inflammatory landscape of multiple stem cell compartments during mammalian aging. Cell Stem Cell [Internet]. 2023 May 4 [cited 2025 Nov 29];30(5):689. Available from: https://pmc.ncbi.nlm.nih.gov/articles/PMC10216894/
5. Wang Q, Zhou W. Roles and molecular mechanisms of physical exercise in cancer prevention and treatment. J Sport Health Sci [Internet]. 2020 Mar 1 [cited 2025 Nov 22];10(2):201. Available from: https://pmc.ncbi.nlm.nih.gov/articles/PMC7987556/
6. Wu G, Chen Y, Chen C, Liu J, Wu Q, Zhang Y, et al. Role and mechanisms of exercise therapy in enhancing drug treatment for glioma: a review. 2025.
7. Barrès R, Yan J, Egan B, Treebak JT, Rasmussen M, Fritz T, et al. Acute exercise remodels promoter methylation in human skeletal muscle. Cell Metab [Internet]. 2012 Mar 7 [cited 2025 Nov 29];15(3):405–11. Available from: https://pubmed.ncbi.nlm.nih.gov/22405075/
8. Simons CCJM, Van Den Brandt PA, Stehouwer CDA, Van Engeland M, Weijenberg MP. Body size, physical activity, early-life energy restriction, and associations with methylated insulin-like growth factor-binding protein genes in colorectal cancer. Cancer Epidemiol Biomarkers Prev [Internet]. 2014 Sep 1 [cited 2025 Nov 29];23(9):1852–62. Available from: https://pubmed.ncbi.nlm.nih.gov/24972776/
9. Epigenetic regulation on gene expression induced by physical exercise—PubMed [Internet]. [cited 2025 Nov 29]. Available from: https://pubmed.ncbi.nlm.nih.gov/23728100/
10. Sanchis-Gomar F, Garcia-Gimenez JL, Perez-Quilis C, Gomez-Cabrera MC, Pallardo F V., Lippi G. Physical exercise as an epigenetic modulator: Eustress, the "positive stress" as an effector of gene expression. J Strength Cond Res [Internet]. 2012 Dec [cited 2025 Nov 29];26(12):3469–72. Available from: https://journals.lww.com/nsca-jscr/fulltext/2012/12000/physical_exercise_as_an_epigenetic_modulator_.38.aspx
11. Sun Y, Keat OB, Rajabi S. The role of physical activity and epigenetic changes in colorectal cancer prevention. Cancer Cell Int [Internet]. 2025 Dec 1 [cited 2025 Nov 29];25(1):227. Available from: https://pmc.ncbi.nlm.nih.gov/articles/PMC12183916/
12. Herman JG, Baylin SB. Gene silencing in cancer in association with promoter hypermethylation. N Engl J Med [Internet]. 2003 Nov 20 [cited 2025 Nov 29];349(21):2042–54. Available from: https://pubmed.ncbi.nlm.nih.gov/14627790/
13. Yuasa Y, Nagasaki H, Akiyama Y, Hashimoto Y, Takizawa T, Kojima K, et al. DNA methylation status is inversely correlated with green tea intake and physical activity in gastric cancer patients. Int J Cancer [Internet]. 2009 Jun 1 [cited 2025 Nov 29];124(11):2677–82. Available from: https://pubmed.ncbi.nlm.nih.gov/19170207/
14. Zeng H, Irwin ML, Lu L, Risch H, Mayne S, Mu L, et al. Physical activity and breast cancer survival: An epigenetic link through reduced methylation of a tumor suppressor gene L3MBTL1. Breast Cancer Res Treat [Internet]. 2012 May [cited 2025 Nov 29];133(1):127–35. Available from: https://pubmed.ncbi.nlm.nih.gov/21837478/
15. Coyle YM, Xie XJ, Lewis CM, Bu D, Milchgrub S, Euhus DM. Role of physical activity in modulating breast cancer risk as defined by APC and RASSF1A

promoter hypermethylation in nonmalignant breast tissue. Cancer Epidemiol Biomarkers Prev [Internet]. 2007 Feb [cited 2025 Nov 29];16(2):192–6. Available from: https://pubmed.ncbi.nlm.nih.gov/17301249/
16. McCullough LE. Gene-specific promoter methylation status in hormone-receptor-positive breast cancer associates with postmenopausal body size and recreational physical activity. Int J Cancer Clin Res. 2015 Feb 28;2(1).
17. Voisin S, Seale K, Jacques M, Landen S, Harvey NR, Haupt LM, et al. Exercise is associated with younger methylome and transcriptome profiles in human skeletal muscle. Aging Cell [Internet]. 2023 Jan 1 [cited 2025 Nov 29];23(1):e13859. Available from: https://pmc.ncbi.nlm.nih.gov/articles/PMC10776126/
18. McGee SL, Hargreaves M. Exercise and skeletal muscle glucose transporter 4 expression: Molecular mechanisms. Clin Exp Pharmacol Physiol [Internet]. 2006 Apr 1 [cited 2025 Nov 29];33(4):395–9. Available from: https://onlinelibrary.wiley.com/doi/full/10.1111/j.1440-1681.2006.04362.x
19. McGee SL, Sparling D, Olson A, Hargreaves M. Exercise increases MEF2- and GEF DNA-binding activity in human skeletal muscle. FASEB J [Internet]. 2006 Feb [cited 2025 Nov 29];20(2):348–9. Available from: https://pubmed.ncbi.nlm.nih.gov/16368714/
20. Vissing K, McGee SL, Roepstorff C, Schjerling P, Hargreaves M, Kiens B. Effect of sex differences on human MEF2 regulation during endurance exercise. Am J Physiol Endocrinol Metab [Internet]. 2008 Feb [cited 2025 Nov 29];294(2). Available from: https://pubmed.ncbi.nlm.nih.gov/18042665/
21. Li B, Carey M, Workman JL. The role of chromatin during transcription. Cell [Internet]. 2007 Feb 23 [cited 2025 Nov 29];128(4):707–19. Available from: https://www.cell.com/action/showFullText?pii=S0092867407001092
22. Hashida R, Matsuse H, Kawaguchi T, Yoshio S, Bekki M, Iwanaga S, et al. Effects of a low-intensity resistance exercise program on serum miR-630, miR-5703, and Fractalkine/CX3CL1 expressions in subjects with No exercise habits: A preliminary study. Hepatology Research [Internet]. 2021 Jul 1 [cited 2025 Nov 29];51(7):823–33. Available from: https://onlinelibrary.wiley.com/doi/full/10.1111/hepr.13670
23. Nakajima K, Takeoka M, Mori M, Hashimoto S, Sakurai A, Nose H, et al. Exercise effects on methylation of ASC gene. Int J Sports Med [Internet]. 2010 [cited 2025 Nov 29];31(9):671–5. Available from: https://pubmed.ncbi.nlm.nih.gov/20200803/
24. Taxman DJ, Zhang J, Champagne C, Bergstralh DT, Iocca HA, Lich JD, et al. Cutting edge: ASC mediates the induction of multiple cytokines by Porphyromonas gingivalis via caspase-1-dependent and -independent pathways. J Immunol [Internet]. 2006 Oct 1 [cited 2025 Nov 29];177(7):4252–6. Available from: https://pubmed.ncbi.nlm.nih.gov/16982856/
25. Vitucci D, Martone D, Alfieri A, Buono P. Muscle-derived exosomes and exercise in cancer prevention. Frontiers in Molecular Medicine. 2023 Jun 6;3:1202190.
26. Saldaña-Meyer R, Recillas-Targa F. Transcriptional and epigenetic regulation of the p53 tumor suppressor gene. Epigenetics [Internet]. 2011 [cited 2025 Nov 29];6(9):1068–77. Available from: https://www.tandfonline.com/action/journalInformation?journalCode=kepi20
27. Cai B, Ma M, Chen B, Li Z, Abdalla BA, Nie Q, et al. MiR-16-5p targets SESN1 to regulate the p53 signaling pathway, affecting myoblast proliferation and apoptosis, and is involved in myoblast differentiation. Cell Death & Disease [Internet]. 2018 Mar 6 [cited 2025 Nov 29];9(3):367. Available from: https://www.nature.com/articles/s41419-018-0403-6

28. Hoene M, Weigert C. The stress response of the liver to physical exercise.
29. Atherton PJ, Babraj J, Smith K, Singh J, Rennie MJ, Wackerhage H. Selective activation of AMPK-PGC-1 or PKB-TSC2-mTOR signaling can explain specific adaptive responses to endurance or resistance training-like electrical muscle stimulation. [cited 2025 Nov 29]. Available from: http://www.fasebj.org/cgi/doi/10.1096/fj.04-2179fje
30. Piguet AC, Saran U, Simillion C, Keller I, Terracciano L, Reeves HL, et al. Regular exercise decreases liver tumors development in hepatocyte-specific PTEN-deficient mice independently of steatosis. J Hepatol. 2015 Jun 1;62(6):1296–303.
31. Theriau CF, Shpilberg Y, Riddell MC, Connor MK. Voluntary physical activity abolishes the proliferative tumor growth microenvironment created by adipose tissue in animals fed a high fat diet. J Appl Physiol (1985) [Internet]. 2016 Jul 1 [cited 2025 Nov 29];121(1):139–53. Available from: https://pubmed.ncbi.nlm.nih.gov/27150834/
32. Panwar V, Singh A, Bhatt M, Tonk RK, Azizov S, Raza AS, et al. Multifaceted role of mTOR (mammalian target of rapamycin) signaling pathway in human health and disease. Signal Transduction and Targeted Therapy 2023 8:1 [Internet]. 2023 Oct 2 [cited 2025 Nov 29];8(1):375. Available from: https://www.nature.com/articles/s41392-023-01608-z
33. De Santi M, Baldelli G, Lucertini F, Natalucci V, Brandi G, Barbieri E. A dataset on the effect of exercise-conditioned human sera in three-dimensional breast cancer cell culture. Data Brief [Internet]. 2019 Dec 1 [cited 2025 Nov 29];27:104704. Available from: https://pmc.ncbi.nlm.nih.gov/articles/PMC6838928/
34. Hojman P, Gehl J, Christensen JF, Pedersen BK. Molecular mechanisms linking exercise to cancer prevention and treatment. Cell Metab [Internet]. 2018 Jan 9 [cited 2019 May 31];27(1):10–21. Available from: https://linkinghub.elsevier.com/retrieve/pii/S1550413117305673
35. Kim J, Kundu M, Viollet B, Guan KL. AMPK and mTOR regulate autophagy through direct phosphorylation of Ulk1. Nat Cell Biol [Internet]. 2011 Feb [cited 2025 Nov 29];13(2):132–41. Available from: https://pubmed.ncbi.nlm.nih.gov/21258367/
36. Egan DF, Shackelford DB, Mihaylova MM, Gelino S, Kohnz RA, Mair W, et al. Phosphorylation of ULK1 (hATG1) by AMP-activated protein kinase connects energy sensing to mitophagy. Science [Internet]. 2011 Jan 28 [cited 2025 Nov 29];331(6016):456–61. Available from: https://pubmed.ncbi.nlm.nih.gov/21205641/
37. Park JM, Lee DH, Kim DH. Redefining the role of AMPK in autophagy and the energy stress response. Nature Communications [Internet]. 2023 May 24 [cited 2025 Nov 29];14(1):2994. Available from: https://www.nature.com/articles/s41467-023-38401-z
38. Chen HY, White E. Role of autophagy in cancer prevention. Cancer Prev Res (Phila) [Internet]. 2011 Jul [cited 2025 Nov 29];4(7):973. Available from: https://pmc.ncbi.nlm.nih.gov/articles/PMC3136921/
39. Wang N, Wang B, Maswikiti EP, Yu Y, Song K, Ma C, et al. AMPK–a key factor in crosstalk between tumor cell energy metabolism and immune microenvironment? Cell Death Discov [Internet]. 2024 Dec 1 [cited 2025 Nov 29];10(1):237. Available from: https://pmc.ncbi.nlm.nih.gov/articles/PMC11102436/
40. Koelwyn GJ, Quail DF, Zhang X, White RM, Jones LW. Exercise-dependent regulation of the tumour microenvironment. Nat Rev Cancer [Internet].

2017 Oct 25 [cited 2019 Dec 6];17(10):620–32. Available from: http://www.nature.com/articles/nrc.2017.78
41. Zhang X, Ashcraft KA, Warner AB, Nair SK, Dewhirst MW. Can exercise-induced modulation of the tumor physiologic microenvironment improve antitumor immunity? Cancer Res [Internet]. 2019 May 15 [cited 2025 Nov 29];79(10):2447–56. Available from: /cancerres/article/79/10/2447/544176/Can-Exercise-Induced-Modulation-of-the-Tumor
42. Burotto M, Chiou VL, Lee JM, Kohn EC. The MAPK pathway across different malignancies: A new perspective. Cancer [Internet]. 2014 Nov 15 [cited 2025 Nov 29];120(22):3446–56. Available from: https://onlinelibrary.wiley.com/doi/full/10.1002/cncr.28864
43. Ryu H, Chung M, Dobrzyński M, Fey D, Blum Y, Lee SS, et al. Frequency modulation of ERK activation dynamics rewires cell fate. Mol Syst Biol [Internet]. 2015 Nov [cited 2025 Nov 29];11(11):838. Available from: https://pmc.ncbi.nlm.nih.gov/articles/PMC4670727/
44. Kiyatkin A, Rosenburgh IK van A van, Klein DE, Lemmon MA. Kinetics of receptor tyrosine kinase activation define ERK signaling dynamics. Sci Signal [Internet]. 2020 Aug 18 [cited 2025 Nov 29];13(645). Available from: https://www.science.org/doi/10.1126/scisignal.aaz5267
45. Sugiura R, Satoh R, Takasaki T. ERK: A double-edged sword in cancer. ERK-dependent apoptosis as a potential therapeutic strategy for cancer. Cells [Internet]. 2021 Oct 1 [cited 2025 Nov 29];10(10):2509. Available from: https://pmc.ncbi.nlm.nih.gov/articles/PMC8533760/
46. Kramer HF, Goodyear LJ. HIGHLIGHTED TOPIC exercise and inflammation exercise, MAPK, and NF-B signaling in skeletal muscle. J Appl Physiol [Internet]. 2007 [cited 2025 Nov 29];103:388–95. Available from: http://www.jap.org388
47. Teng R, Wang Y, Lv N, Zhang D, Williamson RA, Lei L, et al. Hypoxia impairs NK cell cytotoxicity through SHP-1-mediated attenuation of STAT3 and ERK signaling pathways. J Immunol Res [Internet]. 2020 [cited 2025 Nov 29];2020:4598476. Available from: https://pubmed.ncbi.nlm.nih.gov/33123602/
48. Darband SG, Sadighparvar S, Pakdel FG, Naderi S, Majidinia M. Involvement of IGF/IGFBP/Erk axis in the exercise-mediated preventive effects on colorectal cancer in rats. Int J Clin Exp Pathol [Internet]. 2021 [cited 2025 Nov 29];14(5):608. Available from: https://pmc.ncbi.nlm.nih.gov/articles/PMC8167496/
49. Gueritat J, Lefeuvre-Orfila L, Vincent S, Cretual A, Ravanat JL, Gratas-Delamarche A, et al. Exercise training combined with antioxidant supplementation prevents the antiproliferative activity of their single treatment in prostate cancer through inhibition of redox adaptation. Free Radic Biol Med [Internet]. 2014 [cited 2025 Nov 29];77:95–105. Available from: https://pubmed.ncbi.nlm.nih.gov/25236740/
50. Tam SY, Law HKW. JNK in tumor microenvironment: Present findings and challenges in clinical translation. Cancers (Basel) [Internet]. 2021 May 1 [cited 2025 Nov 29];13(9):2196. Available from: https://pmc.ncbi.nlm.nih.gov/articles/PMC8124407/
51. Cui N, Li H, Dun Y, Ripley-Gonzalez JW, You B, Li D, et al. Exercise inhibits JNK pathway activation and lipotoxicity via macrophage migration inhibitory factor in nonalcoholic fatty liver disease. Front Endocrinol (Lausanne). 2022 Sep 6;13:961231.
52. Bulavin D V., Fornace AJ. p38 MAP kinase's emerging role as a tumor suppressor. Adv Cancer Res [Internet]. 2004 [cited 2025 Nov 29];92:95–118. Available from: https://pubmed.ncbi.nlm.nih.gov/15530558/

53. Li X, Cao X, Zhao H, Guo M, Fang X, Li K, et al. Hypoxia activates Notch4 via ERK/JNK/P38 MAPK signaling pathways to promote lung adenocarcinoma progression and metastasis. Front Cell Dev Biol [Internet]. 2021 Dec 20 [cited 2025 Nov 29];9:780121. Available from: https://pmc.ncbi.nlm.nih.gov/articles/PMC8721100/
54. Cheung S, Jain P, So J, Shahidi S, Chung S, Koritzinsky M. p38 MAPK inhibition mitigates hypoxia-induced AR signaling in castration-resistant prostate cancer. Cancers (Basel) [Internet]. 2021 Feb 1 [cited 2025 Nov 29];13(4):831. Available from: https://pmc.ncbi.nlm.nih.gov/articles/PMC7922949/
55. Combes A, Dekerle J, Webborn N, Watt P, Bougault V, Daussin FN. Exercise-induced metabolic fluctuations influence AMPK, p38-MAPK and CaMKII phosphorylation in human skeletal muscle. Physiol Rep [Internet]. 2015 [cited 2025 Nov 29];3(9):e12462. Available from: https://pmc.ncbi.nlm.nih.gov/articles/PMC4600372/
56. Akimoto T, Pohnert SC, Li P, Zhang M, Gumbs C, Rosenberg PB, et al. Exercise stimulates Pgc-1α transcription in skeletal muscle through activation of the p38 MAPK pathway. Journal of Biological Chemistry. 2005 May 20;280(20):19587–93.
57. Irrcher I, Adhihetty PJ, Sheehan T, Joseph AM, Hood DA. PPARγ coactivator-1α expression during thyroid hormone- and contractile activity-induced mitochondrial adaptations. Am J Physiol Cell Physiol [Internet]. 2003 Jun 1 [cited 2025 Nov 29];284(6 53–6). Available from: www.ajpcell.org
58. Gong X, Liu A, Ming X, Deng P, Jiang Y. UV-induced interaction between p38 MAPK and p53 serves as a molecular switch in determining cell fate. FEBS Lett. 2010 Dec 1;584(23):4711–6.
59. Canovas B, Nebreda AR. Diversity and versatility of p38 kinase signalling in health and disease. Nature Reviews Molecular Cell Biology [Internet]. 2021 Jan 27 [cited 2025 Nov 29];22(5):346–66. Available from: https://www.nature.com/articles/s41580-020-00322-w
60. Zonneville J, Colligan S, Grant S, Miller A, Wallace P, Abrams SI, et al. Blockade of p38 kinase impedes the mobilization of pro-tumorigenic myeloid populations to impact breast cancer metastasis. Int J Cancer [Internet]. 2020 Oct 15 [cited 2025 Nov 29];147(8):2279. Available from: https://pmc.ncbi.nlm.nih.gov/articles/PMC7484223/
61. McClung JM, Judge AR, Powers SK, Yan Z. p38 MAPK links oxidative stress to autophagy-related gene expression in cachectic muscle wasting. Am J Physiol Cell Physiol [Internet]. 2009 Mar [cited 2025 Nov 29];298(3):C542. Available from: https://pmc.ncbi.nlm.nih.gov/articles/PMC2838571/
62. Park JA, Kwon YG. Hippo-YAP/TAZ signaling in angiogenesis. BMB Rep [Internet]. 2018 [cited 2025 Nov 29];51(3):157–62. Available from: https://pubmed.ncbi.nlm.nih.gov/29366443/
63. Yu FX, Zhao B, Panupinthu N, Jewell JL, Lian I, Wang LH, et al. Regulation of the Hippo-YAP pathway by G-protein-coupled receptor signaling. Cell. 2012 Aug 17;150(4):780–91.
64. Dethlefsen C, Hansen LS, Lillelund C, Andersen C, Gehl J, Christensen JF, et al. Exercise-induced catecholamines activate the Hippo tumor suppressor pathway to reduce risks of breast cancer development. Cancer Res [Internet]. 2017 Sep 15 [cited 2019 Dec 6];77(18):4894–904. Available from: http://cancerres.aacrjournals.org/lookup/doi/10.1158/0008-5472.CAN-16-3125
65. Baldelli G, De Santi M, Gervasi M, Annibalini G, Sisti D, Højman P, et al. The effects of human sera conditioned by high-intensity exercise sessions and training on the tumorigenic potential of cancer cells. Clin Transl Oncol

[Internet]. 2021 Jan 1 [cited 2025 Nov 16];23(1):22–34. Available from: https://pubmed.ncbi.nlm.nih.gov/32447643/
66. Gabriel BM, Lee Hamilton D, Tremblay AM, Wackerhage H. The Hippo signal transduction network for exercise physiologists. J Appl Physiol [Internet]. 2016 May 15 [cited 2025 Nov 29];120(10):1105. Available from: https://pmc.ncbi.nlm.nih.gov/articles/PMC4867322/
67. Moroishi T, Hansen CG, Guan KL. The emerging roles of YAP and TAZ in cancer. Nat Rev Cancer [Internet]. 2015 Jan 23 [cited 2025 Nov 29];15(2):73. Available from: https://pmc.ncbi.nlm.nih.gov/articles/PMC4562315/
68. Li S, Yang K, Jin Z, Yan P, Wei Y, Li J, et al. Recent advances in bladder cancer stem cells (BCSCs): A descriptive review of emerging therapeutic targets. iScience. 2025 Jul 18;28(7):112720.
69. Zhang Y, Xia H, Ge X, Chen Q, Yuan D, Chen Q, et al. CD44 acts through RhoA to regulate YAP signaling. Cell Signal [Internet]. 2014 [cited 2025 Nov 29];26(11):2504–13. Available from: https://pubmed.ncbi.nlm.nih.gov/25101858/
70. Nguyen CDK, Yi C. YAP/TAZ signaling and resistance to cancer therapy. Trends Cancer [Internet]. 2019 May 1 [cited 2025 Nov 29];5(5):283. Available from: https://pmc.ncbi.nlm.nih.gov/articles/PMC6557283/
71. Guo T, Xu J. Cancer-associated fibroblasts: A versatile mediator in tumor progression, metastasis, and targeted therapy. Cancer Metastasis Rev [Internet]. 2024 Sep 1 [cited 2025 Nov 30];43(3):1095. Available from: https://pmc.ncbi.nlm.nih.gov/articles/PMC11300527/
72. Kim NG, Gumbiner BM. Adhesion to fibronectin regulates Hippo signaling via the FAK–Src–PI3K pathway. J Cell Biol [Internet]. 2015 [cited 2025 Nov 30];210(3):503. Available from: https://pmc.ncbi.nlm.nih.gov/articles/PMC4523609/
73. Nardone G, Oliver-De La Cruz J, Vrbsky J, Martini C, Pribyl J, Skládal P, et al. YAP regulates cell mechanics by controlling focal adhesion assembly. Nat Commun [Internet]. 2017 May 15 [cited 2025 Nov 30];8:15321. Available from: https://pmc.ncbi.nlm.nih.gov/articles/PMC5440673/
74. Dupont S, Morsut L, Aragona M, Enzo E, Giulitti S, Cordenonsi M, et al. Role of YAP/TAZ in mechanotransduction. Nature [Internet]. 2011 Jun 8 [cited 2025 Nov 30];474(7350):179–84. Available from: https://pubmed.ncbi.nlm.nih.gov/21654799/
75. Graham ZA, Gallagher PM, Cardozo CP. Focal adhesion kinase and its role in skeletal muscle. J Muscle Res Cell Motil [Internet]. 2015 Oct 1 [cited 2025 Nov 30];36(0):305. Available from: https://pmc.ncbi.nlm.nih.gov/articles/PMC4659753/
76. Fernández-Sanjurjo M, Díaz-Martínez ÁE, Díez-Robles S, González-González F, De Gonzalo-Calvo D, Rabadán M, et al. Circulating MicroRNA profiling reveals specific subsignatures in response to a maximal incremental exercise test. J Strength Cond Res [Internet]. 2021 Feb 1 [cited 2025 Nov 30];35(2):287–91. Available from: https://journals.lww.com/nsca-jscr/fulltext/2021/02000/circulating_microrna_profiling_reveals_specific.1.aspx
77. An Y, Tan S, Yang J, Gao T, Dong Y. The potential role of Hippo pathway regulates cellular metabolism via signaling crosstalk in disease-induced macrophage polarization. Front Immunol [Internet]. 2024 [cited 2025 Nov 30];14:1344697. Available from: https://pmc.ncbi.nlm.nih.gov/articles/PMC10808647/
78. Huang D, Li X, Sun L, Huang P, Ying H, Wang H, et al. Regulation of Hippo signalling by p38 signalling. J Mol Cell Biol [Internet]. 2016 Aug 19 [cited 2025 Nov 30];8(4):328. Available from: https://pmc.ncbi.nlm.nih.gov/articles/PMC4991669/

79. Severinsen MCK, Pedersen BK. Muscle–organ crosstalk: The emerging roles of myokines. Endocr Rev [Internet]. 2020 Aug 1 [cited 2025 Nov 30];41(4):594–609. Available from: https://dx.doi.org/10.1210/endrev/bnaa016
80. Maggio S, Canonico B, Ceccaroli P, Polidori E, Cioccoloni A, Giacomelli L, et al. Modulation of the circulating extracellular vesicles in response to different exercise regimens and study of their inflammatory effects. Int J Mol Sci [Internet]. 2023 Feb 1 [cited 2025 Nov 30];24(3):3039. Available from: https://pmc.ncbi.nlm.nih.gov/articles/PMC9917742/
81. Chow LS, Gerszten RE, Taylor JM, Pedersen BK, van Praag H, Trappe S, et al. Exerkines in health, resilience and disease. Nature Reviews Endocrinology [Internet]. 2022 Mar 18 [cited 2025 Nov 30];18(5):273–89. Available from: https://www.nature.com/articles/s41574-022-00641-2
82. Walshe I, Robson-Ansley P, St Clair Gibson A, Lawrence C, Thompson KG, Ansley L. The reliability of the IL-6, sIL-6R and sgp130 response to a preloaded time trial. Eur J Appl Physiol [Internet]. 2010 Oct [cited 2025 Nov 30];110(3):619–25. Available from: https://pubmed.ncbi.nlm.nih.gov/20574676/
83. Fischer CP. Interleukin-6 in acute exercise and training: What is the biological relevance? Exerc Immunol Rev. 2006;12:6–33.
84. Benatti FB, Pedersen BK. Exercise as an anti-inflammatory therapy for rheumatic diseases-myokine regulation. Nat Rev Rheumatol [Internet]. 2015 Feb 17 [cited 2025 Nov 30];11(2):86–97. Available from: https://pubmed.ncbi.nlm.nih.gov/25422002/
85. Pedersen BK, Febbraio MA. Muscle as an endocrine organ: Focus on muscle-derived interleukin-6. Physiol Rev [Internet]. 2008 Oct [cited 2025 Nov 30];88(4):1379–406. Available from: https://pubmed.ncbi.nlm.nih.gov/18923185/
86. Docherty S, Harley R, McAuley JJ, Crowe LAN, Pedret C, Kirwan PD, et al. The effect of exercise on cytokines: Implications for musculoskeletal health: A narrative review. BMC Sports Sci Med Rehabil [Internet]. 2022 Dec 1 [cited 2025 Nov 16];14(1):5. Available from: https://pmc.ncbi.nlm.nih.gov/articles/PMC8740100/
87. Hunter CA, Jones SA. IL-6 as a keystone cytokine in health and disease. Nature Immunology [Internet]. 2015 Apr 21 [cited 2025 Nov 30];16(5):448–57. Available from: https://www.nature.com/articles/ni.3153
88. Huang Q, Wu M, Wu X, Zhang Y, Xia Y. Muscle-to-tumor crosstalk: The effect of exercise-induced myokine on cancer progression. Biochimica et Biophysica Acta (BBA)—Reviews on Cancer. 2022 Sep 1;1877(5):188761.
89. Orange ST, Jordan AR, Odell A, Kavanagh O, Hicks KM, Eaglen T, et al. Acute aerobic exercise-conditioned serum reduces colon cancer cell proliferation in vitro through interleukin-6-induced regulation of DNA damage. Int J Cancer [Internet]. 2022 Jul 15 [cited 2025 Nov 30];151(2):265–74. Available from: https://onlinelibrary.wiley.com/doi/full/10.1002/ijc.33982
90. Devin JL, Hill MM, Mourtzakis M, Quadrilatero J, Jenkins DG, Skinner TL. Acute high intensity interval exercise reduces colon cancer cell growth. J Physiol [Internet]. 2019 Apr 1 [cited 2025 Nov 30];597(8):2177–84. Available from: https://onlinelibrary.wiley.com/doi/full/10.1113/JP277648
91. Dethlefsen C, Lillelund C, Midtgaard J, Andersen C, Pedersen BK, Christensen JF, et al. Exercise regulates breast cancer cell viability: Systemic training adaptations versus acute exercise responses. Breast Cancer Res Treat [Internet]. 2016 Oct 1 [cited 2025 Nov 30];159(3):469–79. Available from: https://link.springer.com/article/10.1007/s10549-016-3970-1

92. Celik A, Bakar-Ates F. The confounding effect of interleukin-6 on apoptosis of MCF-7 cells through downregulation of MMP-2/-9 mRNA expression Interlökin-6'nin MMP-2/-9 mRNA Ekspresyonunun Downregülasyonu Yoluyla MCF-7 Hücrelerinin Apoptozisi Üzerindeki Etkisi. Turkish Journal of Biochemistry [Internet]. 2021 Oct 1 [cited 2025 Nov 30];46(5):549–55. Available from: https://www.degruyterbrill.com/document/doi/10.1515/tjb-2020-0508/html
93. Characterization of the role of IL-6 in the progression of prostate cancer [Internet]. [cited 2025 Nov 30]. Available from: https://onlinelibrary.wiley.com/doi/epdf/10.1002/%28SICI%291097-0045%2819990215%2938%3A3%3C199%3A%3AAID-PROS4%3E3.0.CO%3B2-H?saml_referrer
94. Wegiel B, Bjartell A, Culig Z, Persson JL. Interleukin-6 activates PI3K/Akt pathway and regulates cyclin A1 to promote prostate cancer cell survival. Int J Cancer [Internet]. 2008 Apr 1 [cited 2025 Nov 30];122(7):1521–9. Available from: https://pubmed.ncbi.nlm.nih.gov/18027847/
95. Leu CM, Wong FH, Chang C, Huang SF, Hu CP. Interleukin-6 acts as an antiapoptotic factor in human esophageal carcinoma cells through the activation of both STAT3 and mitogen-activated protein kinase pathways. Oncogene [Internet]. 2003 Oct 30 [cited 2025 Nov 30];22(49):7809–18. Available from: https://pubmed.ncbi.nlm.nih.gov/14586407/
96. Hsu JH, Shi Y, Frost P, Yan H, Hoang B, Sharma S, et al. Interleukin-6 activates phosphoinositol-3' kinase in multiple myeloma tumor cells by signaling through RAS-dependent and, separately, through p85-dependent pathways. Oncogene [Internet]. 2004 Apr 22 [cited 2025 Nov 30];23(19):3368–75. Available from: https://pubmed.ncbi.nlm.nih.gov/15021914/
97. Grivennikov S, Karin E, Terzic J, Mucida D, Yu GY, Vallabhapurapu S, et al. IL-6 and Stat3 are required for survival of intestinal epithelial cells and development of colitis-associated cancer. Cancer Cell [Internet]. 2009 Feb 3 [cited 2025 Nov 30];15(2):103–13. Available from: https://pubmed.ncbi.nlm.nih.gov/19185845/
98. Cheteh EH, Sarne V, Ceder S, Bianchi J, Augsten M, Rundqvist H, et al. Interleukin-6 derived from cancer-associated fibroblasts attenuates the p53 response to doxorubicin in prostate cancer cells. Cell Death Discov [Internet]. 2020 Dec 1 [cited 2025 Nov 30];6(1):42. Available from: https://pmc.ncbi.nlm.nih.gov/articles/PMC7265343/
99. Kern L, Mittenbühler MJ, Vesting AJ, Ostermann AL, Wunderlich CM, Wunderlich FT. Obesity-induced TNFα and IL-6 signaling: The missing link between obesity and inflammation—driven liver and colorectal cancers. Cancers (Basel) [Internet]. 2018 Jan 1 [cited 2025 Nov 30];11(1):24. Available from: https://pmc.ncbi.nlm.nih.gov/articles/PMC6356226/
100. Masjedi A, Hashemi V, Hojjat-Farsangi M, Ghalamfarsa G, Azizi G, Yousefi M, et al. The significant role of interleukin-6 and its signaling pathway in the immunopathogenesis and treatment of breast cancer. Biomedicine & Pharmacotherapy. 2018 Dec 1;108:1415–24.
101. Hayashi T, Fujita K, Nojima S, Hayashi Y, Nakano K, Ishizuya Y, et al. High-fat diet-induced inflammation accelerates prostate cancer growth via IL6 signaling. Clinical Cancer Research [Internet]. 2018 Sep 1 [cited 2025 Nov 30];24(17):4309–18. Available from: /clincancerres/article/24/17/4309/80986/High-Fat-Diet-Induced-Inflammation-Accelerates
102. Wu Q, Li B, Li Z, Li J, Sun S, Sun S. Cancer-associated adipocytes: Key players in breast cancer progression. Journal of Hematology & Oncology [Internet]. 2019 Sep 10 [cited 2025 Nov 30];12(1):95. Available from: https://link.springer.com/article/10.1186/s13045-019-0778-6

103. Jones SA, Jenkins BJ. Recent insights into targeting the IL-6 cytokine family in inflammatory diseases and cancer. Nature Reviews Immunology [Internet]. 2018 Sep 25 [cited 2025 Nov 30];18(12):773–89. Available from: https://www.nature.com/articles/s41577-018-0066-7
104. Timper K, Denson JL, Steculorum SM, Heilinger C, Engström-Ruud L, Wunderlich CM, et al. IL-6 improves energy and glucose homeostasis in obesity via enhanced central IL-6 trans-signaling. Cell Rep. 2017 Apr 11;19(2):267–80.
105. Carey AL, Steinberg GR, Macaulay SL, Thomas WG, Holmes AG, Ramm G, et al. Interleukin-6 increases insulin-stimulated glucose disposal in humans and glucose uptake and fatty acid oxidation in vitro via AMP-activated protein kinase. Diabetes [Internet]. 2006 Oct [cited 2025 Nov 30];55(10):2688–97. Available from: https://pubmed.ncbi.nlm.nih.gov/17003332/
106. Pedersen L, Idorn M, Olofsson GH, Lauenborg B, Nookaew I, Hansen RH, et al. Voluntary running suppresses tumor growth through epinephrine- and IL-6-dependent NK cell mobilization and redistribution. Cell Metab 2016 Mar 8;23(3):554–62.
107. Kurz E, Hirsch CA, Dalton T, Shadaloey SA, Khodadadi-Jamayran A, Miller G, et al. Exercise-induced engagement of the IL-15/IL-15Rα axis promotes anti-tumor immunity in pancreatic cancer. Cancer Cell. 2022 Jul 11;40(7):720–737.e5.
108. Carbó N, López-Soriano J, Costelli P, Alvarez B, Busquets S, Baccino FM, et al. Interleukin-15 mediates reciprocal regulation of adipose and muscle mass: A potential role in body weight control. Biochimica et Biophysica Acta (BBA)—General Subjects. 2001 Apr 3;1526(1):17–24.
109. Nielsen AR, Pedersen BK. The biological roles of exercise-induced cytokines: IL-6, IL-8, and IL-15. https://doi.org/101139/H07-054 [Internet]. 2007 Oct [cited 2025 Nov 30];32(5):833–9. Available from: https://cdnsciencepub.com/doi/10.1139/H07-054
110. Quinn LBS, Strait-Bodey L, Anderson BG, Argilés JM, Havel PJ. Interleukin-15 stimulates adiponectin secretion by 3T3-L1 adipocytes: Evidence for a skeletal muscle-to-fat signaling pathway. Cell Biol Int [Internet]. 2005 Jun [cited 2025 Nov 30];29(6):449–57. Available from: https://pubmed.ncbi.nlm.nih.gov/15951205/
111. Alvarez B, Carbó N, López-Soriano J, Drivdahl RH, Busquets S, López-Soriano FJ, et al. Effects of interleukin-15 (IL-15) on adipose tissue mass in rodent obesity models: Evidence for direct IL-15 action on adipose tissue. Biochim Biophys Acta Gen Subj [Internet]. 2002 Feb 15 [cited 2025 Nov 30];1570(1):33–7. Available from: https://pubmed.ncbi.nlm.nih.gov/11960686/
112. Bessard A, Solé V, Bouchaud G, Quéméner A, Jacques Y. High antitumor activity of RLI, an interleukin-15 (IL-15)-IL-15 receptor alpha fusion protein, in metastatic melanoma and colorectal cancer. Mol Cancer Ther [Internet]. 2009 Sep 1 [cited 2025 Nov 30];8(9):2736–45. Available from: https://pubmed.ncbi.nlm.nih.gov/19723883/
113. Desbois M, Le Vu P, Coutzac C, Marcheteau E, Béal C, Terme M, et al. IL-15 trans-signaling with the superagonist RLI promotes effector/memory CD8+ T Cell responses and enhances antitumor activity of PD-1 antagonists. J Immunol [Internet]. 2016 Jul 1 [cited 2025 Nov 30];197(1):168–78. Available from: https://pubmed.ncbi.nlm.nih.gov/27217584/
114. Guo S, Smeltz RB, Nanajian A, Heller R. IL-15/IL-15Rα heterodimeric complex as cancer immunotherapy in murine breast cancer models. Front Immunol [Internet]. 2021 Feb 8 [cited 2025 Nov 30];11. Available from: https://pubmed.ncbi.nlm.nih.gov/33628206/

115. Wrangle JM, Velcheti V, Patel MR, Garrett-Mayer E, Hill EG, Ravenel JG, et al. ALT-803, an IL-15 superagonist, in combination with nivolumab in patients with metastatic non-small cell lung cancer: A non-randomised, open-label, phase 1b trial. Lancet Oncol [Internet]. 2018 May 1 [cited 2025 Nov 30];19(5):694–704. Available from: https://pubmed.ncbi.nlm.nih.gov/29628312/
116. Krolopp JE, Thornton SM, Abbott MJ. IL-15 Activates the Jak3/STAT3 signaling pathway to mediate glucose uptake in skeletal muscle cells. Front Physiol [Internet]. 2016 [cited 2025 Nov 30];7(DEC). Available from: https://pubmed.ncbi.nlm.nih.gov/28066259/
117. Nadeau L, Patten DA, Caron A, Garneau L, Pinault-Masson E, Foretz M, et al. IL-15 improves skeletal muscle oxidative metabolism and glucose uptake in association with increased respiratory chain supercomplex formation and AMPK pathway activation. Biochim Biophys Acta Gen Subj [Internet]. 2019 Feb 1 [cited 2025 Nov 30];1863(2):395–407. Available from: https://pubmed.ncbi.nlm.nih.gov/30448294/
118. Bettariga F, Taaffe DR, Crespo-Garcia C, Clay TD, De Santi M, Baldelli G, et al. A single bout of resistance or high-intensity interval training increases anti-cancer myokines and suppresses cancer cell growth in vitro in survivors of breast cancer. Breast Cancer Res Treat [Internet]. 2025 Aug 1 [cited 2025 Nov 22];213(1):171–80. Available from: https://pubmed.ncbi.nlm.nih.gov/40608178/
119. Nagaraju GP, Dontula R, El-rayes BF, Lakka SS. Molecular mechanisms underlying the divergent roles of SPARC in human carcinogenesis. Carcinogenesis [Internet]. 2014 [cited 2025 Nov 30];35(5):967–73. Available from: https://pubmed.ncbi.nlm.nih.gov/24675529/
120. Shin M, Mizokami A, Kim J, Ofude M, Konaka H, Kadono Y, et al. Exogenous SPARC suppresses proliferation and migration of prostate cancer by interacting with Integrin β1. Prostate [Internet]. 2013 Aug 1 [cited 2025 Nov 30];73(11):1159–70. Available from: https://onlinelibrary.wiley.com/doi/full/10.1002/pros.22664
121. Camacho D, Jesus JP, Palma AM, Martins SA, Afonso A, Peixoto ML, et al. SPARC-p53: The double agents of cancer. Adv Cancer Res. 2020 Jan 1;148:171–99.
122. Podhajcer OL, Benedetti LG, Girotti MR, Prada F, Salvatierra E, Llera AS. The role of the matricellular protein SPARC in the dynamic interaction between the tumor and the host. Cancer and Metastasis Reviews [Internet]. 2008 Dec 10 [cited 2025 Nov 30];27(4):691–705. Available from: https://link.springer.com/article/10.1007/s10555-008-9146-7
123. Nie J, Sage EH. SPARC functions as an inhibitor of adipogenesis. J Cell Commun Signal [Internet]. 2009 [cited 2025 Nov 30];3(3–4):247. Available from: https://pmc.ncbi.nlm.nih.gov/articles/PMC2778584/
124. Dhanesuan N, Sharp JA, Blick T, Price JT, Thompson EW. Doxycycline-inducible expression of SPARC/Osteonectin/BM40 in MDA-MB-231 human breast cancer cells results in growth inhibition. Breast Cancer Res Treat [Internet]. 2002 Sep [cited 2025 Nov 30];75(1):73–85. Available from: https://link.springer.com/article/10.1023/A:1016536725958
125. Yunker CK, Golembieski W, Lemke N, Schultz CR, Cazacu S, Brodie C, et al. SPARC-induced increase in glioma matrix and decrease in vascularity are associated with reduced VEGF expression and secretion. Int J Cancer. 2008 Jun 15;122(12):2735–43.
126. Haber CL, Gottifredi V, Llera AS, Salvatierra E, Prada F, Alonso L, et al. SPARC modulates the proliferation of stromal but not melanoma cells unless endogenous SPARC expression is downregulated. Int J Cancer [Internet].

2008 Apr 1 [cited 2025 Nov 30];122(7):1465–75. Available from: /doi/pdf/10.1002/ijc.23216
127. Arnold S, Mira E, Muneer S, Korpanty G, Beck AW, Holloway SE, et al. Forced expression of MMP9 rescues the loss of angiogenesis and abrogates metastasis of pancreatic tumors triggered by the absence of host SPARC. Exp Biol Med [Internet]. 2008 Jul [cited 2025 Nov 30];233(7):860–73. Available from: /doi/pdf/10.3181/0801-RM-12?download=true
128. Jendraschak E, Sage EH. Regulation of angiogenesis by SPARC and angiostatin: Implications for tumor cell biology. Semin Cancer Biol [Internet]. 1996 Jun 1 [cited 2025 Nov 30];7(3):139–46. Available from: https://www.sciencedirect.com/science/article/abs/pii/S1044579X9690019X
129. Yiu GK, Chan WY, Ng SW, Chan PS, Cheung KK, Berkowitz RS, et al. SPARC (Secreted Protein Acidic and Rich in Cysteine) induces apoptosis in ovarian cancer cells. Am J Pathol [Internet]. 2001 Aug 1 [cited 2025 Nov 30];159(2):609–22. Available from: https://www.sciencedirect.com/science/article/pii/S0002944010617324
130. Yuan Z, Li Y, Zhang S, Wang X, Dou H, Yu X, et al. Extracellular matrix remodeling in tumor progression and immune escape: From mechanisms to treatments. Mol Cancer [Internet]. 2023 Dec 1 [cited 2025 Nov 30];22(1):48. Available from: https://pmc.ncbi.nlm.nih.gov/articles/PMC10007858/
131. Vaz J, Ansari D, Sasor A, Andersson R. SPARC: A potential prognostic and therapeutic target in pancreatic cancer. Pancreas [Internet]. 2015 Oct 1 [cited 2025 Nov 30];44(7):1024. Available from: https://pmc.ncbi.nlm.nih.gov/articles/PMC4568900/
132. Golembieski WA, Ge S, Nelson K, Mikkelsen T, Rempel SA. Increased SPARC expression promotes U87 glioblastoma invasion in vitro. Int J Dev Neurosci [Internet]. 1999 Aug [cited 2025 Nov 30];17(5–6):463–72. Available from: https://pubmed.ncbi.nlm.nih.gov/10571408/
133. Schultz C, Lemke N, Ge S, Golembieski W, Rempel S. Secreted protein acidic and rich in cysteine promotes glioma invasion and delays tumor growth in vivo. Cancer Res. 2002.
134. Matsuo K, Sato K, Suemoto K, Miyamoto-Mikami E, Fuku N, Higashida K, et al. A mechanism underlying preventive effect of high-intensity training on colon cancer. Med Sci Sports Exerc [Internet]. 2017 Sep 1 [cited 2025 Nov 30];49(9):1805–16. Available from: https://pubmed.ncbi.nlm.nih.gov/28463901/
135. Aoi W, Naito Y, Takagi T, Tanimura Y, Takanami Y, Kawai Y, et al. A novel myokine, secreted protein acidic and rich in cysteine (SPARC), suppresses colon tumorigenesis via regular exercise. Gut [Internet]. 2013 Jun 1 [cited 2025 Nov 30];62(6):882–9. Available from: https://gut.bmj.com/content/62/6/882
136. Kim JS, Taaffe DR, Galvão DA, Hart NH, Gray E, Ryan CJ, et al. Exercise in advanced prostate cancer elevates myokine levels and suppresses in-vitro cell growth. Prostate Cancer and Prostatic Diseases [Internet]. 2022 Feb 12 [cited 2025 Nov 30];25(1):86–92. Available from: https://www.nature.com/articles/s41391-022-00504-x
137. Akutsu T, Ito E, Narita M, Ohdaira H, Suzuki Y, Urashima M. Effect of serum SPARC levels on survival in patients with digestive tract cancer: A post hoc analysis of the AMATERASU randomized clinical trial. Cancers [Internet]. 2020 Jun 4 [cited 2025 Nov 30];12(6):1465. Available from: https://www.mdpi.com/2072-6694/12/6/1465/htm
138. Chern YJ, Wong JCT, Cheng GSW, Yu A, Yin Y, Schaeffer DF, et al. The interaction between SPARC and GRP78 interferes with ER stress signaling and

potentiates apoptosis via PERK/eIF2α and IRE1α/XBP-1 in colorectal cancer. Cell Death Dis [Internet]. 2019 Jul 1 [cited 2025 Nov 30];10(7). Available from: https://pubmed.ncbi.nlm.nih.gov/31243264/
139. Chetty C, Dontula R, Ganji PN, Gujrati M, Lakka SS. SPARC expression induces cell cycle arrest via STAT3 signaling pathway in medulloblastoma cells. Biochem Biophys Res Commun [Internet]. 2012 Jan 13 [cited 2025 Nov 30];417(2):874–9. Available from: https://www.sciencedirect.com/science/article/abs/pii/S0006291X11022741
140. Shin M, Mizokami A, Kim J, Ofude M, Konaka H, Kadono Y, et al. Exogenous SPARC suppresses proliferation and migration of prostate cancer by interacting with integrin β1. Prostate [Internet]. 2013 Aug [cited 2025 Nov 30];73(11):1159–70. Available from: https://pubmed.ncbi.nlm.nih.gov/23532895/
141. Neuzillet C, Tijeras-Raballand A, Cros J, Faivre S, Hammel P, Raymond E. Stromal expression of SPARC in pancreatic adenocarcinoma. Cancer and Metastasis Reviews [Internet]. 2013 Dec 21 [cited 2025 Nov 30];32(3–4):585–602. Available from: https://link.springer.com/article/10.1007/s10555-013-9439-3
142. Gannon NP, Vaughan RA, Garcia-Smith R, Bisoffi M, Trujillo KA. Effects of the exercise-inducible myokine irisin on malignant and non-malignant breast epithelial cell behavior in vitro. Int J Cancer [Internet]. 2015 Feb 15 [cited 2025 Nov 16];136(4):E197–202. Available from: https://pubmed.ncbi.nlm.nih.gov/25124080/
143. Anastasilakis AD, Polyzos SA, Saridakis ZG, Kynigopoulos G, Skouvaklidou EC, Molyvas D, et al. Circulating irisin in healthy, young individuals: Day-night rhythm, effects of food intake and exercise, and associations with gender, physical activity, diet, and body composition. J Clin Endocrinol Metab [Internet]. 2014 Sep 1 [cited 2025 Nov 30];99(9):3247–55. Available from: https://pubmed.ncbi.nlm.nih.gov/24915120/
144. Lee P, Linderman JD, Smith S, Brychta RJ, Wang J, Idelson C, et al. Irisin and FGF21 are cold-induced endocrine activators of brown fat function in humans. Cell Metab [Internet]. 2014 Feb 4 [cited 2025 Nov 30];19(2):302–9. Available from: https://pubmed.ncbi.nlm.nih.gov/24506871/
145. Arhire LI, Mihalache L, Covasa M. Irisin: A hope in understanding and managing obesity and metabolic syndrome. Front Endocrinol (Lausanne) [Internet]. 2019 Aug 2 [cited 2025 Nov 30];10. Available from: https://pubmed.ncbi.nlm.nih.gov/31428053/
146. Boström P, Wu J, Jedrychowski MP, Korde A, Ye L, Lo JC, et al. A PGC1-α-dependent myokine that drives brown-fat-like development of white fat and thermogenesis. Nature [Internet]. 2012 Jan 26 [cited 2025 Nov 30];481(7382):463–8. Available from: https://pubmed.ncbi.nlm.nih.gov/22237023/
147. Tsiani E, Tsakiridis N, Kouvelioti R, Jaglanian A, Klentrou P. Current evidence of the role of the myokine irisin in cancer. Cancers (Basel) [Internet]. 2021 Jun 1 [cited 2025 Nov 30];13(11). Available from: https://pubmed.ncbi.nlm.nih.gov/34071869/
148. Fox J, Rioux B V., Goulet EDB, Johanssen NM, Swift DL, Bouchard DR, et al. Effect of an acute exercise bout on immediate post-exercise irisin concentration in adults: A meta-analysis. Scand J Med Sci Sports [Internet]. 2018 Jan 1 [cited 2025 Nov 30];28(1):16–28. Available from: /doi/pdf/10.1111/sms.12904
149. Liu J, Song N, Huang Y, Chen Y. Irisin inhibits pancreatic cancer cell growth via the AMPK-mTOR pathway. Sci Rep [Internet]. 2018 Dec 1 [cited 2025 Nov 30];8(1). Available from: https://pubmed.ncbi.nlm.nih.gov/30323244/
150. Zhang D, Zhang P, Li L, Tang N, Huang F, Kong X, et al. Irisin functions to inhibit malignant growth of human pancreatic cancer cells via downregulation

of the PI3K/AKT signaling pathway. Onco Targets Ther [Internet]. 2019 [cited 2025 Nov 30];12:7243–9. Available from: https://pubmed.ncbi.nlm.nih.gov/31564907/

151. Huang CW, Chang YH, Lee HH, Wu JY, Huang JX, Chung YH, et al. Irisin, an exercise myokine, potently suppresses tumor proliferation, invasion, and growth in glioma. FASEB J [Internet]. 2020 Jul 1 [cited 2025 Nov 30];34(7):9678–93. Available from: https://pubmed.ncbi.nlm.nih.gov/32469121/
152. Shao L, Li H, Chen J, Song H, Zhang Y, Wu F, et al. Irisin suppresses the migration, proliferation, and invasion of lung cancer cells via inhibition of epithelial-to-mesenchymal transition. Biochem Biophys Res Commun [Internet]. 2017 Apr 8 [cited 2025 Nov 30];485(3):598–605. Available from: https://pubmed.ncbi.nlm.nih.gov/27986567/
153. Fan GH, Zhu TY, Huang J. FNDC5 promotes paclitaxel sensitivity of non-small cell lung cancers via inhibiting MDR1. Cell Signal [Internet]. 2020 Aug 1 [cited 2025 Nov 30];72. Available from: https://pubmed.ncbi.nlm.nih.gov/32353410/
154. Kong G, Jiang Y, Sun X, Cao Z, Zhang G, Zhao Z, et al. Irisin reverses the IL-6 induced epithelial-mesenchymal transition in osteosarcoma cell migration and invasion through the STAT3/Snail signaling pathway. Oncol Rep [Internet]. 2017 Nov 1 [cited 2025 Nov 30];38(5):2647–56. Available from: https://pubmed.ncbi.nlm.nih.gov/29048621/
155. Tekin S, Erden Y, Sandal S, Yilmaz B. Is irisin an anticarcinogenic peptide? 2014 [cited 2025 Nov 30]. Available from: www.medicinescience.org|Med-Sciencewww.medicinescience.org|Med-Science
156. Liu J, Huang Y, Liu Y, Chen Y. Irisin enhances doxorubicin-induced cell apoptosis in pancreatic cancer by inhibiting the PI3K/AKT/NF-κB pathway. Med Sci Monit [Internet]. 2019 Aug 14 [cited 2025 Nov 30];25:6085–96. Available from: https://pubmed.ncbi.nlm.nih.gov/31412018/
157. Shi G, Tang N, Qiu J, Zhang D, Huang F, Cheng Y, et al. Irisin stimulates cell proliferation and invasion by targeting the PI3K/AKT pathway in human hepatocellular carcinoma. Biochem Biophys Res Commun [Internet]. 2017 Nov 4 [cited 2025 Nov 30];493(1):585–91. Available from: https://pubmed.ncbi.nlm.nih.gov/28867187/
158. Moon HS, Mantzoros CS. Regulation of cell proliferation and malignant potential by irisin in endometrial, colon, thyroid and esophageal cancer cell lines. Metabolism [Internet]. 2014 Feb [cited 2025 Nov 30];63(2):188–93. Available from: https://pubmed.ncbi.nlm.nih.gov/24268368/
159. Shao L, Li H, Chen J, Song H, Zhang Y, Wu F, et al. Irisin suppresses the migration, proliferation, and invasion of lung cancer cells via inhibition of epithelial-to-mesenchymal transition. Biochem Biophys Res Commun [Internet]. 2017 Apr 8 [cited 2025 Nov 30];485(3):598–605. Available from: https://pubmed.ncbi.nlm.nih.gov/27986567/
160. Kong G, Jiang Y, Sun X, Cao Z, Zhang G, Zhao Z, et al. Irisin reverses the IL-6 induced epithelial-mesenchymal transition in osteosarcoma cell migration and invasion through the STAT3/Snail signaling pathway. Oncol Rep [Internet]. 2017 Nov 1 [cited 2025 Nov 30];38(5):2647–56. Available from: https://pubmed.ncbi.nlm.nih.gov/29048621/
161. Zhang ZP, Zhang XF, Li H, Liu TJ, Zhao QP, Huang LH, et al. Serum irisin associates with breast cancer to spinal metastasis. Medicine [Internet]. 2018 Apr 1 [cited 2025 Nov 30];97(17). Available from: https://pubmed.ncbi.nlm.nih.gov/29703023/
162. Provatopoulou X, Georgiou GP, Kalogera E, Kalles V, Matiatou MA, Papapanagiotou I, et al. Serum irisin levels are lower in patients with breast cancer:

Association with disease diagnosis and tumor characteristics. BMC Cancer 2015 15:1 [Internet]. 2015 Nov 11 [cited 2025 Nov 30];15(1):898. Available from: https://link.springer.com/article/10.1186/s12885-015-1898-1
163. Coletta AM, Agha NH, Baker FL, Niemiro GM, Mylabathula PL, Brewster AM, et al. The impact of high-intensity interval exercise training on NK-cell function and circulating myokines for breast cancer prevention among women at high risk for breast cancer. Breast Cancer Res Treat [Internet]. 2021 Jun 1 [cited 2025 Nov 22];187(2):407–16. Available from: https://link.springer.com/article/10.1007/s10549-021-06111-z
164. Xiong XQ, Geng Z, Zhou B, Zhang F, Han Y, Zhou YB, et al. FNDC5 attenuates adipose tissue inflammation and insulin resistance via AMPK-mediated macrophage polarization in obesity. Metabolism [Internet]. 2018 Jun 1 [cited 2025 Nov 30];83:31–41. Available from: https://pubmed.ncbi.nlm.nih.gov/29374559/
165. Dong J, Dong Y, Dong Y, Chen F, Mitch WE, Zhang L. Inhibition of myostatin in mice improves insulin sensitivity via irisin-mediated cross talk between muscle and adipose tissues. Int J Obes (Lond) [Internet]. 2016 Mar 1 [cited 2025 Nov 30];40(3):434–42. Available from: https://pubmed.ncbi.nlm.nih.gov/26435323/
166. New insight into the direct anti-inflammatory activity of a myokine irisin against proinflammatory activation of adipocytes. Implication for exercise in obesity—PubMed [Internet]. [cited 2025 Nov 30]. Available from: https://pubmed.ncbi.nlm.nih.gov/28614774/
167. Wu F, Song H, Zhang Y, Zhang Y, Mu Q, Jiang M, et al. Irisin induces angiogenesis in human umbilical vein endothelial cells in vitro and in Zebrafish embryos in vivo via activation of the ERK signaling pathway. PLoS One [Internet]. 2015 Aug 4 [cited 2025 Nov 30];10(8):e0134662. Available from: https://journals.plos.org/plosone/article?id=10.1371/journal.pone.0134662
168. Alshanqiti KH, Alomar SF, Alzoman N, Almomen A. Irisin induces apoptosis in metastatic prostate cancer cells and inhibits tumor growth in vivo. Cancers (Basel) [Internet]. 2023 Aug 1 [cited 2025 Nov 30];15(15). Available from: https://pubmed.ncbi.nlm.nih.gov/37568817/
169. Ho MY, Wen MS, Yeh JK, Hsieh IC, Chen CC, Hsieh MJ, et al. Excessive irisin increases oxidative stress and apoptosis in murine heart. Biochem Biophys Res Commun [Internet]. 2018 Sep 18 [cited 2025 Nov 30];503(4):2493–8. Available from: https://pubmed.ncbi.nlm.nih.gov/30208516/
170. Nakamura H, Takada K. Reactive oxygen species in cancer: Current findings and future directions. Cancer Sci [Internet]. 2021 Oct 1 [cited 2025 Nov 30];112(10):3945–52. Available from: https://pubmed.ncbi.nlm.nih.gov/34286881/
171. Yang BC, Leung PS. Irisin is a positive regulator for ferroptosis in pancreatic cancer. Mol Ther Oncolytics [Internet]. 2020 Sep 25 [cited 2025 Nov 30];18:457–66. Available from: https://www.sciencedirect.com/science/article/pii/S2372770520301194
172. Li RL, Wu SS, Wu Y, Wang XX, Chen HY, Xin J juan, et al. Irisin alleviates pressure overload-induced cardiac hypertrophy by inducing protective autophagy via mTOR-independent activation of the AMPK-ULK1 pathway. J Mol Cell Cardiol [Internet]. 2018 Aug 1 [cited 2025 Nov 30];121:242–55. Available from: https://www.sciencedirect.com/science/article/abs/pii/S0022282818306965
173. Pinkowska A, Podhorska-Okołów M, Dzięgiel P, Nowińska K. The role of irisin in cancer disease. Cells [Internet]. 2021 Jun 12 [cited 2025 Nov 30];10(6):1479. Available from: https://www.mdpi.com/2073-4409/10/6/1479/htm
174. Masjedi A, Hajizadeh F, Beigi Dargani F, Beyzai B, Aksoun M, Hojjat-Farsangi M, et al. Oncostatin M: A mysterious cytokine in cancers. Int Immunopharmacol

[Internet]. 2021 Jan 1 [cited 2025 Nov 30];90:107158. Available from: https://www.sciencedirect.com/science/article/abs/pii/S1567576920336250

175. Douglas AM, Goss GA, Sutherland RL, Hilton DJ, Berndt MC, Nicola NA, et al. Expression and function of members of the cytokine receptor superfamily on breast cancer cells. Oncogene [Internet]. 1997 [cited 2025 Nov 30];14(6):661–9. Available from: https://www.nature.com/articles/1200882
176. Scaffidi AK, Mutsaers SE, Moodley YP, McAnulty RJ, Laurent GJ, Thompson PJ, et al. Oncostatin M stimulates proliferation, induces collagen production and inhibits apoptosis of human lung fibroblasts. Br J Pharmacol [Internet]. 2002 [cited 2025 Nov 30];136(5):793. Available from: https://pmc.ncbi.nlm.nih.gov/articles/PMC1573397/
177. Li Q, Zhu J, Sun F, Liu L, Liu X, Yue Y. Oncostatin M promotes proliferation of ovarian cancer cells through signal transducer and activator of transcription 3. Int J Mol Med [Internet]. 2011 Jul [cited 2025 Nov 30];28(1):101–8. Available from: https://www.scopus.com/pages/publications/79955818331
178. Kucia-Tran JA, Tulkki V, Smith S, Scarpini CG, Hughes K, Araujo AM, et al. Overexpression of the oncostatin-M receptor in cervical squamous cell carcinoma is associated with epithelial–mesenchymal transition and poor overall survival. British Journal of Cancer [Internet]. 2016 Jun 28 [cited 2025 Nov 30];115(2):212–22. Available from: https://www.nature.com/articles/bjc2016199
179. Horn D, Fitzpatrick WC, Gompper PT, Ochs V, Bolton-Hansen M, Zarling J, et al. Regulation of cell growth by recombinant Oncostatin M. Growth Factors [Internet]. 1990 [cited 2025 Nov 30];2(2):157–65. Available from: https://www.tandfonline.com/doi/abs/10.3109/08977199009071502
180. Halfter H, Friedrich M, Resch A, Kullmann M, Stögbauer F, Ringelstein EB, et al. Oncostatin M induces growth arrest by inhibition of Skp2, Cks1, and cyclin A expression and induced p21 expression. Cancer Res [Internet]. 2006 Jul 1 [cited 2025 Nov 30];66(13):6530–9. Available from: https://pubmed.ncbi.nlm.nih.gov/16818624/
181. Kan CE, Cipriano R, Jackson MW. c-MYC functions as a molecular switch to alter the response of human mammary epithelial cells to oncostatin M. Cancer Res [Internet]. 2011 Nov 15 [cited 2025 Nov 30];71(22):6930–9. Available from: https://pubmed.ncbi.nlm.nih.gov/21975934/
182. Bryson BL, Junk DJ, Cipriano R, Jackson MW. STAT3-mediated SMAD3 activation underlies Oncostatin M-induced Senescence. Cell Cycle [Internet]. 2017 Feb 16 [cited 2025 Nov 30];16(4):319–34. Available from: https://www.tandfonline.com/doi/pdf/10.1080/15384101.2016.1259037
183. Araujo AM, Abaurrea A, Azcoaga P, López-Velazco JI, Manzano S, Rodriguez J, et al. Stromal oncostatin M cytokine promotes breast cancer progression by reprogramming the tumor microenvironment. J Clin Invest [Internet]. 2022 Apr 1 [cited 2025 Nov 30];132(7):e148667. Available from: https://pmc.ncbi.nlm.nih.gov/articles/PMC8970678/
184. Godoy-Tundidor S, Cavarretta ITR, Fuchs D, Fiechtl M, Steiner H, Friedbichler K, et al. Interleukin-6 and oncostatin M stimulation of proliferation of prostate cancer 22Rv1 cells through the signaling pathways of p38 mitogen-activated protein kinase and phosphatidylinositol 3-kinase. Prostate [Internet]. 2005 Jul 1 [cited 2025 Nov 30];64(2):209–16. Available from: /doi/pdf/10.1002/pros.20235
185. Kim JS, Wilson RL, Taaffe DR, Galvão DA, Gray E, Newton RU. Myokine expression and tumor-suppressive effect of serum after 12 wk of exercise in prostate cancer patients on ADT. Med Sci Sports Exerc [Internet]. 2021 Feb 1 [cited 2025 Nov 30];54(2):197. Available from: https://pmc.ncbi.nlm.nih.gov/articles/PMC8754092/

186. Kim JS, Taaffe DR, Galvão DA, Hart NH, Gray E, Ryan CJ, et al. Exercise in advanced prostate cancer elevates myokine levels and suppresses in-vitro cell growth. Prostate Cancer and Prostatic Diseases [Internet]. 2022 Feb 12 [cited 2025 Nov 30];25(1):86–92. Available from: https://www.nature.com/articles/s41391-022-00504-x
187. Hojman P, Dethlefsen C, Brandt C, Hansen J, Pedersen L, Pedersen BK. Exercise-induced muscle-derived cytokines inhibit mammary cancer cell growth. https://doi.org/101152/ajpendo005202010 [Internet]. 2011 Sep [cited 2025 Nov 30];301(3):504–10. Available from: /doi/pdf/10.1152/ajpendo.00520.2010?download=true
188. Subbotina E, Sierra A, Zhu Z, Gao Z, Koganti SRK, Reyes S, et al. Musclin is an activity-stimulated myokine that enhances physical endurance. Proc Natl Acad Sci USA [Internet]. 2015 Dec 29 [cited 2025 Nov 30];112(52):16042–7. Available from: /doi/pdf/10.1073/pnas.1514250112?download=true
189. Jeremic N, Chaturvedi P, Tyagi SC. Browning of white fat: Novel insight into factors, mechanisms, and therapeutics. J Cell Physiol [Internet]. 2017 Jan 1 [cited 2025 Nov 30];232(1):61–8. Available from: /doi/pdf/10.1002/jcp.25450
190. Re Cecconi AD, Forti M, Chiappa M, Zhu Z, Zingman L V., Cervo L, et al. Musclin, a myokine induced by aerobic exercise, retards muscle atrophy during cancer cachexia in mice. Cancers [Internet]. 2019 Oct 12 [cited 2025 Nov 30];11(10):1541. Available from: https://www.mdpi.com/2072-6694/11/10/1541/htm
191. Fisher FM, Maratos-Flier E. Understanding the physiology of FGF21. Annu Rev Physiol [Internet]. 2016 Feb 10 [cited 2025 Nov 30];78(Volume 78, 2016):223–41. Available from: https://www.annualreviews.org/content/journals/10.1146/annurev-physiol-021115-105339
192. Inagaki T, Dutchak P, Zhao G, Ding X, Gautron L, Parameswara V, et al. Endocrine regulation of the fasting response by PPARα-mediated induction of fibroblast growth factor 21. Cell Metab [Internet]. 2007 Jun 6 [cited 2025 Nov 30];5(6):415–25. Available from: https://pubmed.ncbi.nlm.nih.gov/17550777/
193. Domouzoglou EM, Maratos-Flier E. Fibroblast growth factor 21 is a metabolic regulator that plays a role in the adaptation to ketosis. American Journal of Clinical Nutrition [Internet]. 2011 Apr 1 [cited 2025 Nov 30];93(4). Available from: https://pubmed.ncbi.nlm.nih.gov/21346090/
194. Gälman C, Lundåsen T, Kharitonenkov A, Bina HA, Eriksson M, Hafström I, et al. The circulating metabolic regulator FGF21 is induced by prolonged fasting and PPARα activation in man. Cell Metab [Internet]. 2008 Aug 6 [cited 2025 Nov 30];8(2):169–74. Available from: https://www.sciencedirect.com/science/article/pii/S1550413108002076
195. Izumiya Y, Bina HA, Ouchi N, Akasaki Y, Kharitonenkov A, Walsh K. FGF21 is an Akt-regulated myokine. FEBS Lett [Internet]. 2008 Nov 12 [cited 2025 Nov 30];582(27):3805–10. Available from: https://www.sciencedirect.com/science/article/pii/S0014579308008296
196. Rosales-Soto G, Diaz-Vegas A, Casas M, Contreras-Ferrat A, Jaimovich E. Fibroblast growth factor-21 potentiates glucose transport in skeletal muscle fibers. J Mol Endocrinol [Internet]. 2020 Oct 1 [cited 2025 Nov 30];65(3):85–95. Available from: https://jme.bioscientifica.com/view/journals/jme/65/3/JME-19-0210.xml
197. Kharitonenkov A, Shiyanova TL, Koester A, Ford AM, Micanovic R, Galbreath EJ, et al. FGF-21 as a novel metabolic regulator. J Clin Invest [Internet]. 2005 Jun [cited 2025 Nov 30];115(6):1627–35. Available from: https://pubmed.ncbi.nlm.nih.gov/15902306/

198. Mashili FL, Austin RL, Deshmukh AS, Fritz T, Caidahl K, Bergdahl K, et al. Direct effects of FGF21 on glucose uptake in human skeletal muscle: Implications for type 2 diabetes and obesity. Diabetes Metab Res Rev [Internet]. 2011 Mar 1 [cited 2025 Nov 30];27(3):286–97. Available from: /doi/pdf/10.1002/dmrr.1177
199. Järvinen TAH, Prince S. Decorin: A growth factor antagonist for tumor growth inhibition. Biomed Res Int [Internet]. 2015 [cited 2025 Nov 30];2015:654765. Available from: https://pmc.ncbi.nlm.nih.gov/articles/PMC4677162/
200. Sofeu Feugaing DD, Götte M, Viola M. More than matrix: The multifaceted role of decorin in cancer. Eur J Cell Biol [Internet]. 2013 Jan 1 [cited 2025 Nov 30];92(1):1–11. Available from: https://www.sciencedirect.com/science/article/abs/pii/S0171933512001264
201. Kanzleiter T, Rath M, Görgens SW, Jensen J, Tangen DS, Kolnes AJ, et al. The myokine decorin is regulated by contraction and involved in muscle hypertrophy. Biochem Biophys Res Commun [Internet]. 2014 Jul 25 [cited 2025 Nov 30];450(2):1089–94. Available from: https://www.sciencedirect.com/science/article/abs/pii/S0006291X14011978
202. Bekki M, Hashida R, Kawaguchi T, Goshima N, Yoshiyama T, Otsuka T, et al. The association between sarcopenia and decorin, an exercise-induced myokine, in patients with liver cirrhosis: A pilot study. JCSM Rapid Commun [Internet]. 2018 Jul 1 [cited 2025 Nov 30];1(2):1–10. Available from: /doi/pdf/10.1002/j.2617-1619.2018.tb00009.x
203. Bozoky B, Savchenko A, Guven H, Ponten F, Klein G, Szekely L. Decreased decorin expression in the tumor microenvironment. Cancer Med [Internet]. 2014 Jun 1 [cited 2025 Nov 30];3(3):485–91. Available from: /doi/pdf/10.1002/cam4.231
204. Hu Y, Sun H, Owens RT, Wu J, Chen YQ, Berquin IM, et al. Decorin suppresses prostate tumor growth through inhibition of epidermal growth factor and androgen receptor pathways. Neoplasia [Internet]. 2009 Oct 1 [cited 2025 Nov 30];11(10):1042–53. Available from: https://www.sciencedirect.com/science/article/pii/S1476558609800079
205. Seidler DG, Goldoni S, Agnew C, Cardi C, Thakur ML, Owens RT, et al. Decorin protein core inhibits in vivo cancer growth and metabolism by hindering epidermal growth factor receptor function and triggering apoptosis via caspase-3 activation. Journal of Biological Chemistry [Internet]. 2006 Sep 8 [cited 2025 Nov 30];281(36):26408–18. Available from: https://pubmed.ncbi.nlm.nih.gov/16835231/
206. Merline R, Moreth K, Beckmann J, Nastase M V., Zeng-Brouwers J, Tralhão JG, et al. Signaling by the matrix proteoglycan decorin controls inflammation and cancer through PDCD4 and microRNA-21. Sci Signal [Internet]. 2011 Nov 15 [cited 2025 Nov 30];4(199):ra75. Available from: https://pmc.ncbi.nlm.nih.gov/articles/PMC5029092/
207. Soria-Valles C, Gutiérrez-Fernández A, Guiu M, Mari B, Fueyo A, Gomis RR, et al. The anti-metastatic activity of collagenase-2 in breast cancer cells is mediated by a signaling pathway involving decorin and miR-21. Oncogene [Internet]. 2013 Jul 15 [cited 2025 Nov 30];33(23):3054–63. Available from: https://www.nature.com/articles/onc2013267
208. Liang S, Xu JF, Cao WJ, Li HP, Hu CP. Human decorin regulates proliferation and migration of human lung cancer A549 cells. Chin Med J (Engl) [Internet]. 2013 [cited 2025 Nov 30];126(24):4736–41. Available from: https://journals.lww.com/cmj/fulltext/2013/12200/human_decorin_regulates_proliferation_and.26.aspx

209. Horváth Z, Reszegi A, Szilák L, Dankó T, Kovalszky I, Baghy K. Tumor-specific inhibitory action of decorin on different hepatoma cell lines. Cell Signal [Internet]. 2019 Oct 1 [cited 2025 Nov 30];62:109354. Available from: https://www.sciencedirect.com/science/article/abs/pii/S0898656819301500
210. Lee JH, Jun HS. Role of myokines in regulating skeletal muscle mass and function. Front Physiol [Internet]. 2019 [cited 2025 Nov 30];10(JAN):42. Available from: https://pmc.ncbi.nlm.nih.gov/articles/PMC6363662/
211. Kazemi F. The correlation of resistance exercise-induced myostatin with insulin resistance and plasma cytokines in healthy young men. Journal of Endocrinological Investigation [Internet]. 2015 Aug 18 [cited 2025 Nov 30];39(4):383–8. Available from: https://link.springer.com/article/10.1007/s40618-015-0373-9
212. McPherron AC, Lawler AM, Lee SJ. Regulation of skeletal muscle mass in mice by a new TGF-beta superfamily member. Nature [Internet]. 1997 May 1 [cited 2025 Nov 30];387(6628):83–90. Available from: https://pubmed.ncbi.nlm.nih.gov/9139826/
213. Loumaye A, De Barsy M, Nachit M, Lause P, Frateur L, Van Maanen A, et al. Role of activin A and myostatin in human cancer cachexia. J Clin Endocrinol Metab [Internet]. 2015 May 1 [cited 2025 Nov 30];100(5):2030–8. Available from: https://dx.doi.org/10.1210/jc.2014-4318
214. Amthor H, Hoogaars WMH. Interference with myostatin/ActRIIB signaling as a therapeutic strategy for duchenne muscular dystrophy. Curr Gene Ther [Internet]. 2012 Jun 13 [cited 2025 Nov 30];12(3):245–59. Available from: https://www.eurekaselect.com/article/43569
215. Lee SJ, McPherron AC. Regulation of myostatin activity and muscle growth. Proc Natl Acad Sci USA [Internet]. 2001 Jul 31 [cited 2025 Nov 30];98(16):9306–11. Available from: https://pubmed.ncbi.nlm.nih.gov/11459935/
216. Matzuk MM, Nalfang L, Vogel H, Sellheyer K, Roop DR, Bradley A. Multiple defects and perinatal death in mice deficient in follistatin. Nature [Internet]. 1995 Mar 23 [cited 2025 Nov 30];374(6520):360–3. Available from: https://pubmed.ncbi.nlm.nih.gov/7885475/
217. Sandri M, Sandri C, Gilbert A, Skurk C, Calabria E, Picard A, et al. Foxo transcription factors induce the atrophy-related ubiquitin ligase atrogin-1 and cause skeletal muscle atrophy. Cell [Internet]. 2004 Apr 30 [cited 2025 Nov 30];117(3):399–412. Available from: https://www.sciencedirect.com/science/article/pii/S0092867404004003
218. Rodriguez J, Vernus B, Chelh I, Cassar-Malek I, Gabillard JC, Hadj Sassi A, et al. Myostatin and the skeletal muscle atrophy and hypertrophy signaling pathways. Cellular and Molecular Life Sciences [Internet]. 2014 Jul 31 [cited 2025 Nov 30];71(22):4361–71. Available from: https://link.springer.com/article/10.1007/s00018-014-1689-x
219. McFarlane C, Plummer E, Thomas M, Hennebry A, Ashby M, Ling N, et al. Myostatin induces cachexia by activating the ubiquitin proteolytic system through an NF-κB-independent, FoxO1-dependent mechanism. J Cell Physiol [Internet]. 2006 Nov 1 [cited 2025 Nov 30];209(2):501–14. Available from: /doi/pdf/10.1002/jcp.20757
220. Han HQ, Zhou X, Mitch WE, Goldberg AL. Myostatin/activin pathway antagonism: Molecular basis and therapeutic potential. Int J Biochem Cell Biol [Internet]. 2013 Oct 1 [cited 2025 Nov 30];45(10):2333–47. Available from: https://www.sciencedirect.com/science/article/abs/pii/S1357272513001635
221. White GE, Greaves DR. Fractalkine: A survivor's guide chemokines as antiapoptotic mediators. Arterioscler Thromb Vasc Biol [Internet]. 2012 Mar

[cited 2025 Nov 30];32(3):589–94. Available from: /doi/pdf/10.1161/ATVBAHA.111.237412?download=true
222. Ferretti E, Pistoia V, Corcione A. Role of Fractalkine/CX3CL1 and its receptor in the pathogenesis of inflammatory and malignant diseases with emphasis on B cell malignancies. Mediators Inflamm [Internet]. 2014 Jan 1 [cited 2025 Nov 30];2014(1):480941. Available from: /doi/pdf/10.1155/2014/480941
223. Hashida R, Matsuse H, Kawaguchi T, Yoshio S, Bekki M, Iwanaga S, et al. Effects of a low-intensity resistance exercise program on serum miR-630, miR-5703, and Fractalkine/CX3CL1 expressions in subjects with no exercise habits: A preliminary study. Hepatology Research [Internet]. 2021 Jul 1 [cited 2025 Nov 30];51(7):823–33. Available from: /doi/pdf/10.1111/hepr.13670
224. Ohta M, Tanaka F, Yamaguchi H, Sadanaga N, Inoue H, Mori M. The high expression of Fractalkine results in a better prognosis for colorectal cancer patients. Int J Oncol [Internet]. 2005 Jan 1 [cited 2025 Nov 30];26(1):41–7. Available from: http://www.spandidos-publications.com/10.3892/ijo.26.1.41/abstract
225. Hyakudomi M, Matsubara T, Hyakudomi R, Yamamoto T, Kinugasa S, Yamanoi A, et al. Increased expression of fractalkine is correlated with a better prognosis and an increased number of both CD8+ T cells and natural killer cells in gastric adenocarcinoma. Ann Surg Oncol [Internet]. 2008 Jun [cited 2025 Nov 30];15(6):1775–82. Available from: https://pubmed.ncbi.nlm.nih.gov/18363071/
226. Park MH, Lee JS, Yoon JH. High expression of CX3CL1 by tumor cells correlates with a good prognosis and increased tumor-infiltrating CD8+ T cells, natural killer cells, and dendritic cells in breast carcinoma. J Surg Oncol [Internet]. 2012 Sep 15 [cited 2025 Nov 30];106(4):386–92. Available from: https://pubmed.ncbi.nlm.nih.gov/22422195/
227. Chaudhri A, Bu X, Wang Y, Gomez M, Torchia JA, Hua P, et al. The CX3CL1-CX3CR1 chemokine axis can contribute to tumor immune evasion and blockade with a novel CX3CR1 monoclonal antibody enhances response to anti-PD-1 immunotherapy. Front Immunol. 2023 Sep 13;14:1237715.
228. Whitham M, Parker BL, Friedrichsen M, Hingst JR, Hjorth M, Hughes WE, et al. Extracellular vesicles provide a means for tissue crosstalk during exercise. Cell Metab [Internet]. 2018 Jan 9 [cited 2025 Nov 30];27(1):237–251.e4. Available from: https://www.cell.com/action/showFullText?pii=S1550413117307118
229. Silvestri M, Grazioli E, Duranti G, Sgrò P, Dimauro I. Exploring the impact of exercise-derived extracellular vesicles in cancer biology. Biology [Internet]. 2024 Sep 6 [cited 2025 Nov 30];13(9):701. Available from: https://www.mdpi.com/2079-7737/13/9/701/htm
230. Llorente A, Brokāne A, Mlynska A, Puurand M, Sagini K, Folkmane S, et al. From sweat to hope: The role of exercise-induced extracellular vesicles in cancer prevention and treatment. J Extracell Vesicles [Internet]. 2024 Aug 1 [cited 2025 Nov 30];13(8):e12500. Available from: /doi/pdf/10.1002/jev2.12500
231. Pinto AC, Tavares P, Neves B, Oliveira PF, Vitorino R, Moreira-Gonçalves D, et al. Exploiting the therapeutic potential of contracting skeletal muscle-released extracellular vesicles in cancer: Current insights and future directions. Journal of Molecular Medicine 2024 102:5 [Internet]. 2024 Mar 7 [cited 2025 Nov 30];102(5):617–28. Available from: https://link.springer.com/article/10.1007/s00109-024-02427-7
232. Ni J, Zhang L. Cancer cachexia: Definition, staging, and emerging treatments. Cancer Manag Res [Internet]. 2020 [cited 2025 Nov 30];12:5597. Available from: https://pmc.ncbi.nlm.nih.gov/articles/PMC7358070/

233. Guney Eskiler G, Bezdegumeli E, Ozman Z, Deveci Ozkan A, Bilir C, Kucukakca BN, et al. IL-6 mediated JAK/STAT3 signaling pathway in cancer patients with cachexia. Bratisl Lek Listy [Internet]. 2019 [cited 2025 Nov 30];66(11): 819–26. Available from: https://pubmed.ncbi.nlm.nih.gov/31747761/
234. Iwase S, Murakami T, Saito Y, Nakagawa K. Steep elevation of blood interleukin-6 (IL-6) associated only with late stages of cachexia in cancer patients. Eur Cytokine Netw [Internet]. 2004 Oct 1 [cited 2025 Nov 30];15(4):312–6. Available from: https://www.jle.com/fr/revues/ecn/e-docs/steep_elevation_of_blood_interleukin_6_il_6_associated_only_with_late_stages_of_cachexia_in_cancer_patients_264242/article.phtml?tab=texte
235. Carson JA, Baltgalvis KA. Interleukin-6 as a key regulator of muscle mass during cachexia. Exerc Sport Sci Rev [Internet]. 2010 Oct [cited 2025 Nov 30];38(4):168. Available from: https://pmc.ncbi.nlm.nih.gov/articles/PMC3065300/
236. O'Leary MF, Wallace GR, Bennett AJ, Tsintzas K, Jones SW. IL-15 promotes human myogenesis and mitigates the detrimental effects of TNFα on myotube development. Scientific Reports [Internet]. 2017 Oct 11 [cited 2025 Nov 30];7(1):12997. Available from: https://www.nature.com/articles/s41598-017-13479-w
237. Carbó N, López-Soriano J, Costelli P, Busquets S, Alvarez B, Baccino FM, et al. Interleukin-15 antagonizes muscle protein waste in tumour-bearing rats. Br J Cancer [Internet]. 2000 [cited 2025 Nov 30];83(4):526–31. Available from: https://pubmed.ncbi.nlm.nih.gov/10945502/
238. Quinn LBS, Anderson BG, Drivdahl RH, Alvarez B, Argilés JM. Overexpression of Interleukin-15 induces skeletal muscle hypertrophy in vitro: Implications for treatment of muscle wasting disorders. Exp Cell Res [Internet]. 2002 Oct 15 [cited 2025 Nov 30];280(1):55–63. Available from: https://www.sciencedirect.com/science/article/abs/pii/S0014482702956247
239. Franz K, Ost M, Otten L, Herpich C, Coleman V, Endres AS, et al. Higher serum levels of fibroblast growth factor 21 in old patients with cachexia. Nutrition [Internet]. 2019 Jul 1 [cited 2025 Nov 30];63–64:81–6. Available from: https://www.sciencedirect.com/science/article/abs/pii/S0899900718306348
240. Jung HW, Park JH, Kim DA, Jang IY, Park SJ, Lee JY, et al. Association between serum FGF21 level and sarcopenia in older adults. Bone [Internet]. 2021 Apr 1 [cited 2025 Nov 30];145:115877. Available from: https://www.sciencedirect.com/science/article/abs/pii/S8756328221000399
241. Oost LJ, Kustermann M, Armani A, Blaauw B, Romanello V. Fibroblast growth factor 21 controls mitophagy and muscle mass. J Cachexia Sarcopenia Muscle [Internet]. 2019 Jun 1 [cited 2025 Nov 30];10(3):630–42. Available from: https://pubmed.ncbi.nlm.nih.gov/30895728/
242. Paajanen J, Ilonen I, Lauri H, Järvinen T, Sutinen E, Ollila H, et al. Elevated circulating activin A levels in patients with malignant pleural mesothelioma are related to cancer cachexia and reduced response to platinum-based chemotherapy. Clin Lung Cancer [Internet]. 2020 May 1 [cited 2025 Nov 30];21(3):e142–50. Available from: https://www.sciencedirect.com/science/article/pii/S1525730419302876
243. Zhou X, Wang JL, Lu J, Song Y, Kwak KS, Jiao Q, et al. Reversal of cancer cachexia and muscle wasting by ActRIIB antagonism leads to prolonged survival. Cell [Internet]. 2010 Aug 20 [cited 2025 Nov 30];142(4):531–43. Available from: https://www.sciencedirect.com/science/article/pii/S0092867410007804
244. Gallot YS, Durieux AC, Castells J, Desgeorges MM, Vernus B, Plantureux L, et al. Myostatin gene inactivation prevents skeletal muscle wasting in cancer.

Cancer Res [Internet]. 2014 Dec 15 [cited 2025 Nov 30];74(24):7344–56. Available from: https://pubmed.ncbi.nlm.nih.gov/25336187/
245. Hatakeyama S, Summermatter S, Jourdain M, Melly S, Minetti GC, Lach-Trifilieff E. ActRII blockade protects mice from cancer cachexia and prolongs survival in the presence of anti-cancer treatments. Skelet Muscle [Internet]. 2016 Jul 26 [cited 2025 Nov 30];6(1). Available from: https://pubmed.ncbi.nlm.nih.gov/27462398/
246. Pin F, Bonewald LF, Bonetto A. Role of myokines and osteokines in cancer cachexia. Exp Biol Med [Internet]. 2021 Oct 1 [cited 2025 Nov 30];246(19):2118. Available from: https://pmc.ncbi.nlm.nih.gov/articles/PMC8524772/
247. Manole E, Ceafalan LC, Popescu BO, Dumitru C, Bastian AE. Myokines as possible therapeutic targets in cancer cachexia. J Immunol Res [Internet]. 2018 [cited 2025 Nov 30];2018. Available from: https://pubmed.ncbi.nlm.nih.gov/30426026/
248. Pérez-Tomás R, Pérez-Guillén I. Lactate in the tumor microenvironment: An essential molecule in cancer progression and treatment. Cancers (Basel) [Internet]. 2020 Nov 1 [cited 2025 Nov 30];12(11):3244. Available from: https://pmc.ncbi.nlm.nih.gov/articles/PMC7693872/
249. Małkowska P. Positive effects of physical activity on insulin signaling. Curr Issues Mol Biol [Internet]. 2024 Jun 1 [cited 2025 Nov 30];46(6):5467. Available from: https://pmc.ncbi.nlm.nih.gov/articles/PMC11202552/
250. Colleluori G, Viola V, Bathina S, Armamento-Villareal R, Qualls C, Giordano A, et al. Effect of aerobic or resistance exercise, or both on insulin secretion, ciliary neurotrophic factor, and insulin-like growth factor-1 in dieting older adults with obesity. Clinical Nutrition [Internet]. 2025 Aug 1 [cited 2025 Nov 30];51:50–62. Available from: https://www.clinicalnutritionjournal.com/action/showFullText?pii=S026156142500144X
251. Liu H, Wang S, Wang J, Guo X, Song Y, Fu K, et al. Energy metabolism in health and diseases. Signal Transduction and Targeted Therapy [Internet]. 2025 Feb 18 [cited 2025 Nov 30];10(1):69. Available from: https://www.nature.com/articles/s41392-025-02141-x
252. Bettariga F, Taaffe DR, Galvão DA, Bishop C, Kim JS, Newton RU. Suppressive effects of exercise-conditioned serum on cancer cells: A narrative review of the influence of exercise mode, volume, and intensity. J Sport Health Sci [Internet]. 2024 Jul 1 [cited 2025 Nov 30];13(4):484–98. Available from: https://www.sciencedirect.com/science/article/pii/S2095254623001175
253. Clemente-Suárez VJ, Martín-Rodríguez A, Redondo-Flórez L, Ruisoto P, Navarro-Jiménez E, Ramos-Campo DJ, et al. Metabolic health, mitochondrial fitness, physical activity, and cancer. Cancers (Basel) [Internet]. 2023 Feb 1 [cited 2025 Nov 22];15(3):814. Available from: https://pmc.ncbi.nlm.nih.gov/articles/PMC9913323/
254. Hofmann P. Cancer and exercise: Warburg hypothesis, tumour metabolism and high-intensity anaerobic exercise. Sports [Internet]. 2018 Mar 1 [cited 2025 Nov 30];6(1):10. Available from: https://pmc.ncbi.nlm.nih.gov/articles/PMC5969185/
255. Arena SK, Doherty DJ, Bellford A, Hayman G. Effects of aerobic exercise on oxidative stress in patients diagnosed with cancer: A narrative review. Cureus [Internet]. 2019 Aug 13 [cited 2025 Nov 30];11(8):e5382. Available from: https://pmc.ncbi.nlm.nih.gov/articles/PMC6786842/
256. Chen X, Zhang J, Gao F, Liu N, Du H, Li J, et al. Exercise therapy: An effective approach to mitigate the risk of cancer metastasis. World J Surg Oncol [Internet]. 2025 Dec 1 [cited 2025 Nov 30];23(1):192. Available from: https://pmc.ncbi.nlm.nih.gov/articles/PMC12082867/

257. Spaulding HR, Yan Z. AMPK and the adaptation to exercise. Annu Rev Physiol [Internet]. 2022 [cited 2025 Nov 30];84:209. Available from: https://pmc.ncbi.nlm.nih.gov/articles/PMC8919726/
258. Matuszewska K, Pereira M, Petrik D, Lawler J, Petrik J. Normalizing tumor vasculature to reduce hypoxia, enhance perfusion, and optimize therapy uptake. Cancers (Basel) [Internet]. 2021 Sep 1 [cited 2025 Nov 30];13(17):4444. Available from: https://pmc.ncbi.nlm.nih.gov/articles/PMC8431369/
259. Xiong X, Wen YA, Fairchild R, Zaytseva YY, Weiss HL, Evers BM, et al. Upregulation of CPT1A is essential for the tumor-promoting effect of adipocytes in colon cancer. Cell Death Dis [Internet]. 2020 Sep 1 [cited 2025 Nov 30];11(9):736. Available from: https://pmc.ncbi.nlm.nih.gov/articles/PMC7484798/
260. Huang K, Han Y, Chen Y, Shen H, Zeng S, Cai C. Tumor metabolic regulators: Key drivers of metabolic reprogramming and the promising targets in cancer therapy. Molecular Cancer [Internet]. 2025 Jan 9 [cited 2025 Nov 30];24(1):7. Available from: https://link.springer.com/article/10.1186/s12943-024-02205-6
261. Stolarczyk E. Adipose tissue inflammation in obesity: A metabolic or immune response? Curr Opin Pharmacol [Internet]. 2017 Dec 1 [cited 2025 Nov 30];37:35–40. Available from: https://pubmed.ncbi.nlm.nih.gov/28843953/
262. Liu S, Wu D, Fan Z, Yang J, Li Y, Meng Y, et al. FABP4 in obesity-associated carcinogenesis: Novel insights into mechanisms and therapeutic implications. Front Mol Biosci [Internet]. 2022 Aug 19 [cited 2025 Nov 30];9:973955. Available from: https://pmc.ncbi.nlm.nih.gov/articles/PMC9438896/
263. Calabrese C, Miserocchi G, De Vita A, Spadazzi C, Cocchi C, Vanni S, et al. Lipids and adipocytes involvement in tumor progression with a focus on obesity and diet. Obesity Reviews [Internet]. 2024 Dec 1 [cited 2025 Nov 30];25(12):e13833. Available from: /doi/pdf/10.1111/obr.13833
264. Velez-Bonet E, Gumpper-Fedus K, Cruz-Monserrate Z. Exploring the role of hyperinsulinemia in obesity-associated tumor development. Cancer Res [Internet]. 2024 Feb 1 [cited 2025 Nov 30];84(3):351. Available from: https://pmc.ncbi.nlm.nih.gov/articles/PMC11472301/
265. Larson EA, Dalamaga M, Magkos F. The role of exercise in obesity-related cancers: Current evidence and biological mechanisms. Semin Cancer Biol [Internet]. 2023 Jun 1 [cited 2025 Nov 30];91:16–26. Available from: https://pubmed.ncbi.nlm.nih.gov/36871634/
266. Feng Y, Feng X, Wan R, Luo Z, Qu L, Wang Q. Impact of exercise on cancer: mechanistic perspectives and new insights. Front Immunol [Internet]. 2024 [cited 2025 Nov 22];15. Available from: https://pubmed.ncbi.nlm.nih.gov/39346906/
267. Perego S, Sansoni V, Ziemann E, Lombardi G. Another weapon against cancer and metastasis: Physical-activity-dependent effects on adiposity and adipokines. Int J Mol Sci [Internet]. 2021 Feb 2 [cited 2025 Nov 30];22(4):1–31. Available from: https://pubmed.ncbi.nlm.nih.gov/33670492/
268. Mika A, Macaluso F, Barone R, Di Felice V, Sledzinski T. Effect of exercise on fatty acid metabolism and adipokine secretion in adipose tissue. Front Physiol [Internet]. 2019 [cited 2025 Nov 30];10(JAN):26. Available from: https://pmc.ncbi.nlm.nih.gov/articles/PMC6360148/
269. Sun X, Sui W, Mu Z, Xie S, Deng J, Li S, et al. Mirabegron displays anticancer effects by globally browning adipose tissues. Nat Commun [Internet]. 2023 Dec 1 [cited 2025 Nov 30];14(1):7610. Available from: https://pmc.ncbi.nlm.nih.gov/articles/PMC10665320/

270. Idorn M, thor Straten P. Exercise and cancer: From "healthy" to "therapeutic"? Cancer Immunol Immunother [Internet]. 2017 May 1 [cited 2025 Nov 16];66(5):667–71. Available from: https://pubmed.ncbi.nlm.nih.gov/28324125/
271. Gao K, Su Z, Meng J, Yao Y, Li LG, Su Y, et al. Effect of exercise training on some anti-inflammatory adipokines, high sensitivity C-reactive protein, and clinical outcomes in sedentary adults with metabolic syndrome. Biol Res Nurs [Internet]. 2024 Jan 1 [cited 2025 Nov 30];26(1):125–38. Available from: https://journals.sagepub.com/doi/10.1177/10998004231195541
272. Sirico F, Bianco A, D'Alicandro G, Castaldo C, Montagnani S, Spera R, et al. Effects of physical exercise on adiponectin, leptin, and inflammatory markers in childhood obesity: Systematic review and meta-analysis. Childhood Obesity [Internet]. 2018 May 1 [cited 2025 Nov 30];14(4):207. Available from: https://pmc.ncbi.nlm.nih.gov/articles/PMC5994661/
273. Bird SR, Hawley JA. Update on the effects of physical activity on insulin sensitivity in humans. BMJ Open Sport—Exercise Medicine [Internet]. 2017 Mar 1 [cited 2025 Nov 30];2(1):e000143. Available from: https://pmc.ncbi.nlm.nih.gov/articles/PMC5569266/
274. Lin Y, Fan R, Hao Z, Li J, Yang X, Zhang Y, et al. The association between physical activity and insulin level under different levels of lipid indices and serum uric acid. Front Physiol [Internet]. 2022 Feb 2 [cited 2025 Nov 30];13:809669. Available from: http://www.cdc.gov/nchs/nhanes/.
275. Winder WW, Hardie DG. Inactivation of acetyl-CoA carboxylase and activation of AMP-activated protein kinase in muscle during exercise. Am J Physiol [Internet]. 1996 [cited 2025 Nov 30];270(2 Pt 1). Available from: https://pubmed.ncbi.nlm.nih.gov/8779952/
276. Ruderman NB, Carling D, Prentki M, Cacicedo JM. AMPK, insulin resistance, and the metabolic syndrome. J Clin Invest [Internet]. 2013 Jul 1 [cited 2025 Nov 30];123(7):2764. Available from: https://pmc.ncbi.nlm.nih.gov/articles/PMC3696539/
277. Iyengar NM, Zhou XK, Mendieta H, Giri DD, El-Hely O, Winston L, et al. Effects of adiposity and exercise on breast tissue and systemic metabo-inflammatory factors in women at high risk or diagnosed with breast cancer. Cancer Prev Res (Phila) [Internet]. 2021 May 1 [cited 2025 Nov 30];14(5):541. Available from: https://pmc.ncbi.nlm.nih.gov/articles/PMC8102399/
278. Min SY, Learnard H, Kant S, Gealikman O, Rojas-Rodriguez R, Desouza T, et al. Exercise rescues gene pathways involved in vascular expansion and promotes functional angiogenesis in subcutaneous white adipose tissue. International Journal of Molecular Sciences [Internet]. 2019 Apr 25 [cited 2025 Nov 30];20(8):2046. Available from: https://www.mdpi.com/1422-0067/20/8/2046/htm
279. Garritson JD, Boudina S. The effects of exercise on white and brown adipose tissue cellularity, metabolic activity and remodeling. Front Physiol [Internet]. 2021 Nov 2 [cited 2025 Nov 30];12:772894. Available from: www.frontiersin.org
280. Trayhurn P. Hypoxia and adipose tissue function and dysfunction in obesity. https://doi.org/101152/physrev000172012 [Internet]. 2013 Jan 1 [cited 2025 Nov 30];93(1):1–21. Available from: /doi/pdf/10.1152/physrev.00017.2012?download=true
281. Pellegata NS, Berriel Diaz M, Rohm M, Herzig S. Obesity and cancer—extracellular matrix, angiogenesis, and adrenergic signaling as unusual suspects linking the two diseases. Cancer and Metastasis Reviews [Internet].

2022 Sep 8 [cited 2025 Nov 30];41(3):517–47. Available from: https://link.springer.com/article/10.1007/s10555-022-10058-y
282. Liu ZL, Chen HH, Zheng LL, Sun LP, Shi L. Angiogenic signaling pathways and anti-angiogenic therapy for cancer. Signal Transduction and Targeted Therapy [Internet]. 2023 May 11 [cited 2025 Nov 30];8(1):198. Available from: https://www.nature.com/articles/s41392-023-01460-1
283. Schadler KL, Thomas NJ, Galie PA, Bhang DH, Roby KC, Addai P, et al. Tumor vessel normalization after aerobic exercise enhances chemotherapeutic efficacy. Oncotarget [Internet]. 2016 [cited 2025 Nov 14];7(40):65429. Available from: https://pmc.ncbi.nlm.nih.gov/articles/PMC5323166/
284. Philippou A, Tryfonos A, Theos A, Nezos A, Halapas A, Maridaki M, et al. Expression of tissue remodelling, inflammation- and angiogenesis-related factors after eccentric exercise in humans. Molecular Biology Reports [Internet]. 2021 May 24 [cited 2025 Nov 30];48(5):4047–54. Available from: https://link.springer.com/article/10.1007/s11033-021-06412-y
285. Yao Z, Lafage-Proust MH, Plouët J, Bloomfield S, Alexandre C, Vico L. Increase of both angiogenesis and bone mass in response to exercise depends on VEGF. Journal of Bone and Mineral Research [Internet]. 2004 Sep 1 [cited 2025 Nov 30];19(9):1471–80. Available from: https://dx.doi.org/10.1359/JBMR.040517
286. Katoh K. Effects of mechanical stress on endothelial cells in situ and in vitro. Int J Mol Sci [Internet]. 2023 Nov 1 [cited 2025 Nov 30];24(22):16518. Available from: https://pmc.ncbi.nlm.nih.gov/articles/PMC10671803/
287. Liu Z ji, Semenza GL, Zhang H feng. Hypoxia-inducible factor 1 and breast cancer metastasis. J Zhejiang Univ Sci B [Internet]. 2015 [cited 2025 Nov 30];16(1):32–43. Available from: https://pubmed.ncbi.nlm.nih.gov/25559953/
288. van Doorslaer de Ten Ryen S, Deldicque L. The regulation of the metastatic cascade by physical activity: A narrative review. Cancers (Basel) [Internet]. 2020 Jan 8 [cited 2025 Jan 10];12(1):153. Available from: http://www.ncbi.nlm.nih.gov/pubmed/31936342
289. Jones LW, Viglianti BL, Tashjian JA, Kothadia SM, Keir ST, Freedland SJ, et al. Effect of aerobic exercise on tumor physiology in an animal model of human breast cancer. J Appl Physiol [Internet]. 2010 Feb [cited 2019 May 31];108(2):343–8. Available from: http://www.ncbi.nlm.nih.gov/pubmed/19959769
290. Jones LW, Antonelli J, Masko EM, Broadwater G, Lascola CD, Fels D, et al. Exercise modulation of the host-tumor interaction in an orthotopic model of murine prostate cancer. https://doi.org/101152/japplphysiol015752011 [Internet]. 2012 Jul 15 [cited 2025 Nov 30];113(2):263–72. Available from: /doi/pdf/10.1152/japplphysiol.01575.2011?download=true
291. Rehman J, Li J, Parvathaneni L, Karlsson G, Panchal VR, Temm CJ, et al. Exercise acutely increases circulating endothelial progenitor cells and monocyte-/macrophage-derived angiogenic cells. J Am Coll Cardiol [Internet]. 2004 Jun 16 [cited 2025 Nov 30];43(12):2314–8. Available from: https://www.sciencedirect.com/science/article/pii/S073510970400676X
292. Kaplan RN, Riba RD, Zacharoulis S, Bramley AH, Vincent L, Costa C, et al. VEGFR1-positive haematopoietic bone marrow progenitors initiate the pre-metastatic niche. Nature [Internet]. 2005 Dec 8 [cited 2025 Nov 30];438(7069):820–7. Available from: https://pubmed.ncbi.nlm.nih.gov/16341007/
293. Faustino-Rocha AI, Silva A, Gabriel J, Gil da Costa RM, Moutinho M, Oliveira PA, et al. Long-term exercise training as a modulator of mammary

cancer vascularization. Biomedicine & Pharmacotherapy [Internet]. 2016 Jul 1 [cited 2025 Nov 30];81:273–80. Available from: https://www.sciencedirect.com/science/article/abs/pii/S0753332216301639?via%3Dihub
294. Tsai MS, Kuo ML, Chang CC, Wu YT. The effects of exercise training on levels of vascular endothelial growth factor in tumor-bearing mice. Cancer Biomark [Internet]. 2013 [cited 2025 Nov 22];13(5):307–13. Available from: https://pubmed.ncbi.nlm.nih.gov/24440969/
295. Yan L, Demars LC. Effects of non-motorized voluntary running on experimental and spontaneous metastasis in mice.
296. Fukumura D, Kashiwagi S, Jain RK. The role of nitric oxide in tumour progression. Nature Reviews Cancer [Internet]. 2006 Jul [cited 2025 Nov 30];6(7):521–34. Available from: https://www.nature.com/articles/nrc1910
297. Smeda M, Przyborowski K, Proniewski B, Zakrzewska A, Kaczor D, Stojak M, et al. Breast cancer pulmonary metastasis is increased in mice undertaking spontaneous physical training in the running wheel; a call for revising beneficial effects of exercise on cancer progression. Am J Cancer Res [Internet]. 2017 [cited 2025 Nov 30];7(9):1926. Available from: https://pmc.ncbi.nlm.nih.gov/articles/PMC5622226/
298. Yan H, Jiang A, Huang Y, Zhang J, Yang W, Zhang W, et al. Exercise sensitizes PD-1/PD-L1 immunotherapy as a hypoxia modulator in the tumor microenvironment of melanoma. Front Immunol. 2023 Oct 9;14:1265914.
299. Henke E, Nandigama R, Ergün S. Extracellular matrix in the tumor microenvironment and its impact on cancer therapy. Front Mol Biosci [Internet]. 2020 Jan 31 [cited 2025 Nov 30];6:160. Available from: https://pmc.ncbi.nlm.nih.gov/articles/PMC7025524/
300. Luo Z, Mei J, Wang X, Wang R, He Z, Geffen Y, et al. Voluntary exercise sensitizes cancer immunotherapy via the collagen inhibition-orchestrated inflammatory tumor immune microenvironment. Cell Rep [Internet]. 2024 Sep 24 [cited 2025 Nov 30];43(9). Available from: https://pubmed.ncbi.nlm.nih.gov/39217611/
301. Walker C, Mojares E, Del Río Hernández A. Role of extracellular matrix in development and cancer progression. Int J Mol Sci [Internet]. 2018 [cited 2025 Nov 30];19(10):3028. Available from: https://pmc.ncbi.nlm.nih.gov/articles/PMC6213383/
302. Xiao Q, Ge G. Lysyl oxidase, extracellular matrix remodeling and cancer metastasis. Cancer Microenvironment [Internet]. 2012 Dec 1 [cited 2025 Nov 30];5(3):261. Available from: https://pmc.ncbi.nlm.nih.gov/articles/PMC3460045/
303. Khalil AA, Smits D, Haughton PD, Koorman T, Jansen KA, Verhagen MP, et al. A YAP-centered mechanotransduction loop drives collective breast cancer cell invasion. Nature Communications [Internet]. 2024 Jun 7 [cited 2025 Nov 30];15(1):4866. Available from: https://www.nature.com/articles/s41467-024-49230-z
304. Karagiannis GS, Poutahidis T, Erdman SE, Kirsch R, Riddell RH, Diamandis EP. Cancer-associated fibroblasts drive the progression of metastasis through both paracrine and mechanical pressure on cancer tissue. Mol Cancer Res [Internet]. 2012 Nov [cited 2025 Nov 30];10(11):1403. Available from: https://pmc.ncbi.nlm.nih.gov/articles/PMC4399759/
305. Luo Z, Wan R, Liu S, Feng X, Peng Z, Wang Q, et al. Mechanisms of exercise in the treatment of lung cancer—a mini-review. Front Immunol [Internet]. 2023 [cited 2025 Nov 30];14:1244764. Available from: https://pmc.ncbi.nlm.nih.gov/articles/PMC10483406/

306. Ren Y, Zhang J, Wang M, Bi J, Wang T, Qiu M, et al. Identification of irisin as a therapeutic agent that inhibits oxidative stress and fibrosis in a murine model of chronic pancreatitis. Biomedicine & Pharmacotherapy [Internet]. 2020 Jun 1 [cited 2025 Nov 30];126:110101. Available from: https://www.sciencedirect.com/science/article/pii/S0753332220302936
307. Trombetta-eSilva J, Bradshaw AD. The function of SPARC as a mediator of fibrosis. Open Rheumatol J [Internet]. 2012 Jun 22 [cited 2025 Nov 30];6(1):146. Available from: https://pmc.ncbi.nlm.nih.gov/articles/PMC3395844/
308. Tan M, Song B, Zhao X, Du J. The role and mechanism of compressive stress in tumor. Front Oncol [Internet]. 2024 [cited 2025 Nov 30];14:1459313. Available from: https://pmc.ncbi.nlm.nih.gov/articles/PMC11439826/
309. Verma VK, Singh V, Singh MP, Singh SM. Effect of physical exercise on tumor growth regulating factors of tumor microenvironment: Implications in exercise-dependent tumor growth retardation. Immunopharmacol Immunotoxicol [Internet]. 2009 [cited 2025 Nov 30];31(2):274–82. Available from: https://pubmed.ncbi.nlm.nih.gov/19235538/
310. Hoon JL, Tan MH, Koh CG. The regulation of cellular responses to mechanical cues by Rho GTPases. Cells [Internet]. 2016 Apr 6 [cited 2025 Nov 30];5(2):17. Available from: https://pmc.ncbi.nlm.nih.gov/articles/PMC4931666/
311. Park JH, Shin JE, Park HW. The role of Hippo pathway in cancer stem cell biology. Mol Cells [Internet]. 2018 [cited 2025 Nov 30];41(2):83. Available from: https://pmc.ncbi.nlm.nih.gov/articles/PMC5824027/
312. Zhang M, Zhang B. Extracellular matrix stiffness: mechanisms in tumor progression and therapeutic potential in cancer. Exp Hematol Oncol [Internet]. 2025 Dec 1 [cited 2025 Nov 30];14(1):54. Available from: https://pmc.ncbi.nlm.nih.gov/articles/PMC11984264/
313. Panciera T, Azzolin L, Cordenonsi M, Piccolo S. Mechanobiology of YAP and TAZ in physiology and disease. Nat Rev Mol Cell Biol [Internet]. 2017 Dec 1 [cited 2025 Nov 30];18(12):758–70. Available from: https://pubmed.ncbi.nlm.nih.gov/28951564/
314. Mohri Z, Rio Hernandez A Del, Krams R. The emerging role of YAP/TAZ in mechanotransduction. J Thorac Dis [Internet]. 2017 May 1 [cited 2025 Nov 30];9(5):E507. Available from: https://pmc.ncbi.nlm.nih.gov/articles/PMC5465147/
315. Li H, Raghunathan VK, Stamer WD, Ganapathy PS, Herberg S. Extracellular matrix stiffness and TGFβ2 regulate YAP/TAZ activity in human trabecular meshwork cells. Front Cell Dev Biol [Internet]. 2022 Mar 1 [cited 2025 Nov 30];10:844342. Available from: https://pmc.ncbi.nlm.nih.gov/articles/PMC8923257/
316. Scott KE, Fraley SI, Rangamani P. A spatial model of YAP/TAZ signaling reveals how stiffness, dimensionality, and shape contribute to emergent outcomes. Proceedings of the National Academy of Sciences [Internet]. 2021 May 18 [cited 2025 Nov 30];118(20):e2021571118. Available from: /doi/pdf/10.1073/pnas.2021571118?download=true
317. Cheng H, Zhong W, Wang L, Zhang Q, Ma X, Wang Y, et al. Effects of shear stress on vascular endothelial functions in atherosclerosis and potential therapeutic approaches. Biomedicine & Pharmacotherapy [Internet]. 2023 Feb 1 [cited 2025 Nov 30];158:114198. Available from: https://www.sciencedirect.com/science/article/pii/S0753332222015876
318. Song Y, Jia H, Hua Y, Wu C, Li S, Li K, et al. The molecular mechanism of aerobic exercise improving vascular remodeling in hypertension. Front Physiol [Internet]. 2022 Feb 28 [cited 2025 Nov 30];13:792292. Available from: https://pmc.ncbi.nlm.nih.gov/articles/PMC8919036/

319. Kourek C, Briasoulis A, Zouganeli V, Karatzanos E, Nanas S, Dimopoulos S. Exercise training effects on circulating endothelial and progenitor cells in heart failure. Journal of Cardiovascular Development and Disease [Internet]. 2022 Jul 10 [cited 2025 Nov 30];9(7):222. Available from: https://www.mdpi.com/2308-3425/9/7/222/htm
320. Bellafiore M, Battaglia G, Bianco A, Farina F, Palma A, Paoli A. The involvement of MMP-2 and MMP-9 in heart exercise-related angiogenesis. J Transl Med [Internet]. 2013 Nov 7 [cited 2025 Nov 30];11(1). Available from: https://pubmed.ncbi.nlm.nih.gov/24195673/
321. Rullman E, Norrbom J, Strömberg A, Wågsäter D, Rundqvist H, Haas T, et al. Endurance exercise activates matrix metalloproteinases in human skeletal muscle. https://doi.org/101152/japplphysiol908722008 [Internet]. 2009 Mar [cited 2025 Nov 30];106(3):804–12. Available from: /doi/pdf/10.1152/japplphysiol.90872.2008?download=true
322. Jaoude J, Koh Y. Matrix metalloproteinases in exercise and obesity. Vasc Health Risk Manag [Internet]. 2016 Jul 14 [cited 2025 Nov 30];12:287–95. Available from: https://www.dovepress.com/matrix-metalloproteinases-in-exercise-and-obesity-peer-reviewed-fulltext-article-VHRM
323. Zhang CX, Huang RYJ, Sheng G, Thiery JP. Epithelial-mesenchymal transition. Cell [Internet]. 2025 Oct 2 [cited 2025 Nov 30];188(20):5436–86. Available from: https://www.sciencedirect.com/science/article/abs/pii/S0092867425010256
324. Massagué J, Sheppard D. TGF-β signaling in health and disease. Cell [Internet]. 2023 Sep 14 [cited 2025 Nov 30];186(19):4007. Available from: https://pmc.ncbi.nlm.nih.gov/articles/PMC10772989/
325. Oh A, Pardo M, Rodriguez A, Yu C, Nguyen L, Liang O, et al. NF-κB signaling in neoplastic transition from epithelial to mesenchymal phenotype. Cell Commun Signal [Internet]. 2023 Dec 1 [cited 2025 Nov 30];21(1):291. Available from: https://pmc.ncbi.nlm.nih.gov/articles/PMC10585759/
326. Zhang QB, Zhang BH, Zhang KZ, Meng XT, Jia QA, Bu Y, et al. Moderate swimming suppressed the growth and metastasis of the transplanted liver cancer in mice model: with reference to nervous system. Oncogene [Internet]. 2016 [cited 2025 Nov 30];35:4122–31. Available from: www.nature.com/onc
327. Wang JS, Chang CY, Chow SE, Chen YW, Yang CM, J-s W, et al. Exercise modulates platelet-nasopharyngeal carcinoma cell aggregation and subsequent tissue factor and matrix metalloproteinase activities. https://doi.org/101152/japplphysiol001652007 [Internet]. 2007 Sep [cited 2025 Nov 30];103(3):763–70. Available from: /doi/pdf/10.1152/japplphysiol.00165.2007?download=true
328. Wolff G, Davidson SJ, Wrobel JK, Toborek M. Exercise maintains blood–brain barrier integrity during early stages of brain metastasis formation. Biochem Biophys Res Commun [Internet]. 2015 Aug 7 [cited 2025 Nov 30];463(4):811–7. Available from: https://www.sciencedirect.com/science/article/pii/S0006291X1530070X?via%3Dihub
329. Westley RL, May FEB. A twenty-first century cancer epidemic caused by obesity: The involvement of insulin, diabetes, and insulin-like growth factors. Int J Endocrinol [Internet]. 2013 [cited 2025 Nov 30];2013:632461. Available from: https://pmc.ncbi.nlm.nih.gov/articles/PMC3747439/
330. Zhou Y, Jia N, Ding M, Yuan K. Effects of exercise on inflammatory factors and IGF system in breast cancer survivors: A meta-analysis. BMC Womens Health [Internet]. 2022 Dec 1 [cited 2025 Nov 16];22(1):507. Available from: https://bmcwomenshealth.biomedcentral.com/articles/10.1186/s12905-022-02058-5

331. Brown JC, Winters-Stone K, Lee A, Schmitz KH. Cancer, physical activity, and exercise. Compr Physiol [Internet]. 2012 Oct [cited 2024 Jul 25];2(4): 2775–809. Available from: http://www.ncbi.nlm.nih.gov/pubmed/23720265
332. Bulun SE, Chen D, Moy I, Brooks DC, Zhao H. Aromatase, breast cancer and obesity: A complex interaction. Trends Endocrinol Metab [Internet]. 2011 Feb [cited 2025 Nov 30];23(2):83. Available from: https://pmc.ncbi.nlm.nih.gov/articles/PMC3428377/
333. Bhardwaj P, Brown KA. Obese adipose tissue as a driver of breast cancer growth and development: Update and emerging evidence. Front Oncol [Internet]. 2021 Mar 30 [cited 2025 Nov 30];11:638918. Available from: https://pmc.ncbi.nlm.nih.gov/articles/PMC8042134/
334. Thomas GA, Cartmel B, Harrigan M, Fiellin M, Capozza S, Zhou Y, et al. The effect of exercise on body composition and bone mineral density in breast cancer survivors taking aromatase inhibitors. Obesity (Silver Spring) [Internet]. 2016 Feb 1 [cited 2025 Nov 30];25(2):346. Available from: https://pmc.ncbi.nlm.nih.gov/articles/PMC5450163/
335. Garcia-Unciti M, Palacios Samper N, Méndez-Sandoval S, Idoate F, Ibáñez-Santos J. Effect of combining impact-aerobic and strength exercise, and dietary habits on body composition in breast cancer survivors treated with aromatase inhibitors. Int J Environ Res Public Health [Internet]. 2023 Mar 1 [cited 2025 Nov 30];20(6):4872. Available from: https://www.mdpi.com/1660-4601/20/6/4872/htm
336. Wiggs AG, Chandler JK, Aktas A, Sumner SJ, Stewart DA. The effects of diet and exercise on endogenous estrogens and subsequent breast cancer risk in postmenopausal women. Front Endocrinol (Lausanne) [Internet]. 2021 Sep 20 [cited 2025 Nov 30];12:732255. Available from: www.frontiersin.org
337. Cespedes P, Martínez-Arnau FM, Torregrosa MD, Cauli O, Buigues C. Impact of a physical exercise and health education program on metabolic syndrome and quality of life in postmenopausal breast cancer women undergoing adjuvant treatment with aromatase inhibitors. Medicina (Lithuania) [Internet]. 2024 Nov 1 [cited 2025 Nov 30];60(11):1893. Available from: https://www.mdpi.com/1648-9144/60/11/1893/htm
338. Zhang F, Luo Z, Xue Q, Guo X, Zhang W, Xiong Y, et al. The impact of exercise on prostate-specific antigen and testosterone in prostate cancer: a systematic review and meta-analysis. Aging Male [Internet]. 2025 [cited 2025 Nov 30];28(1). Available from: https://pubmed.ncbi.nlm.nih.gov/40842180/
339. Taaffe DR, Buffart LM, Newton RU, Spry N, Denham J, Joseph D, et al. Time on androgen deprivation therapy and adaptations to exercise: Secondary analysis from a 12-month randomized controlled trial in men with prostate cancer. BJU Int [Internet]. 2018 Feb 1 [cited 2025 Nov 30];121(2):194–202. Available from: https://pubmed.ncbi.nlm.nih.gov/28872752/
340. De Nys L, Anderson K, Ofosu EF, Ryde GC, Connelly J, Whittaker AC. The effects of physical activity on cortisol and sleep: A systematic review and meta-analysis. Psychoneuroendocrinology [Internet]. 2022 Sep 1 [cited 2025 Nov 30];143. Available from: https://pubmed.ncbi.nlm.nih.gov/35777076/
341. Moyers SA, Hagger MS. Physical activity and cortisol regulation: A meta-analysis ☆. Biol Psychol [Internet]. 2023 [cited 2025 Nov 30];179:108548. Available from: https://doi.org/10.1016/j.biopsycho.2023.108548
342. Langley RR, Fidler IJ. The seed and soil hypothesis revisited—the role of tumor-stroma interactions in metastasis to different organs. International Journal of Cancer Journal International du Cancer [Internet]. 2011 Jun 1 [cited 2025 Nov 30];128(11):2527. Available from: https://pmc.ncbi.nlm.nih.gov/articles/PMC3075088/

343. Yang L, Morielli AR, Heer E, Kirkham AA, Cheung WY, Usmani N, et al. Effects of exercise on cancer treatment efficacy: A systematic review of preclinical and clinical studies. Cancer Res [Internet]. 2021 Oct 1 [cited 2025 Nov 30];81(19):4889. Available from: https://pmc.ncbi.nlm.nih.gov/articles/PMC9397632/
344. Hapuarachi B, Danson S, Wadsley J, Muthana M. Exercise to transform tumours from cold to hot and improve immunotherapy responsiveness. Front Immunol. 2023 Dec 12;14:1335256.
345. An KY, Min J, Lee DH, Kang DW, Courneya KS, Jeon JY. Exercise across the phases of cancer survivorship: A narrative review. Yonsei Med J [Internet]. 2024 Jun 1 [cited 2025 Nov 23];65(6):315–23. Available from: https://doi.org/10.3349/ymj.2023.0638
346. Courneya KS, Booth CM. Exercise as cancer treatment: A clinical oncology framework for exercise oncology research. Front Oncol. 2022 Sep 2;12:957135.

PART II

FITT for life

5

TYPES OF EXERCISE AND THEIR BENEFITS

5.1 Introduction

The previous chapters explored the cellular, molecular and systemic mechanisms through which physical activity and exercise influence cancer biology. These examined how exercise modulates signalling pathways, immune surveillance, metabolic regulation and the TME, laying the scientific foundation for why exercise matters in cancer prevention and survivorship.

In this chapter, the focus shifts from "why" to "how," specifically exploring the different types of exercise: What they are, how they work and what benefits they confer across the cancer continuum. This approach is anchored in the FITT framework (Frequency, Intensity, Time, Type): A cornerstone of exercise prescription. While frequency, intensity and duration are critical variables, the emphasis in this chapter is on type: Aerobic, resistance and endurance exercise, as well as everyday physical activity and mind-body therapies. Each type elicits distinct physiological responses and offers unique benefits for people living with and beyond cancer.

5.2 Aerobic exercise

Aerobic exercise, often referred to as cardiorespiratory endurance or cardiovascular exercise, encompasses any physical activity that increases heart rate and breathing while using large muscle groups repetitively and uses oxygen to produce energy for the muscles (1). Common modalities include walking, jogging, cycling, swimming and dancing. Aerobic exercise is

DOI: 10.4324/9781003511519-7

characterised by sustained movement over time and primarily relies on oxidative phosphorylation for energy production, making it a potent stimulus for cardiovascular and pulmonary adaptations.

5.2.1 *Physiological mechanisms of aerobic exercise*

At the physiological level, aerobic exercise stimulates a cascade of acute and chronic responses. Acutely, it increases cardiac output, ventilatory rate and oxygen delivery to working muscles. Chronically, regular aerobic training induces adaptations such as increased mitochondrial density, capillarisation, cardiac stroke volume and improved VO_2max (2). These systemic changes translate into enhanced oxygen utilisation, improved metabolic flexibility and reduced systemic inflammation, all of which are pertinent in the context of cancer prevention and survivorship. Aerobic exercise also engages numerous molecular pathways implicated in tumour biology. Notably, it improves insulin sensitivity and modulates levels of insulin-like growth factor-1 (IGF-1), both of which are associated with cancer risk and progression (3). Moreover, aerobic activity influences adipokine secretion, reducing leptin and increasing adiponectin levels, thereby mitigating pro-inflammatory signalling within the TME (4).

5.2.2 *Cardiovascular benefits in cancer prevention and survivorship*

Cardiovascular health is a key determinant of cancer outcomes, with cardiorespiratory fitness serving as a prognostic indicator in several cancer types (5). Aerobic exercise contributes to reduced blood pressure, improved lipid profiles and lower resting heart rate, thereby enhancing overall cardiovascular resilience (6). In cancer survivors, these adaptations are particularly beneficial given the cardiotoxic potential of many chemotherapeutic agents (e.g., anthracyclines, HER2-targeted therapies). Aerobic exercise has been shown to mitigate treatment-induced declines in cardiac function and reduce the risk of CVD, which is a leading cause of non-cancer mortality among cancer survivors (7–9). Importantly, large-scale epidemiological studies support a dose-response relationship between leisure-time physical activity and reduced cancer incidence. Moore et al. (2016) demonstrated that higher levels of aerobic activity were associated with reduced risk across 13 cancer types, including breast, colon and endometrial cancers (10). These benefits are attributed not only to direct physiological effects but also to exercise-mediated reductions in obesity and systemic inflammation.

5.2.3 Evidence for aerobic exercise during and after treatment

A growing body of RCTs, systematic reviews and meta-analyses has confirmed the feasibility, safety and efficacy of aerobic exercise during active treatment (11–19). Meta-analyses indicate that moderate-intensity aerobic training undertaken two to five times per week for 20–60 minutes per session is associated with improvements in physical functioning, treatment tolerance and psychological wellbeing (14). During chemotherapy or radiotherapy, aerobic exercise can alleviate common side effects such as fatigue, nausea and sleep disturbance (20). Post-treatment aerobic training supports recovery of cardiorespiratory fitness, muscle function and QoL (21). In breast cancer patients, for instance, supervised aerobic programmes have demonstrated significant improvements in VO_2max, walking distance and fatigue scores (16,22,23). Similarly, in colorectal cancer survivors, structured walking interventions have been linked to improved physical function and reduced recurrence risk (24,25).

5.2.4 Impact on fatigue, aerobic capacity and immune modulation

Cancer-related fatigue is one of the most prevalent and debilitating side effects of cancer and its treatment (26). Aerobic exercise is among the most effective non-pharmacological interventions for cancer-related fatigue (27). By improving mitochondrial efficiency, reducing systemic inflammation and enhancing sleep quality, aerobic activity can reduce fatigue severity and improve daily functioning (28). In terms of aerobic capacity, studies consistently show that cancer patients experience marked declines in VO_2max—up to 25–30% during treatment (29,30). Aerobic training can restore or even exceed pre-treatment levels, thereby improving functional independence and resilience against future health challenges. Aerobic exercise has also been shown to increase the mobilisation and cytotoxic potential of NK cells, enhance T cell function and shift cytokine profiles towards an anti-inflammatory state (31,32). These changes may play a role in tumour surveillance and immunoediting, potentially contributing to delayed progression or recurrence.

Emerging evidence also suggests that exercise intensity may play a key role in shaping immune responses. For example, Coletta et al. (2021) found that high-intensity interval training (HIIT) produced the strongest correlations between changes in NK cell function and alterations in circulating myokines in breast cancer patients (33). These results point towards a synergistic effect of vigorous-intensity exercise in enhancing both immune surveillance and tumour-suppressive signalling. While still preliminary, such findings provide mechanistic support for the observed associations between vigorous exercise and reduced breast cancer risk (34). The differential effects of exercise intensity will be discussed in more detail in Chapter 6. Collectively, these findings affirm that aerobic exercise represents an essential element of supportive care in oncology. Its multi-systemic effects offer a multitude of benefits, not only for cardiovascular health but also for metabolic regulation and immune competence.

5.3 Resistance exercise

Resistance exercise, also known as strength or resistance training, involves the use of external resistance to induce muscular contraction, with the goal of improving muscular strength, power and endurance (35,36). Modalities include free weights, resistance machines, resistance bands and bodyweight exercises such as squats and push-ups. Unlike aerobic training, which primarily targets cardiorespiratory systems, resistance exercise specifically stimulates neuromuscular and musculoskeletal adaptations. While both aerobic and resistance training contribute to overall health and cancer survivorship, their physiological mechanisms and primary adaptations differ: Aerobic training enhances cardiovascular and metabolic function; resistance training builds and preserves skeletal muscle mass, improves bone density and supports neuromuscular coordination (37). Crucially, resistance training plays a unique role in counteracting the muscle-wasting effects of cancer and its treatments. Resistance exercise induces mechanical tension and metabolic stress in muscle fibres, leading to muscle protein synthesis and hypertrophy (38). It activates anabolic signalling pathways such as mTOR and IGF-1, promoting muscle regeneration and satellite cell activity (39). These responses are vital in preserving lean body mass, which has been positively associated with survival in multiple cancer types (40).

5.3.1 Role in preserving and improving muscle mass, strength and bone density

Cancer treatments such as chemotherapy, radiotherapy and ADT can lead to significant losses in muscle and bone mass (41). Sarcopenia, a loss of skeletal muscle mass and strength, is associated with poorer treatment outcomes, increased toxicity and reduced survival (42). Resistance training has been shown to mitigate these effects by promoting muscle hypertrophy, improving functional strength and preserving bone mineral density. In prostate cancer patients undergoing ADT, resistance exercise improves lean body mass, reduces fat mass and enhances physical function (43). Similarly, postmenopausal women with breast cancer benefit from increased bone strength and reduced osteopenia risk with regular resistance training (44).

5.3.2 Prevention and management of cancer cachexia and sarcopenia

Cachexia is a complex metabolic syndrome characterised by systemic inflammation, involuntary weight loss and muscle wasting (see Chapter 4, Section 4.5). It is particularly prevalent in advanced cancers, notably gastrointestinal and lung malignancies (45). Resistance training offers a non-pharmacological strategy to counteract cachexia by stimulating muscle protein synthesis and reducing catabolic signalling (46). Although exercise alone may not reverse cachexia in its most severe stages, it can attenuate its progression and improve functional capacity and QoL (47). Early integration of resistance training into cancer care, particularly in patients at high risk of muscle loss, may help maintain physical independence and reduce hospitalisation. Moreover, resistance training combined with nutritional support, particularly adequate protein intake, has demonstrated synergistic effects on muscle mass preservation and recovery (48,49).

5.3.3 Specific benefits for lymphoedema, particularly in breast cancer patients

Lymphoedema is a chronic and often debilitating condition characterised by the accumulation of lymphatic fluid, most commonly following lymph node dissection or radiotherapy in breast cancer treatment (50). Historically, resistance training was contraindicated in individuals with or at risk of lymphoedema due to fears of exacerbating the condition (51). However, multiple RCTs now support the safety and efficacy of supervised, progressive resistance training in women with breast cancer-related lymphoedema (52–54). Studies show improvements in arm strength and body image, with no increase in lymphoedema incidence or severity. Indeed, resistance training may improve lymphatic flow and reduce limb swelling through the pump-like action of rhythmic skeletal muscle contractions during exercise (55,56). Importantly, programmes should be individualised and monitored, beginning with low-load exercise and gradually progressing to higher intensities. Emphasis on proper technique and symptom awareness is essential. The benefits of resistance exercise for muscle health, bone strength and lymphatic function are summarised in Figure 5.1.

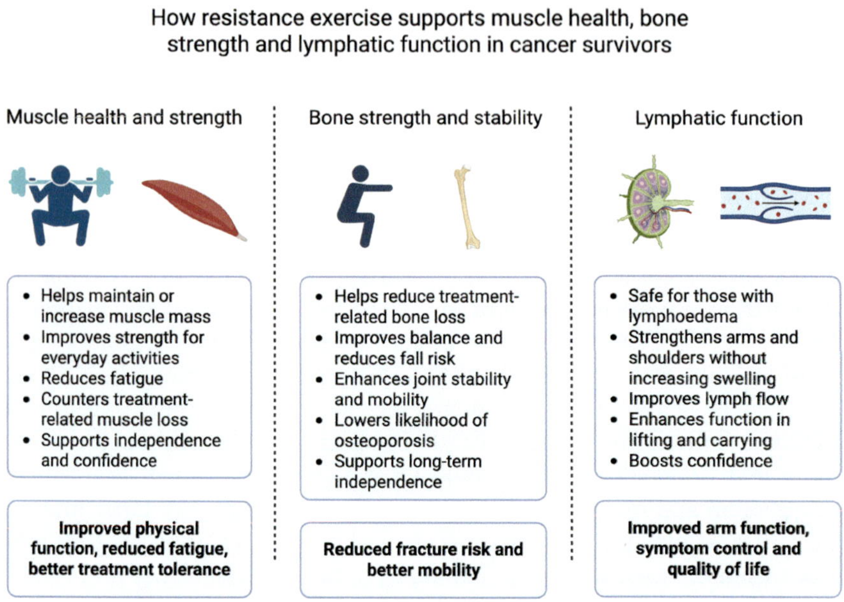

FIGURE 5.1 Benefits of resistance exercise for muscle health, bone strength and lymphatic function in cancer survivors. Regular, progressive resistance training helps maintain or increase muscle mass, improves strength for everyday activities and reduces treatment-related fatigue. It also supports bone density, balance and joint stability, lowering fracture risk and enhancing long-term mobility. For individuals with or at risk of lymphoedema, resistance exercise is safe when appropriately prescribed, improving arm strength, lymphatic flow and confidence in using the affected limb. Together, these effects contribute to better physical functioning, symptom control and quality of life during and after cancer treatment. Created in Biorender.com.

5.4 Endurance training and mental toughness

Endurance training refers to sustained, prolonged bouts of physical activity designed to improve the body's ability to perform at moderate-to-high intensity over extended periods of time (57,58). While it overlaps substantially with aerobic training, endurance exercise places particular emphasis on metabolic efficiency, psychological resilience and the capacity to withstand physical and mental stressors. Both aerobic and endurance exercise rely heavily on oxidative metabolism and share adaptations such as improved VO_2max, increased mitochondrial density and enhanced cardiovascular efficiency. However, endurance training is distinguished by its duration and cumulative physical demands. Examples include distance running, long-distance cycling, open-water swimming and triathlon training. In the oncology setting, endurance exercise may not always be feasible during treatment, yet its principles of sustained activity, progressive overload and resilience can be adapted to patient capacity. For survivors and those in remission, endurance training offers a pathway to rebuild stamina, restore confidence and cultivate a sense of mastery over the body (59).

5.4.1 Psychological resilience, mood regulation and cognitive benefits

Beyond its physiological effects, endurance training exerts numerous psychological and neurocognitive benefits. Sustained physical effect challenges the individual not only physically but also mentally, cultivating perseverance, discipline and emotional resilience (60,61). Cancer survivors often report that endurance training helps them regain a sense of control and identity, counteracting the loss of autonomy experienced during treatment (62,63)

BOX-OUT 5.1 CASE STUDY: RECLAIMING A SENSE OF SELF AFTER BREAST CANCER

Context and intervention

Five female breast cancer survivors (aged 41–57) completed a 12-week structured resistance training protocol (EFICAN—Exercise and Cancer), involving both individual and small group sessions. The intervention was supervised by exercise instructors, whose perspectives were also gathered during the study in a group interview.

Reported outcomes and personal impact

1. Empowerment and recovery: Participants described the exercise programme as a catalyst for reclaiming control over their bodies and their lives after cancer treatment, helping them mitigate physical side effects and rebuild strength.
2. Social bonds and psychological support: Group-based exercise fostered social connections and peer support, reducing feelings of isolation, promoting shared resilience and improving emotional wellbeing.
3. Body perception and self-acceptance: Many participants reported altered body image after treatment. Exercise helped them renegotiate their

relationship with their bodies, restoring a sense of normalcy, agency and confidence.

4. Broader QoL benefits: Improved physical strength and function translated into better ability to perform everyday tasks, greater autonomy and a sense of regained normality in daily living. Instructors corroborated these changes, noting visible improvements in emotional expression, confidence and social engagement among participants.

Source: Resilience and renewal: The personal impact of physical activity in breast cancer survivors (64).

Mechanistically, endurance activity stimulates the release of endorphins and endocannabinoids, contributing to improved mood and reduced perception of pain (65). It also enhances neuroplasticity via brain-derived neurotrophic factor (BDNF), supporting cognitive flexibility, memory and learning (66). These effects are particularly relevant in addressing cancer-related cognitive impairment—commonly referred to as "chemo brain." Furthermore, endurance training may act as a behavioural intervention to mitigate symptoms of anxiety and depression. Evidence suggests that structured endurance programmes reduce treatment-related distress, improve self-efficacy and foster a greater sense of purpose (67).

5.4.2 Evidence linking long-term exercise engagement to better coping and reduced recurrence anxiety

Observational and interventional studies indicate that individuals who engage in sustained endurance activity after cancer diagnosis demonstrate better psychological coping strategies, lower perceived stress and reduced fear of recurrence (68). For instance, a systematic review and meta-analysis of women with breast cancer demonstrated that those who participated in structured exercise interventions saw a moderate improvement in QoL (as measured by the Functional Assessment of Cancer Therapy-Breast Cancer, FACT-B) and showed small improvements in mental wellbeing domains, such as anxiety, body image, depression and emotional function compared to control counterparts (69). Similarly, a meta-analysis of people with non-advanced colorectal cancer also showed positive effects of physical activity interventions on health-related QoL, but no significant effect on disease-related mental health (70). In another network meta-analysis, mind-body exercise, resistance training and aerobic exercise all significantly decreased levels of anxiety and depression among individuals with cancer (71). Longitudinal studies further support the notion that consistent engagement in combined aerobic and endurance exercise is associated with improved overall survival and reduced secondary recurrence risk in cancer survivors (72,73). These benefits may arise from a combination of biological effects, such as reduced systemic inflammation and improved immune surveillance, and psychological benefits, including strengthened social networks often built through group-based endurance activities. From a practical standpoint, endurance training should be tailored to the individual's treatment history, comorbidities and preferences. For some, this may mean structured long walks; for others, participation in community endurance events may provide both physical and psychosocial reinforcement.

5.5 Mind-body therapies

Mind-body therapies (MBTs) occupy a unique space within supportive cancer care, bridging physical movement with psychological and emotional regulation. Typically encompassing practices such as yoga, Tai chi, Qigong, mindfulness meditation, breathing exercises and relaxation-based modalities, MBTs aim to modulate the interaction between cognitive-emotional processes and physiological function. Although often less physically demanding than traditional exercise modes, MBTs can improve both physical and psychosocial outcomes, making them particularly accessible for individuals experiencing fatigue, pain or functional limitations during and after treatment.

5.5.1 Physiological and psychological rationale

MBTs operate through integrated pathways involving autonomic regulation, neuroendocrine function and inflammation. Techniques that emphasise slow, controlled movement and paced breathing, such as yoga, Tai chi and Qigong, activate parasympathetic activity, reduce sympathetic arousal and improve heart rate variability (74). Complementary psychological mechanisms, including enhanced mindfulness, emotional regulation and reduced rumination, may further reduce anxiety and stress, while promoting cognitive clarity and self-efficacy (75,76). In the context of cancer survivorship, these mechanisms are particularly relevant given the high prevalence of anxiety, sleep disturbance, emotional distress and treatment-related fatigue. MBTs may provide gentler alternatives for individuals who struggle to meet aerobic or resistance exercise guidelines, while still offering clinically meaningful benefits.

5.5.2 Evidence from systematic reviews and meta-analyses

A growing body of high-quality reviews supports the role of MBTs in managing symptoms and improving QoL among people living with and beyond cancer. A systematic review by Danon et al. (2022) found that MBTs, including yoga, meditation, Tai chi and mind-body therapies, may reduce cancer-related pain, anxiety and insomnia, although the evidence base remains heterogeneous and many studies were limited by methodological quality (77). Nonetheless, the review concluded that these therapies show promise as adjunctive interventions for symptom relief. Stronger evidence comes from interventions delivered alongside active treatment. A meta-analysis of MBTs used as adjuvants to chemotherapy across breast, lung and colorectal cancers demonstrated that participation in MBTs led to significant improvements in fatigue, particularly among colorectal cancer patients, and improved health-related QoL (78). These findings position MBTs as effective, low risk complements to chemotherapeutic treatment. Among cancer survivors, a focused systematic review and meta-analysis of 22 trials showed that MBTs were associated with improvements in cancer-related fatigue, QoL and emotional wellbeing (79).

However, findings are not uniformly positive. In a study comparing MBTs alone or in combination with physical training on depressive symptoms, while combined interventions showed moderate benefits, MBTs alone did not show any significant improvements in depression scores when isolated from general exercise. This nuance highlights that MBTs may be most effective when embedded within broader lifestyle interventions (80). Similarly, a meta-analysis investigating MBTs for cancer-related dyspnoea (shortness of breath) reported no significant improvements in breathlessness, QoL or anxiety (81). Such findings underline that MBTs may be better suited to addressing psychosocial symptoms (e.g., anxiety, stress, sleep disturbance) rather than specific physiological impairments such as dyspnoea. However, overall the evidence suggests that MBTs are feasible, safe and moderately effective for improving emotional wellbeing, sleep quality, fatigue and overall QoL in cancer populations. Their gentleness and adaptability make them particularly suitable for individuals with limited physical capacity, those early in recovery or those who prefer a holistic or low-impact approach to movement (Figure 5.2).

5.5.3 Clinical and practical applications

MBTs may be integrated into cancer care as a low-intensity movement for people unable to engage in aerobic or resistance training, or as complementary stress-management tools, to help address anxiety, fear of recurrence and emotional distress. They may be integrated as part of group-based supportive care, providing opportunities for social connection, shared experience and community, or as a method to support sleep hygiene, especially for survivors experiencing insomnia or dysregulated circadian rhythms. Importantly, MBTs offer survivors a sense of agency and calm, often counteracting feelings of loss of control that accompany diagnosis and

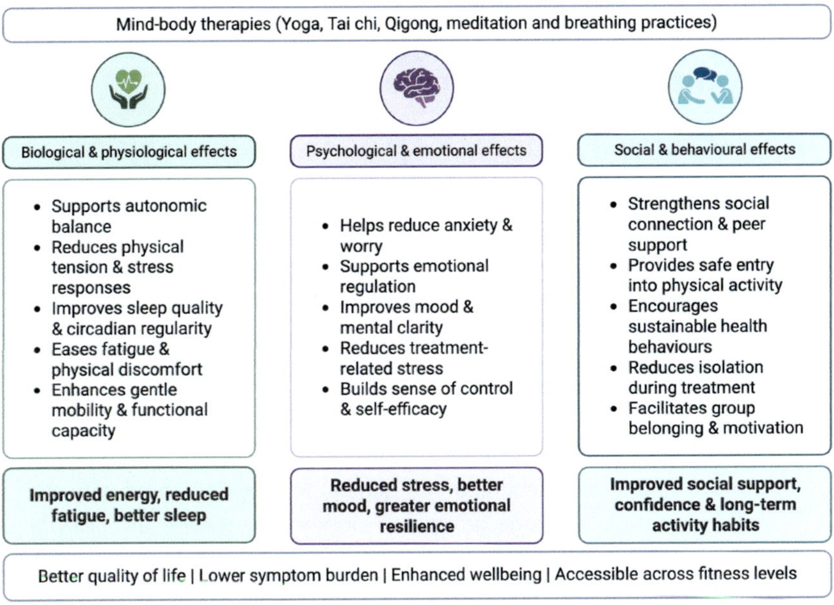

FIGURE 5.2 Biopsychosocial mechanisms of mind-body therapies. Mind-body therapies exert their benefits through interconnected biological, psychological and social pathways. Together, these biopsychosocial effects contribute to improved energy, reduced anxiety and enhanced quality of life for people living with and beyond cancer. Created in Biorender.com.

treatment. Qualitative research frequently highlights themes of grounding, empowerment and emotional restoration, outcomes that are deeply valued by participants, even if not easily quantified.

PATIENT VIGNETTE 5.1 "Claire"—finding light in movement

Claire, a 56-year-old breast cancer survivor, remembers how overwhelming chemotherapy felt. "There were days when keeping down water was the only goal," she recalled. Exercise was the last thing on her mind. But once her nausea subsided, gentle stretching and slow walks gave her a sense of accomplishment. "I felt like I was reclaiming something," she wrote. Claire had not received any advice about exercise from her consultant and only discovered yoga classes through a Macmillan Facebook group. Looking back, she says movement gave her "a bit of myself back."

BOX-OUT 5.2 CASE STUDY: YOGA DURING RADIOTHERAPY FOR BREAST CANCER

Context and intervention

Women with stage 0-III breast cancer undergoing 6 weeks of adjuvant radiotherapy were randomly assigned to a yoga intervention (three times per week), a stretching control, or a wait-list control group. Outcomes measured included QoL, fatigue, physical functioning, general health perception, sleep quality, depressive symptoms, and salivary cortisol (as a stress biomarker), collected at baseline, the end of treatment and 1, 3 and 6 months after radiotherapy ended.

Reported outcomes

1. Improved physical functioning and general health: Compared with the wait-list control, the yoga group had significantly greater increases in physical component scores at 1- and 3-months post-radiotherapy.
2. Reduced fatigue during treatment: Both the yoga and the stretching groups reported reductions in fatigue by the end of radiotherapy compared with baseline, suggesting that even gentle physical postures or movements plus breathing/relaxation might mitigate treatment burden.
3. Sustained benefit over time: Gains in physical functioning persisted at least 3 months post-treatment in the yoga group.
4. Physiological stress regulation: The yoga group demonstrated a steeper (healthier) diurnal cortisol slope at the end of treatment and 1 month after radiotherapy compared with controls, potentially indicating improved stress regulation.

Source: Randomized controlled trial of yoga in women with breast cancer undergoing radiotherapy (82).

PATIENT VIGNETTE 5.2 "Fatima"—cultural and personal motivation

Fatima, 45, struggled with isolation and fatigue during chemotherapy for ovarian cancer. She noted the lack of culturally sensitive resources and exercise spaces. Eventually, she adapted yoga into her daily prayer routine, finding both physical and spiritual relief. "Some days I didn't want to move, but I found peace in slow stretching during prayer. It became part of my healing." She advocates for more inclusive and adaptable exercise options for diverse communities.

5.6 Broader benefits of physical activity and exercise

While the preceding sections have highlighted the physiological and performance-specific effects of distinct exercise modalities, it is equally important to acknowledge the broader benefits of physical activity and exercise across the cancer continuum. These extend beyond measurable biomedical endpoints, encompassing domains of QoL, sleep hygiene, physical functioning, social connection and psychological wellbeing.

5.6.1 Quality of life, sleep hygiene and physical function

QoL is a multidimensional construct incorporating physical, psychological and social aspects of health (83). Cancer and its treatments often diminish QoL through fatigue, pain, impaired mobility and emotional distress (84). Exercise has consistently emerged as one of the most effective non-pharmacological interventions to improve overall QoL in survivors (85–88). Exercise also improves physical functioning, enabling patients to maintain independence in activities of daily living such as walking, dressing and household tasks. These gains translate into greater self-efficacy and confidence, which in turn reinforce continued engagement in physical activity and exercise (89).

Sleep disturbance, including insomnia and fragmented sleep, are highly prevalent in cancer populations (90), often exacerbated by steroid therapy, anxiety or menopausal symptoms, where relevant. Aerobic and resistance training interventions have been shown to improve sleep quality assessed by the Pittsburgh Sleep Quality Index (PSQI), wake after sleep onset and circadian rhythm as assessed by salivary cortisol levels, but no significant effect on sleep efficiency, sleep onset latency, total sleep time and circadian rhythm as assessed by accelerometry values (91). These effects may be mediated by reduced inflammation, lowered anxiety and reduced hyperarousal. Even light-to-moderate exercise, such as walking or yoga, has demonstrated positive effects on sleep hygiene, with walking being more effective than yoga (92).

5.6.2 Managing chemotherapy-induced peripheral neuropathy

Chemotherapy-induced peripheral neuropathy (CIPN) is a common and often debilitating side effect of neurotoxic agents such as taxanes, platinum compounds, vinca alkaloids and bortezomib. Damage to sensory neurons within the dorsal root ganglia produces symptoms including pain, numbness, tingling, burning sensations and altered thermal sensitivity, with motor impairment occurring less frequently (93). CIPN affects approximately 30–40% of patients receiving neurotoxic chemotherapy and is strongly associated with reduced QoL, functional limitation, and in severe cases, dose reduction or discontinuation of treatment, thereby potentially compromising cancer outcomes (93,94). Moreover, evidence suggests substantially higher healthcare costs in individuals with CIPN.

Emerging evidence suggests that structured exercise offers a promising non-pharmacological intervention for CIPN (95). Aerobic, resistance and balance-focused training appear to improve both sensory and motor symptoms through mechanisms including enhanced proprioception, neuromuscular control and improved peripheral circulation (96). In a multicentre randomised controlled trial, a combined programme of aerobic and resistance training during chemotherapy reduced key sensory symptoms, including numbness/tingling and thermal sensitivity, when compared with standard care (97). Complementary evidence demonstrates that endurance and balance training improved functional performance and alleviated neuropathic symptoms in survivors with established CIPN (98). Improvements in gait speed, dynamic balance and patient-reported outcomes suggest that neuromuscular retraining may play a key role in restoring sensorimotor function. These findings reinforce the value of incorporating lower-intensity, proprioceptive-rich modalities such as balance boards, targeted foot-ankle exercises and controlled stepping drills to support neural adaptation.

5.6.3 Social connection and psychological wellbeing

Cancer is often described as an isolating experience, with many patients reporting feelings of loneliness, anxiety and depression (99). Physical activity, especially when undertaken in group or community settings, provides opportunities for social interaction, peer support and collective motivation. Group-based exercise classes, walking groups and survivorship programmes create safe spaces where individuals can share experiences while engaging in health-promoting behaviours. Psychologically, exercise enhances mood and emotional wellbeing through neurochemical pathways involving endorphins, serotonin and dopamine. It also promotes resilience by reinforcing an individual's sense of agency and control over their body. Studies demonstrate reductions in depressive symptoms, improved anxiety management and enhanced coping strategies in survivors who regularly participate in physical activity and exercise (100). Moreover, exercise can serve as a meaningful ritual of recovery, symbolising progression beyond illness. For many survivors, the act of exercising is a tangible reminder of regained strength and vitality.

BOX-OUT 5.3 CASE STUDY: "FINDING MY OWN MOTIVATION" THROUGH EXERCISE DURING TREATMENT

Profile

Participants were adults with breast, colorectal or prostate cancer undergoing oncological treatment who completed a 6-month supervised exercise programme combining resistance and endurance training plus behaviour-change support.

Experience and process

Many participants described a motivational journey, catalysed by the early experience of "health gains and mastery." After even a single session, sometimes when they felt unwell, completing planned exercise could bring a sense of alertness, improved mood and improved comfort when warmed up. One participant recalled, "Even just one exercise . . . made it all feel better."

Over time, participants reported increased energy, improved sleep quality and better functional capacity, adding to feelings of competence and increasing their intrinsic motivation to continue. Some characterised the exercise as a way of asserting agency in the face of cancer: "I sort of wanted to . . . spit in the face of cancer . . . so that I was really motivated."

Support and behaviour change elements

The study highlighted that certain behaviour change techniques were critical to maintaining adherence during treatment. Scheduled, supervised sessions provided structure and accountability, self-monitoring (e.g., training logs, heart rate feedback) which allowed participants to track progress and visualise gains was a positive motivator, and peer and coach support (group-based training) fostered a sense of affinity, since participants valued exercising with others going through similar challenges. This reduced isolation and enhanced relatedness.

Outcomes and participants' reflections

Enhanced psychological resilience, improved mood, better sense of control and improved coping with treatment stress were all reported outcomes. Participants also reported greater physical comfort in respect of reduced tingling/numbness after chemotherapy infusions, and better tolerance of side effects, as well as preserved functional capacity. Many participants reported that the initial improvements and supportive environment motivated them to maintain activity beyond the study period, even when symptoms fluctuated or during difficult phases.

Source: "Finding my own motivation"—A mixed methods study of exercise and behaviour change support during oncological treatment (101).

5.7 Making every step count: Everyday physical activity

While structured exercise programmes confer well-documented benefits, everyday physical activity plays an equally important role in cancer prevention and survivorship. This concept emphasises the value of small incremental movements accumulated throughout the day, often referred to as non-exercise activity thermogenesis (NEAT) (102).

5.7.1 The importance of non-exercise activity thermogenesis

NEAT encompasses the energy expended in activities other than deliberate exercise, such as walking between rooms, fidgeting, carrying shopping bags or gardening. These activities may seem trivial, but cumulatively they contribute substantially to daily energy expenditure. In the context of cancer survivorship, higher levels of NEAT have been associated with reduced risk of weight gain, metabolic dysfunction and secondary comorbidities (103). Given that sedentary behaviour independently increases cancer incidence and mortality risk (104,105), encouraging NEAT is essential. Breaking up prolonged sitting periods with short bouts of movement—even standing or light stretching—can significantly impact cardiometabolic health and reduce systemic inflammation (106).

5.7.2 Role of walking, gardening, housework and active commuting

Everyday tasks that require moderate effort provide accessible means of incorporating physical activity without requiring specialised equipment or gym access. Walking remains the most studied and universally applicable activity. For cancer survivors, regular walking improves functional mobility, reduces fatigue and supports weight management (100). Gardening, housework and active commuting (e.g., cycling or walking to work) also provide opportunities for moderate-intensity activity (107). These behaviours can be integrated into daily routines relatively easily, making them highly sustainable and culturally adaptable forms of physical activity. For individuals experiencing treatment-related side effects such as neuropathy or fatigue, these activities can be tailored to include shorter bouts, lighter tasks or use of assistive devices, to ensure safety while still reaping benefits.

PATIENT VIGNETTE 5.3 "Linda"—the power of routine

Linda, 62, found that exercise helped not just physically but mentally. "It made me feel normal again." After finishing radiotherapy for uterine cancer, she started going to a local walking group. Her mood lifted, her energy slowly returned, and she felt supported. "It wasn't just about movement—it was connection," she shared. For Linda, group activity was key: "We weren't just walking. We were talking. Laughing. Coping."

5.7.3 Accessible strategies for reducing sedentary time

Strategies to increase NEAT and reduce sedentary behaviour should prioritise accessibility and individual preference. Examples include:

- Standing or walking meetings
- Taking stairs instead of lifts
- Using a step counter or wearable device to monitor daily activity
- Setting reminders to stand or move every 30–60 minutes
- Incorporating short walks into lunch breaks or television viewing

These small behavioural changes, while seemingly modest, accumulate into meaningful physiological benefits over weeks and months. A novel approach to motivating individuals to be physically active is the notion of "Snacktivity™," which promotes shorter (2–5 minutes) and more frequent bouts, or "snacks" of physical activity throughout the day, something participants have found easy to implement, raising awareness of opportunities to incorporate more activity throughout their day (108).

5.7.4 Benefits for those unable or unwilling to do structured exercise

Not all cancer survivors are able or willing to participate in structured exercise programmes due to treatment side effects, comorbidities, financial constraints or psychological barriers (109). For these individuals, everyday physical activity offers a non-threatening entry point to movement.

Even light activities such as stretching, slow walking or tidying the house can support mobility, circulation and mood. With evidence suggesting that "every step counts," incremental increases in step count are associated with reduced all-cause and cancer-specific mortality, even in those who do not meet formal exercise guidelines. A recent study demonstrated that the more steps you take each day, the lower your chances of developing up to 13 different types of cancer; however, these risk-reducing benefits levelled off at 9,000 steps and beyond (110). This reinforces the message that perfection is not required; consistent small actions provide real health benefits. In public health and clinical messaging, emphasising the importance of everyday movement helps dismantle the misconception that only vigorous or structured exercise is worthwhile. Instead, an inclusive framework highlights that all movement matters in the fight against cancer.

5.8 Practical strategies and behaviour change

While the evidence for exercise and physical activity in cancer prevention and survivorship is compelling, translating knowledge into sustained behaviour remains a challenge. Practical strategies, grounded in behavioural science, are essential to help patients, survivors and clinicians move from intention to action.

5.8.1 Actionable tips to integrate movement into daily life

Simple, achievable strategies can empower individuals to incorporate more movement into daily routines:

- Breaking up long periods of sitting with 2–3 minutes of walking or stretching.
- Pairing activity with routine tasks, for example, light stretching while watching television or walking during phone calls.
- Using environmental cues, such as leaving walking shoes by the door to encourage spontaneous activity.
- Starting small: Even 5–10 minutes of movement daily can build confidence and momentum.

These strategies emphasis that exercise does not have to be time-consuming or intimidating. Instead, consistent, incremental steps lay the foundation for sustainable change.

5.8.2 Role of goal setting, self-monitoring and support networks

Behavioural frameworks such as Social Cognitive Theory and the Transtheoretical Model highlight the importance of self-efficacy, feedback and social reinforcement (111,112). The transtheoretical model proposes six stages of health behaviour change: Precontemplation, contemplation, preparation, action, maintenance and termination. Using stage-matched interventions and proactive recruitment procedures have been found to elicit dramatic improvements in recruitment, retention and progress (112). This emphasises the importance of goal setting with patients in an individualised, targeted approach using step counts, minutes of activity or participation in specific classes, which can provide structure and motivation. Self-monitoring, through activity diaries or wearable devices, allows individuals to track progress and adjust behaviours. Evidence shows that patients who monitor their activity are more likely to sustain long-term engagement (113–116). Support networks, including family, peers or structured programmes, offer accountability, encouragement and shared experiences. Group-based interventions or buddy systems can increase adherence while reducing feelings of isolation (117,120).

5.8.3 How technology can support behaviour change

Technology offers novel opportunities to support exercise oncology. Mobile apps, wearable devices or sensors and online platforms enable real-time tracking, personalised feedback and remote coaching. These digital tools can also facilitate virtual communities, connecting survivors across geographic boundaries. For example, step counters and motivational apps have been associated with increased physical activity adherence in cancer populations (118,121). Ultimately, behaviour change strategies must be personalised, context-sensitive and empowering (119). Integrating practical tips, behavioural techniques and digital tools maximises the likelihood that survivors will embrace physical activity as a sustainable part of their lifestyle.

5.9 Summary and key takeaways

Exercise is not a single intervention but a spectrum of behaviours, each with unique physiological, psychological and social benefits. Aerobic exercise enhances cardiovascular health, reduces cancer recurrence risk and strengthens immune function. Resistance training preserves muscle mass, supports bone density and can safely benefit those at risk of lymphoedema. Endurance training cultivates stamina, psychological resilience and coping strategies that are vital for long-term survivorship. Beyond structured exercise, everyday physical activity such as walking, gardening and active commuting, contributes meaningfully to reducing sedentary time and improving overall health. Across all types, the benefits extend beyond physical function. Exercise alleviates common treatment side effects, enhances sleep, improves mood and fosters social connection. Importantly, there is no single "correct" mode or dose. The principle that *all movement matters* underscores the importance of tailoring activity to individual needs, preferences and capacities. Behaviour change strategies, including goal setting, self-monitoring and the use of digital tools, can help embed activity into everyday life, making it sustainable beyond clinical settings.

This chapter illustrates that exercise is both a medical adjunct and a lifestyle medicine. Its diverse modalities offer patients, survivors and clinicians a toolkit to address not only cancer biology but also quality of life, recovery and long-term wellbeing. The following chapter will build on this foundation by exploring how varying exercise intensities influence cancer cells and the TME, with particular focus on immune regulation.

Chapter 5 Test your understanding question bank

1. What are the primary physiological adaptations induced by aerobic exercise?
2. How does aerobic exercise contribute to reduced cancer recurrence risk?
3. Why is aerobic exercise considered beneficial during chemotherapy?
4. What distinguishes resistance training from aerobic training in cancer care?
5. How can resistance training mitigate the effects of sarcopenia and cachexia?
6. What are the key considerations for prescribing resistance training to patients with lymphoedema?
7. How does endurance training differ from general aerobic exercise in its goals and adaptations?
8. What neurobiological mechanisms underpin the mental health benefits of endurance training?
9. In what ways might endurance training reduce cancer recurrence anxiety?
10. How does exercise improve sleep hygiene in cancer survivors?
11. Which forms of exercise are particularly helpful for managing chemotherapy-induced neuropathy?
12. In what ways can group-based exercise enhance psychological wellbeing and social connection?
13. What is NEAT, and why is it important in cancer prevention and survivorship?
14. Which everyday activities can contribute meaningfully to physical activity levels?
15. How can NEAT benefit individuals unable to engage in structured exercise programmes?

16. Why is self-monitoring an effective strategy for sustaining exercise behaviour?
17. What role do support networks play in exercise adherence for cancer survivors?
18. How can digital tools complement traditional behaviour change strategies?

References

1. And physical activity president's council on physical fitness and sports. Research Digest Definitions [Internet]. [cited 2025 Nov 18]. Available from: http://mmfitness.gov/activity/activity2/digest_mar2000/digest_mar2000.html
2. Caspersen C, Powell K, Gregory C. Physical activity, exercise, and physical fitness: Definitions and distinctions for health-related research. Public Health Rep [Internet]. 1985 [cited 2025 Nov 18];100(2):126. Available from: https://pmc.ncbi.nlm.nih.gov/articles/PMC1424733/
3. Dasso NA. How is exercise different from physical activity? A concept analysis. Nurs Forum (Auckl) [Internet]. 2019 Jan 1 [cited 2025 Nov 18];54(1):45–52. Available from: https://pubmed.ncbi.nlm.nih.gov/30332516/
4. ACSM's guidelines for exercise testing and prescription—ACSM [Internet]. [cited 2025 Nov 18]. Available from: https://acsm.org/education-resources/books/guidelines-exercise-testing-prescription/
5. Normal versus chronic adaptations to aerobic exercise—StatPearls—NCBI bookshelf [Internet]. [cited 2025 Nov 18]. Available from: https://www.ncbi.nlm.nih.gov/books/NBK572066/
6. Hojman P, Gehl J, Christensen JF, Pedersen BK. Molecular mechanisms linking exercise to cancer prevention and treatment. Cell Metab. 2018 Jan 9;27(1):10–21.
7. Golbidi S, Laher I. Exercise induced adipokine changes and the metabolic syndrome. J Diabetes Res [Internet]. 2014 Jan 1 [cited 2025 Nov 18];2014(1):726861. Available from: https://onlinelibrary.wiley.com/doi/full/10.1155/2014/726861
8. Kunutsor SK, Kaminsky LA, Lehoczki A, Laukkanen JA. Unraveling the link between cardiorespiratory fitness and cancer: A state-of-the-art review. Geroscience [Internet]. 2024 Dec 1 [cited 2025 Nov 18];46(6):5559. Available from: https://pmc.ncbi.nlm.nih.gov/articles/PMC11493895/
9. Nystoriak MA, Bhatnagar A. Cardiovascular effects and benefits of exercise. Front Cardiovasc Med [Internet]. 2018 Sep 28 [cited 2025 Nov 22];5:135. Available from: https://pmc.ncbi.nlm.nih.gov/articles/PMC6172294/
10. Scott JM, Khakoo A, MacKey JR, Haykowsky MJ, Douglas PS, Jones LW. Modulation of anthracycline-induced cardiotoxicity by aerobic exercise in breast cancer: Current evidence and underlying mechanisms. Circulation [Internet]. 2011 Aug 2 [cited 2025 Nov 22];124(5):642–50. Available from: https://pubmed.ncbi.nlm.nih.gov/21810673/
11. Jones LW, Alfano CM. Exercise-oncology research: Past, present, and future. Acta Oncol [Internet]. 2013 Feb [cited 2025 Nov 22];52(2):195–215. Available from: https://pubmed.ncbi.nlm.nih.gov/23244677/
12. Wilson RL, Christopher CN, Yang EH, Barac A, Adams SC, Scott JM, et al. Incorporating exercise training into cardio-oncology care: Current evidence and opportunities: JACC: CardioOncology state-of-the-art review. JACC CardioOncol. 2023 Oct 1;5(5):553–69.

13. Moore SC, Lee IM, Weiderpass E, Campbell PT, Sampson JN, Kitahara CM, et al. Association of leisure-time physical activity with risk of 26 types of cancer in 1.44 million adults. JAMA Intern Med [Internet]. 2016 Jun 1 [cited 2025 Nov 22];176(6):816–25. Available from: https://pubmed.ncbi.nlm.nih.gov/27183032/
14. Stout NL, Baima J, Swisher AK, Winters-Stone KM, Welsh J. A systematic review of exercise systematic reviews in the cancer literature. (2005–2017). PM R [Internet]. 2017 Sep 1 [cited 2025 Nov 22];9(9 Suppl 2):S347. Available from: https://pmc.ncbi.nlm.nih.gov/articles/PMC5679711/
15. Juvet LK, Thune I, Elvsaas IKØ, Fors EA, Lundgren S, Bertheussen G, et al. The effect of exercise on fatigue and physical functioning in breast cancer patients during and after treatment and at 6 months follow-up: A meta-analysis. Breast [Internet]. 2017 Jun 1 [cited 2025 Nov 22];33:166–77. Available from: https://pubmed.ncbi.nlm.nih.gov/28415013/
16. De Lazzari N, Niels T, Tewes M, Götte M. A systematic review of the safety, feasibility and benefits of exercise for patients with advanced cancer. Cancers [Internet]. 2021 Sep 6 [cited 2025 Nov 22];13(17):4478. Available from: https://www.mdpi.com/2072-6694/13/17/4478/htm
17. Buffart LM, Kalter J, Sweegers MG, Courneya KS, Newton RU, Aaronson NK, et al. Effects and moderators of exercise on quality of life and physical function in patients with cancer: An individual patient data meta-analysis of 34 RCTs. Cancer Treat Rev. 2017 Jan 1;52:91–104.
18. Courneya KS, Sellar CM, Stevinson C, McNeely ML, Peddle CJ, Friedenreich CM, et al. Randomized controlled trial of the effects of aerobic exercise on physical functioning and quality of life in lymphoma patients. J Clin Oncol [Internet]. 2009 Sep 20 [cited 2025 Nov 22];27(27):4605–12. Available from: https://ascopubs.org/doi/10.1200/JCO.2008.20.0634
19. Singh B, Spence RR, Steele ML, Sandler CX, Peake JM, Hayes SC. A systematic review and meta-analysis of the safety, feasibility, and effect of exercise in women with stage II+ breast cancer. Arch Phys Med Rehabil [Internet]. 2018 Dec 1 [cited 2025 Nov 22];99(12):2621–36. Available from: https://www.archives-pmr.org/action/showFullText?pii=S0003999318302806
20. Scott JM, Iyengar NM, Nilsen TS, Michalski M, Thomas SM, Herndon J, et al. Feasibility, safety, and efficacy of aerobic training in pretreated patients with metastatic breast cancer: A randomized controlled trial. Cancer [Internet]. 2018 Jun 15 [cited 2025 Nov 22];124(12):2552–60. Available from: https://onlinelibrary.wiley.com/doi/full/10.1002/cncr.31368
21. Mizrahi D, Broderick C, Friedlander M, Ryan M, Harrison M, Pumpa K, et al. An exercise intervention during chemotherapy for women with recurrent ovarian cancer: A feasibility study. Int J Gynecol Cancer. 2015 Jul 1;25(6):985–92.
22. Park SE, Kim DH, Kim DK, Ha JY, Jang JS, Choi JH, et al. Feasibility and safety of exercise during chemotherapy in people with gastrointestinal cancers: A pilot study. Supportive Care in Cancer [Internet]. 2023 Oct 1 [cited 2025 Nov 22];31(10):561. Available from: https://pmc.ncbi.nlm.nih.gov/articles/PMC10480261/
23. Mustian KM, Sprod LK, Palesh OG, Peppone LJ, Janelsins MC, Mohile SG, et al. Exercise for the management of side effects and quality of life among cancer survivors. Curr Sports Med Rep [Internet]. 2009 Nov [cited 2025 Nov 22];8(6):325. Available from: https://pmc.ncbi.nlm.nih.gov/articles/PMC2875185/
24. Grønset C, Bech MN, Jarden M, Høgdal N, Hutchings M, Suetta C, et al. The effectiveness of exercise-based interventions on muscle mass, muscle strength,

functional performance, aerobic capacity, and health-related quality of life in adults with malignant lymphoma undergoing chemotherapy: A systematic review of randomized controlled trials. Acta Oncol (Madr) [Internet]. 2025 Jan 28 [cited 2025 Nov 22];64:129–42. Available from: https://medicaljournalssweden.se/actaoncologica/article/view/42056/49067
25. Casla S, López-Tarruella S, Jerez Y, Marquez-Rodas I, Galvão DA, Newton RU, et al. Supervised physical exercise improves VO_2max, quality of life, and health in early stage breast cancer patients: A randomized controlled trial. Breast Cancer Res Treat [Internet]. 2015 Sep 7 [cited 2025 Nov 22];153(2):371–82. Available from: https://pubmed.ncbi.nlm.nih.gov/26293147/
26. Hiraoui M, Al-Haddabi B, Gmada N, Doutrellot PL, Mezlini A, Ahmaidi S. Effects of combined supervised intermittent aerobic, muscle strength and home-based walking training programs on cardiorespiratory responses in women with breast cancer. Bull Cancer. 2019 Jun 1;106(6):527–37.
27. Haydon AMM, MacInnis RJ, English DR, Giles GG. Effect of physical activity and body size on survival after diagnosis with colorectal cancer. Gut [Internet]. 2006 Jan [cited 2025 Nov 22];55(1):62–7. Available from: https://pubmed.ncbi.nlm.nih.gov/15972299/
28. Courneya KS, Vardy JL, O'Callaghan CJ, Gill S, Friedenreich CM, Wong RKS, et al. Structured exercise after adjuvant chemotherapy for colon cancer. N Engl J Med [Internet]. 2025 Jul 3 [cited 2025 Nov 22];393(1):13–25. Available from: https://pubmed.ncbi.nlm.nih.gov/40450658/
29. Hofman M, Ryan JL, Figueroa-Moseley CD, Jean-Pierre P, Morrow GR. Cancer-related fatigue: The scale of the problem. Oncologist [Internet]. 2007 May 1 [cited 2025 Nov 22];12 Suppl 1(S1):4–10. Available from: https://pubmed.ncbi.nlm.nih.gov/17573451/
30. Chen X, Li J, Chen C, Zhang Y, Zhang S, Zhang Y, et al. Effects of exercise interventions on cancer-related fatigue and quality of life among cancer patients: A meta-analysis. BMC Nursing [Internet]. 2023 Jun 13 [cited 2025 Nov 22];22(1):200. Available from: https://bmcnurs.biomedcentral.com/articles/10.1186/s12912-023-01363-0
31. Clemente-Suárez VJ, Martín-Rodríguez A, Redondo-Flórez L, Ruisoto P, Navarro-Jiménez E, Ramos-Campo DJ, et al. Metabolic health, mitochondrial fitness, physical activity, and cancer. Cancers (Basel) [Internet]. 2023 Feb 1 [cited 2025 Nov 22];15(3):814. Available from: https://pmc.ncbi.nlm.nih.gov/articles/PMC9913323/
32. Ceseiko R, Tomsone S, Majevska L, Vetra A. Aerobic capacity for breast cancer survivors 2 to 3 years after breast surgery. [cited 2025 Nov 22]. Available from: https://doi.org/10.1051/shsconf/20196802009
33. Johansen SH, Wisløff T, Edvardsen E, Kollerud ST, Jensen JSS, Agwu G, et al. Effects of systemic anticancer treatment on cardiorespiratory fitness: A systematic review and meta-analysis. JACC CardioOncol [Internet]. 2025 Feb 1 [cited 2025 Nov 22];7(2):96. Available from: https://pmc.ncbi.nlm.nih.gov/articles/PMC11866419/
34. Pedersen L, Idorn M, Olofsson GH, Lauenborg B, Nookaew I, Hansen RH, et al. Voluntary running suppresses tumor growth through epinephrine- and IL-6-dependent NK cell mobilization and redistribution. Cell Metab [Internet]. 2016 Mar 8 [cited 2025 Nov 22];23(3):554–62. Available from: https://pubmed.ncbi.nlm.nih.gov/26895752/
35. Idorn M, thor Straten P. Exercise and cancer: From "healthy" to "therapeutic"? Cancer Immunol Immunother [Internet]. 2017 May 1 [cited 2025 Nov 22];66(5):667–71. Available from: https://pubmed.ncbi.nlm.nih.gov/28324125/

36. Coletta AM, Agha NH, Baker FL, Niemiro GM, Mylabathula PL, Brewster AM, et al. The impact of high-intensity interval exercise training on NK-cell function and circulating myokines for breast cancer prevention among women at high risk for breast cancer. Breast Cancer Res Treat [Internet]. 2021 Jun 1 [cited 2025 Nov 22];187(2):407–16. Available from: https://link.springer.com/article/10.1007/s10549-021-06111-z
37. Sprague BL, Trentham-Dietz A, Newcomb PA, Titus-Ernstoff L, Hampton JM, Egan KM. Lifetime recreational and occupational physical activity and risk of in situ and invasive breast cancer. Cancer Epidemiology, Biomarkers & Prevention [Internet]. 2007 Feb 1 [cited 2025 Nov 22];16(2):236–43. Available from: /cebp/article/16/2/236/275623/Lifetime-Recreational-and-Occupational-Physical
38. ACSM's foundations of strength training and conditioning—Nicholas ratamess—Google books [Internet]. [cited 2025 Nov 22]. Available from: https://books.google.co.uk/books?hl=en&lr=&id=8VYkEAAAQBAJ&oi=fnd&pg=PT24&dq=ratamess+na+2012+acsm%27s+foundations+of+strength+training+and+conditioning&ots=aoeSoxryRT&sig=jLY8lBOluaaK_rPnbumOgNNIbpc#v=onepage&q=ratamess%20na%202012%20acsm's%20foundations%20of%20strength%20training%20and%20conditioning&f=false
39. Kraemer WJ, Ratamess NA. Fundamentals of resistance training: Progression and exercise prescription. Med Sci Sports Exerc [Internet]. 2004 Apr [cited 2025 Nov 22];36(4):674–88. Available from: https://pubmed.ncbi.nlm.nih.gov/15064596/
40. Westcott WL. Resistance training is medicine: Effects of strength training on health. Curr Sports Med Rep [Internet]. 2012 [cited 2025 Nov 22];11(4):209–16. Available from: https://pubmed.ncbi.nlm.nih.gov/22777332/
41. Curovic I. The role of resistance exercise-induced local metabolic stress in mediating systemic health and functional adaptations: Could condensed training volume unlock greater benefits beyond time efficiency? Front Physiol [Internet]. 2025 [cited 2025 Nov 22];16:1549609. Available from: https://pmc.ncbi.nlm.nih.gov/articles/PMC12045103/
42. Egerman MA, Glass DJ. Signaling pathways controlling skeletal muscle mass. Crit Rev Biochem Mol Biol [Internet]. 2013 Jan [cited 2025 Nov 22];49(1):59. Available from: https://pmc.ncbi.nlm.nih.gov/articles/PMC3913083/
43. Liu C, Zhang Q, Liu T, Zhang Q, Song M, Ruan G, et al. Predicted lean body mass trajectories, and cancer risk and cancer-specific and all-cause mortality: A prospective cohort study. J Cachexia Sarcopenia Muscle [Internet]. 2023 Dec 1 [cited 2025 Nov 22];14(6):2916. Available from: https://pmc.ncbi.nlm.nih.gov/articles/PMC10751432/
44. Sturgeon KM, Mathis KM, Rogers CJ, Schmitz KH, Waning DL. Cancer- and chemotherapy-induced musculoskeletal degradation. JBMR Plus [Internet]. 2019 Mar 1 [cited 2025 Nov 22];3(3):e10187. Available from: https://pmc.ncbi.nlm.nih.gov/articles/PMC6419610/
45. Anjanappa M, Corden M, Green A, Roberts D, Hoskin P, McWilliam A, et al. Sarcopenia in cancer: Risking more than muscle loss. Tech Innov Patient Support Radiat Oncol [Internet]. 2020 Dec 1 [cited 2025 Nov 22];16:50. Available from: https://pmc.ncbi.nlm.nih.gov/articles/PMC7769854/
46. Houben LHP, Overkamp M, Van Kraaij P, Trommelen J, Van Roermund JGH, De Vries P, et al. Resistance exercise training increases muscle mass and dtrength in prostate cancer patients on androgen deprivation therapy. Med Sci Sports Exerc [Internet]. 2022 Apr 1 [cited 2025 Nov 22];55(4):614. Available from: https://pmc.ncbi.nlm.nih.gov/articles/PMC9997646/

47. Winters-Stone KM, Dobek J, Nail L, Bennett JA, Leo MC, Naik A, et al. Strength training stops bone loss and builds muscle in postmenopausal breast cancer survivors: A randomized, controlled trial. Breast Cancer Res Treat [Internet]. 2011 [cited 2025 Nov 22];127(2):447. Available from: https://pmc.ncbi.nlm.nih.gov/articles/PMC3124708/
48. Ni J, Zhang L. Cancer cachexia: Definition, staging, and emerging treatments. Cancer Manag Res [Internet]. 2020 [cited 2025 Nov 22];12:5597. Available from: https://pmc.ncbi.nlm.nih.gov/articles/PMC7358070/
49. Tsitkanou S, Murach KA, Washington TA, Greene NP. Exercise counteracts the deleterious effects of cancer cachexia. Cancers (Basel) [Internet]. 2022 May 1 [cited 2025 Nov 22];14(10):2512. Available from: https://pmc.ncbi.nlm.nih.gov/articles/PMC9139714/
50. Tamayo-Torres E, Garrido A, de Cabo R, Carretero J, Gómez-Cabrera MC. Molecular mechanisms of cancer cachexia: Role of exercise training. Mol Aspects Med. 2024 Oct 1;99:101293.
51. Guimarães-Ferreira L, Cholewa JM, Naimo MA, Zhi XIA, Magagnin D, Dal Ponte de Sá RB, et al. Synergistic effects of resistance training and protein intake: Practical aspects. Nutrition [Internet]. 2014 [cited 2025 Nov 22];30(10):1097–103. Available from: https://pubmed.ncbi.nlm.nih.gov/24751198/
52. Pradhan R, Dieterich W, Natarajan A, Schwappacher R, Reljic D, Herrmann HJ, et al. Influence of amino acids and exercise on muscle protein turnover, particularly in cancer cachexia. Cancers (Basel) [Internet]. 2024 May 1 [cited 2025 Nov 22];16(10):1921. Available from: https://pmc.ncbi.nlm.nih.gov/articles/PMC11119313/
53. Sharifi N, Ahmad S. Breast cancer-related lymphedema: A critical review on recent progress. Surg Oncol. 2024 Oct 1;56:102124.
54. Paramanandam VS, Roberts D. Weight training is not harmful for women with breast cancer-related lymphoedema: A systematic review. J Physiother [Internet]. 2014 [cited 2025 Nov 22];60(3):136–43. Available from: https://pubmed.ncbi.nlm.nih.gov/25086730/
55. Schmitz KH, Troxel AB, Cheville A, Grant LL, Bryan CJ, Gross CR, et al. Physical Activity and Lymphedema (The PAL trial): Assessing the safety of progressive strength training in breast cancer survivors. Contemp Clin Trials [Internet]. 2009 May [cited 2025 Nov 22];30(3):233. Available from: https://pmc.ncbi.nlm.nih.gov/articles/PMC2730488/
56. Cormie P, Pumpa K, Galvão DA, Turner E, Spry N, Saunders C, et al. Is it safe and efficacious for women with lymphedema secondary to breast cancer to lift heavy weights during exercise: A randomised controlled trial. J Cancer Surviv [Internet]. 2013 Sep [cited 2025 Nov 22];7(3):413–24. Available from: https://pubmed.ncbi.nlm.nih.gov/23604998/
57. Buchan J, Janda M, Box R, Schmitz K, Hayes S. A randomized trial on the effect of exercise mode on breast cancer-related lymphedema. Med Sci Sports Exerc [Internet]. 2016 Oct 1 [cited 2025 Nov 22];48(10):1866–74. Available from: https://pubmed.ncbi.nlm.nih.gov/27187092/
58. Wittenkamp MC, Christensen J, Vinther A, Juhl CB. The effect of exercise in patients with lower limb lymphedema: A systematic review. Acta Oncol [Internet]. 2025 [cited 2025 Nov 22];64:484–98. Available from: https://pubmed.ncbi.nlm.nih.gov/40165003/
59. Hsu YY, Nguyen TT, Chou YJ, Ho CL. Effects of exercise on lower limb lymphedema in gynecologic cancer: A systematic review and meta-analysis. Eur J Oncol Nurs [Internet]. 2024 Jun 1 [cited 2025 Nov 22];70. Available from: https://pubmed.ncbi.nlm.nih.gov/38554614/

60. Hughes DC, Ellefsen S, Baar K. Adaptations to endurance and strength training. Cold Spring Harb Perspect Med [Internet]. 2018 Jun 1 [cited 2025 Nov 22];8(6):a029769. Available from: https://pmc.ncbi.nlm.nih.gov/articles/PMC5983157/
61. Morici G, Gruttad'Auria CI, Baiamonte P, Mazzuca E, Castrogiovanni A, Bonsignore MR. Endurance training: Is it bad for you? Breathe (Sheff) [Internet]. 2016 Jun 1 [cited 2025 Nov 22];12(2):140–7. Available from: https://pubmed.ncbi.nlm.nih.gov/27408632/
62. Campbell KL, Winters-Stone KM, Wiskemann J, May AM, Schwartz AL, Courneya KS, et al. Exercise guidelines for cancer survivors: Consensus statement from international multidisciplinary roundtable. Med Sci Sports Exerc [Internet]. 2019 Nov 1 [cited 2025 Nov 22];51(11):2375. Available from: https://pmc.ncbi.nlm.nih.gov/articles/PMC8576825/
63. Arida RM, Teixeira-Machado L. The contribution of physical exercise to brain resilience. Front Behav Neurosci [Internet]. 2021 Jan 20 [cited 2025 Nov 22];14:626769. Available from: https://pmc.ncbi.nlm.nih.gov/articles/PMC7874196/
64. Martín-Rodríguez A, Gostian-Ropotin LA, Beltrán-Velasco AI, Belando-Pedreño N, Simón JA, López-Mora C, et al. Sporting mind: The interplay of physical activity and psychological health. Sports [Internet]. 2024 Jan 1 [cited 2025 Nov 22];12(1):37. Available from: https://pmc.ncbi.nlm.nih.gov/articles/PMC10819297/
65. Lirola MJ, Hernández-Rodríguez AI, Cuenca-Piqueras C, Prados-Megías ME. Resilience and renewal: The personal impact of physical activity in breast cancer survivors. BMC Womens Health [Internet]. 2025 Dec 1 [cited 2025 Nov 22];25(1):257. Available from: https://pmc.ncbi.nlm.nih.gov/articles/PMC12107817/
66. Mazzoni AS, Carlsson M, Berntsen S, Nordin K, Demmelmaier I. "Finding my own motivation"—A mixed methods study of exercise and behaviour change support during oncological treatment. Int J Behav Med [Internet]. 2019 Oct 1 [cited 2025 Nov 22];26(5):499. Available from: https://pmc.ncbi.nlm.nih.gov/articles/PMC6785591/
67. Lirola MJ, Hernández-Rodríguez AI, Cuenca-Piqueras C, Prados-Megías ME. Resilience and renewal: The personal impact of physical activity in breast cancer survivors. BMC Womens Health [Internet]. 2025 Dec 1 [cited 2025 Nov 30];25(1):257. Available from: https://pmc.ncbi.nlm.nih.gov/articles/PMC12107817/
68. Matei D, Trofin D, Iordan DA, Onu I, Condurache I, Ionite C, et al. The endocannabinoid system and physical exercise. Int J Mol Sci [Internet]. 2023 Jan 19 [cited 2025 Nov 22];24(3):1989. Available from: https://www.mdpi.com/1422-0067/24/3/1989/htm
69. De Sousa Fernandes MS, Ordônio TF, Santos GCJ, Santos LER, Calazans CT, Gomes DA, et al. Effects of physical exercise on neuroplasticity and brain function: A systematic review in human and animal studies. Neural Plast [Internet]. 2020 [cited 2025 Nov 22];2020:8856621. Available from: https://pmc.ncbi.nlm.nih.gov/articles/PMC7752270/
70. Chen Y jing, Li X xia, Ma H kun, Zhang X, Wang B wei, Guo T tao, et al. Exercise training for improving patient-reported outcomes in patients with advanced-stage cancer: A systematic review and meta-analysis. J Pain Symptom Manage [Internet]. 2020 Mar 1 [cited 2025 Nov 22];59(3):734-749.e10. Available from: https://pubmed.ncbi.nlm.nih.gov/31546002/
71. Seiler A, Jenewein J. Resilience in cancer patients. Front Psychiatry [Internet]. 2019 Apr 1 [cited 2025 Nov 22];10:208. Available from: https://pmc.ncbi.nlm.nih.gov/articles/PMC6460045/

72. Ramírez-vélez R, Zambom-ferraresi F, García-hermoso A, Kievisiene J, Rauckiene-michealsson A, Agostinis-sobrinho C. Evidence-based exercise recommendations to improve mental wellbeing in women with breast cancer during active treatment: A systematic review and meta-analysis. Cancers (Basel) [Internet]. 2021 Jan 2 [cited 2025 Nov 22];13(2):264. Available from: https://pmc.ncbi.nlm.nih.gov/articles/PMC7828164/
73. McGettigan M, Cardwell CR, Cantwell MM, Tully MA. Physical activity interventions for disease-related physical and mental health during and following treatment in people with non-advanced colorectal cancer. Cochrane Database Syst Rev [Internet]. 2020 May 3 [cited 2025 Nov 22];2020(5):CD012864. Available from: https://pmc.ncbi.nlm.nih.gov/articles/PMC7196359/
74. Wu P, Qian M, Chen X, Zhu M, Liu J. Impact of different exercise types on depression and anxiety in individuals with cancer: A systematic review and network meta-analysis of randomized controlled trials. J Psychosom Res. 2025 May 1;192:112107.
75. Courneya KS, Segal RJ, McKenzie DC, Dong H, Gelmon K, Friedenreich CM, et al. Effects of exercise during adjuvant chemotherapy on breast cancer outcomes. Med Sci Sports Exerc [Internet]. 2014 [cited 2025 Nov 22];46(9): 1744–51. Available from: https://journals.lww.com/acsm-msse/fulltext/2014/09000/effects_of_exercise_during_adjuvant_chemotherapy.9.aspx
76. Chen H, Zhou H, Wu B, Lu H, Zhang J, Zhang Y, et al. Physical activity and exercise in liver cancer. Liver Res. 2024 Mar 1;8(1):22–33.
77. Zaccaro A, Piarulli A, Laurino M, Garbella E, Menicucci D, Neri B, et al. How breath-control can change your life: A systematic review on psycho-physiological correlates of slow breathing. Front Hum Neurosci [Internet]. 2018 Sep 7 [cited 2025 Nov 22];12:353. Available from: https://pmc.ncbi.nlm.nih.gov/articles/PMC6137615/
78. Keng SL, Smoski MJ, Robins CJ. Effects of mindfulness on psychological health: A review of empirical studies. Clin Psychol Rev [Internet]. 2011 Aug [cited 2025 Nov 22];31(6):1041. Available from: https://pmc.ncbi.nlm.nih.gov/articles/PMC3679190/
79. Desrosiers A, Vine V, Klemanski DH, Nolen-Hoeksema S. Mindfulness and emotion regulation in depression and anxiety: Common and distinct mechanisms of action. Depress Anxiety [Internet]. 2013 Jul [cited 2025 Nov 22];30(7):654. Available from: https://pmc.ncbi.nlm.nih.gov/articles/PMC4012253/
80. Danon N, Al-Gobari M, Burnand B, Rodondi PY. Are mind-body therapies effective for relieving cancer-related pain in adults? A systematic review and meta-analysis. Psychooncology [Internet]. 2022 Mar 1 [cited 2025 Nov 22];31(3):345–71. Available from: https://pubmed.ncbi.nlm.nih.gov/34545984/
81. Bailey LE, Morris MA. Mind-body therapies adjuvant to chemotherapy improve quality of life and fatigue in top cancers: A systematic review and meta-analysis. Complement Ther Clin Pract [Internet]. 2024 Feb 1 [cited 2025 Nov 22];54. Available from: https://pubmed.ncbi.nlm.nih.gov/38029633/
82. Duan L, Xu Y, Li M. Effects of mind-body exercise in cancer survivors: A systematic review and meta-analysis. Evid Based Complement Alternat Med [Internet]. 2020 [cited 2025 Nov 22];2020:7607161. Available from: https://pmc.ncbi.nlm.nih.gov/articles/PMC7487122/
83. Zeng Y, Huang R, Zhao L, He X, Mao S. The effectiveness of mind-body therapy and physical training in alleviating depressive symptoms in adult cancer patients: A meta-analysis. J Cancer Res Clin Oncol [Internet]. 2024 Jun 1 [cited 2025 Nov 22];150(6):289. Available from: https://link.springer.com/article/10.1007/s00432-024-05813-3

84. Papurcu A, Tang C, Cheema BS, Smith SM. Mind-body interventions for cancer-related dyspnoea: A systematic review and meta-analysis of randomised controlled trials. Support Care Cancer [Internet]. 2025 Dec 1 [cited 2025 Nov 22];33(12). Available from: https://pubmed.ncbi.nlm.nih.gov/41247541/
85. Chandwani KD, Perkins G, Nagendra HR, Raghuram NV., Spelman A, Nagarathna R, et al. Randomized, controlled trial of yoga in women with breast cancer undergoing radiotherapy. J Clin Oncol [Internet]. 2014 Apr 1 [cited 2025 Nov 30];32(10):1058. Available from: https://pmc.ncbi.nlm.nih.gov/articles/PMC3965260/
86. Löchner J, Moshe I, Schiepek G, Schuller BW, Schoedel R, Rodgar M, et al. Tracking health-related quality of life dynamics: Advances in ambulatory assessment methods. Brain Behavior and Immunity Integrative. 2024 Apr 1;6:100061.
87. Stein KD, Syrjala KL, Andrykowski MA. Physical and psychological long-term and late effects of cancer. Cancer [Internet]. 2008 Jun 1 [cited 2025 Nov 22];112(11 Suppl):2577. Available from: https://pmc.ncbi.nlm.nih.gov/articles/PMC7047657/
88. Ferrer RA, Huedo-Medina TB, Johnson BT, Ryan S, Pescatello LS. Exercise interventions for cancer survivors: A meta-analysis of quality of life outcomes. Ann Behav Med [Internet]. 2011 Feb [cited 2025 Nov 22];41(1):32. Available from: https://pmc.ncbi.nlm.nih.gov/articles/PMC3712334/
89. Chen X, Li J, Chen C, Zhang Y, Zhang S, Zhang Y, et al. Effects of exercise interventions on cancer-related fatigue and quality of life among cancer patients: A meta-analysis. BMC Nursing [Internet]. 2023 Jun 13 [cited 2025 Nov 22];22(1):200. Available from: https://bmcnurs.biomedcentral.com/articles/10.1186/s12912-023-01363-0
90. Bailey LE, Morris MA. Mind-body therapies adjuvant to chemotherapy improve quality of life and fatigue in top cancers: A systematic review and meta-analysis. Complement Ther Clin Pract [Internet]. 2024 Feb 1 [cited 2025 Nov 22];54. Available from: https://pubmed.ncbi.nlm.nih.gov/38029633/
91. Mok J, Brown MJ, Akam EC, Morris MA. The lasting effects of resistance and endurance exercise interventions on breast cancer patient mental wellbeing and physical fitness. Sci Rep [Internet]. 2022 Dec 1 [cited 2025 Nov 22];12(1). Available from: https://pubmed.ncbi.nlm.nih.gov/35241723/
92. Mcauley E, Szabo A, Gothe N, Olson EA. Self-efficacy: Implications for physical activity, function, and functional limitations in older adults. Am J Lifestyle Med [Internet]. 2011 [cited 2025 Nov 22];5(4):10.1177/1559827610392704. Available from: https://pmc.ncbi.nlm.nih.gov/articles/PMC3864698/
93. Liu L, Ancoli-Israel S. Sleep disturbances in cancer. Psychiatr Ann [Internet]. 2008 Sep [cited 2025 Nov 22];38(9):627. Available from: https://pmc.ncbi.nlm.nih.gov/articles/PMC3021374/
94. Gururaj R, Samuel SR, Kumar KV, Nagaraja R, Keogh JWL. Effect of exercise based interventions on sleep and circadian rhythm in cancer survivors—A systematic review and meta-analysis. PeerJ [Internet]. 2024 [cited 2025 Nov 22];12:e17053. Available from: https://pmc.ncbi.nlm.nih.gov/articles/PMC10926908/
95. Tang MF, Chiu HY, Xu X, Kwok JY, Cheung DST, Chen CY, et al. Walking is more effective than yoga at reducing sleep disturbance in cancer patients: A systematic review and meta-analysis of randomized controlled trials. Sleep Med Rev [Internet]. 2019 Oct 1 [cited 2025 Nov 22];47:1–8. Available from: https://pubmed.ncbi.nlm.nih.gov/31207341/

96. Staff NP, Grisold A, Grisold W, Windebank AJ. Chemotherapy-induced peripheral neuropathy: A current review. Ann Neurol [Internet]. 2017 Jun 1 [cited 2025 Nov 22];81(6):772. Available from: https://pmc.ncbi.nlm.nih.gov/articles/PMC5656281/
97. Stubblefield MD, McNeely ML, Alfano CM, Mayer DK. A prospective surveillance model for physical rehabilitation of women with breast cancer: Chemotherapy-induced peripheral neuropathy. Cancer [Internet]. 2012 Apr 15 [cited 2025 Nov 22];118(8 Suppl):2250–60. Available from: https://pubmed.ncbi.nlm.nih.gov/22488699/
98. Huang Y, Tan T, Liu L, Yan Z, Deng Y, Li G, et al. Exercise for reducing chemotherapy-induced peripheral neuropathy: A systematic review and meta-analysis of randomized controlled trials. Front Neurol [Internet]. 2023 [cited 2025 Nov 22];14:1252259. Available from: https://pmc.ncbi.nlm.nih.gov/articles/PMC10813204/
99. Kneis S, Wehrle A, Müller J, Maurer C, Ihorst G, Gollhofer A, et al. It's never too late—Balance and endurance training improves functional performance, quality of life, and alleviates neuropathic symptoms in cancer survivors suffering from chemotherapy-induced peripheral neuropathy: Results of a randomized controlled trial. BMC Cancer [Internet]. 2019 May 2 [cited 2025 Nov 22];19(1):414. Available from: https://pmc.ncbi.nlm.nih.gov/articles/PMC6498676/
100. Kleckner IR, Kamen C, Gewandter JS, Mohile NA, Heckler CE, Culakova E, et al. Effects of exercise during chemotherapy on chemotherapy-induced peripheral neuropathy: A multicenter, randomized controlled trial. Support Care Cancer [Internet]. 2018 Apr 1 [cited 2025 Nov 22];26(4):1019–28. Available from: https://pubmed.ncbi.nlm.nih.gov/29243164/
101. Kneis S, Wehrle A, Müller J, Maurer C, Ihorst G, Gollhofer A, et al. It's never too late—Balance and endurance training improves functional performance, quality of life, and alleviates neuropathic symptoms in cancer survivors suffering from chemotherapy-induced peripheral neuropathy: Results of a randomized controlled trial. BMC Cancer [Internet]. 2019 May 2 [cited 2025 Nov 22];19(1). Available from: https://pubmed.ncbi.nlm.nih.gov/31046719/
102. Wang C, Qiu X, Yang X, Mao J, Li Q. Factors influencing social isolation among cancer patients: A systematic review. Healthcare [Internet]. 2024 May 1 [cited 2025 Nov 22];12(10):1042. Available from: https://pmc.ncbi.nlm.nih.gov/articles/PMC11120751/
103. Misiąg W, Piszczyk A, Szymańska-Chabowska A, Chabowski M. Physical activity and cancer care—A review. Cancers (Basel) [Internet]. 2022 Sep 1 [cited 2025 Nov 22];14(17):4154. Available from: https://pmc.ncbi.nlm.nih.gov/articles/PMC9454950/
104. Mazzoni AS, Carlsson M, Berntsen S, Nordin K, Demmelmaier I. "Finding my own motivation"—A mixed methods study of exercise and behaviour change support during oncological treatment. Int J Behavi Med [Internet]. 2019 Aug 22 [cited 2025 Dec 1];26(5):499–511. Available from: https://link.springer.com/article/10.1007/s12529-019-09809-z
105. Chung N, Park MY, Kim J, Park HY, Hwang H, Lee CH, et al. Non-Exercise Activity Thermogenesis (NEAT): A component of total daily energy expenditure. J Exerc Nutrition Biochem [Internet]. 2018 Jun 30 [cited 2025 Nov 22];22(2):23. Available from: https://pmc.ncbi.nlm.nih.gov/articles/PMC6058072/
106. Loeffelholz C von, Birkenfeld AL. Non-exercise activity thermogenesis in human energy homeostasis. Endotext [Internet]. 2022 Nov 25 [cited 2025 Nov 22]. Available from: https://www.ncbi.nlm.nih.gov/sites/books/NBK279077/

107. Katzmarzyk PT, Church TS, Craig CL, Bouchard C. Sitting time and mortality from all causes, cardiovascular disease, and cancer. Med Sci Sports Exerc [Internet]. 2009 May [cited 2025 Nov 22];41(5):998–1005. Available from: https://pubmed.ncbi.nlm.nih.gov/19346988/
108. Aicr, WCRF. Diet, nutrition, physical activity and cancer: A global perspective a summary of the third expert report. [cited 2025 Nov 22]. Available from: http://gco.iarc.fr/today
109. Buffey AJ, Herring MP, Langley CK, Donnelly AE, Carson BP. The acute effects of interrupting prolonged sitting time in adults with standing and light-intensity walking on biomarkers of cardiometabolic health in adults: A systematic review and meta-analysis. Sports Med [Internet]. 2022 Aug 1 [cited 2025 Nov 22];52(8):1765–87. Available from: https://pubmed.ncbi.nlm.nih.gov/35147898/
110. Raza W, Krachler B, Forsberg B, Sommar JN. Health benefits of leisure time and commuting physical activity: A meta-analysis of effects on morbidity. J Transp Health. 2020 Sep 1;18:100873.
111. Tyldesley-Marshall N, Greenfield SM, Parretti HM, Gokal K, Greaves C, Jolly K, et al. SnacktivityTM to promote physical activity: A qualitative study. Int J Behav Med [Internet]. 2022 Oct 1 [cited 2025 Nov 22];29(5):553–64. Available from: https://link.springer.com/article/10.1007/s12529-021-10040-y
112. Doughty HC, Hill RA, Riley A, Midgley AW, Patterson JM, Boddy LM, et al. Barriers to and facilitators of physical activity in adults living with and beyond cancer, with special emphasis on head and neck cancer: A systematic review of qualitative and mixed methods studies. Supportive Care in Cancer [Internet]. 2023 Aug 1 [cited 2025 Nov 22];31(8):471. Available from: https://pmc.ncbi.nlm.nih.gov/articles/PMC10352410/
113. Shreves AH, Small SR, Walmsley R, Chan S, Saint-Maurice PF, Moore SC, et al. Amount and intensity of daily total physical activity, step count and risk of incident cancer in the UK Biobank. Br J Sports Med [Internet]. 2025 Jun 1 [cited 2025 Nov 22];59(12):839–47. Available from: https://bjsm.bmj.com/content/59/12/839
114. Bandura A. Social cognitive theory. Handbook of Theories of Social Psychology. 2012 Jan 1;1:349–74.
115. Prochaska JO, Velicer WF. The transtheoretical model of health behavior change. Am J Health Promot [Internet]. 1997 [cited 2025 Nov 22];12(1):38–48. Available from: https://pubmed.ncbi.nlm.nih.gov/10170434/
116. Friel CP, Cornelius T, Diaz KM. Factors associated with long-term wearable physical activity monitor user engagement. Transl Behav Med [Internet]. 2019 Jan 1 [cited 2025 Nov 22];11(1):262. Available from: https://pmc.ncbi.nlm.nih.gov/articles/PMC7982124/
117. Tudor-Locke C, Lutes L. Why do pedometers work?: A reflection upon the factors related to successfully increasing physical activity. Sports Med [Internet]. 2009 [cited 2025 Nov 22];39(12):981–93. Available from: https://pubmed.ncbi.nlm.nih.gov/19902981/
118. Lee K, Kwon H, Lee B, Lee G, Lee JH, Park YR, et al. Effect of self-monitoring on long-term patient engagement with mobile health applications. PLoS One [Internet]. 2018 Jul 1 [cited 2025 Nov 22];13(7):e0201166. Available from: https://pmc.ncbi.nlm.nih.gov/articles/PMC6062090/
119. Jones LW, Eves ND, Scott JM. Bench-to-bedside approaches for personalized exercise therapy in cancer. Am Soc Clin Oncol Educ Book [Internet]. 2017 May [cited 2025 Nov 22];37(37):684–94. Available from: https://pubmed.ncbi.nlm.nih.gov/28561646/

120. Ranes M, Wiestad TH, Thormodsen I, Arving C. Determinants of exercise adherence and maintenance for cancer survivors: Implementation of a community-based group exercise program: A qualitative feasibility study. PEC Innovation [Internet]. 2022 Dec 1 [cited 2025 Nov 22];1:100088. Available from: https://pmc.ncbi.nlm.nih.gov/articles/PMC10194213/
121. Singh B, Zopf EM, Howden EJ. Effect and feasibility of wearable physical activity trackers and pedometers for increasing physical activity and improving health outcomes in cancer survivors: A systematic review and meta-analysis. J Sport Health Sci [Internet]. 2021 Mar 1 [cited 2025 Nov 22];11(2):184. Available from: https://pmc.ncbi.nlm.nih.gov/articles/PMC9068515/

6

DIFFERENTIAL EFFECTS OF EXERCISE INTENSITIES

6.1 Introduction

The previous chapter explored the distinct physiological effects and clinical benefits of different types of exercise, including aerobic, resistance, endurance and incidental activity, as well as mind-body therapies across the cancer continuum. Aerobic training enhances cardiovascular and immune function, resistance training serves to preserve muscle and bone health, and endurance activity can support psychological resilience and reduce recurrence-related anxiety. The role of everyday physical activity, such as walking, gardening or active commuting, was also highlighted as an important contributor to reducing sedentary time and improving survivorship outcomes. While each type of activity elicits unique adaptations, this chapter will explore how these effects are strongly influenced by the intensity at which exercise is performed.

Exercise intensity refers to the relative effort or physiological demand of a given activity (1). It can be quantified objectively using measures such as heart rate, oxygen uptake (VO_2max), or lactate threshold, or subjectively through the rating of perceived exertion (RPE) (2). Among the components of the FITT framework, intensity is considered a critical driver of biological adaptation. Many of the cellular and systemic responses that underpin the anti-cancer effects of exercise, including mitochondrial biogenesis, insulin sensitivity, immune cell mobilisation and cytokine signalling, are modulated by exercise intensity (3). However, the relationship between exercise intensity and cancer outcomes is complex. In the field of exercise immunology, immune function follows a biphasic, or J-shaped, curve whereby sedentary behaviour or very high exercise workload is associated with reduced

DOI: 10.4324/9781003511519-8

immune function and increased rates of upper respiratory tract infections, whereas moderate exercise is associated with lower rates of infections (4,5).

It stands to reason, then, that in the field of exercise oncology, where it is well known that anti-tumour immunity plays an important role in reducing cancer incidence, a similar pattern would apply (Figure 6.1). Evidence

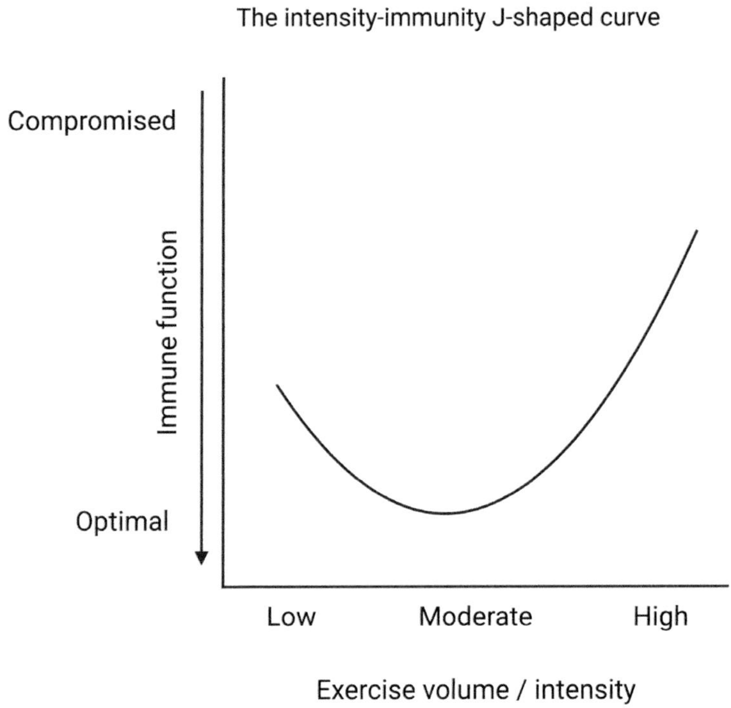

FIGURE 6.1 The J-shaped relationship between exercise intensity and immune function. This conceptual model, adapted from Nieman (1994), illustrates the biphasic or J-shaped curve describing the relationship between exercise intensity and immune function (4). Sedentary behaviour (left side) is associated with low immune competence and elevated systemic inflammation. Regular moderate-intensity exercise enhances immune surveillance, reduces inflammation, and supports anti-tumour immune activity, representing the optimal zone for immunological benefit. In contrast, excessive, high-intensity exercise performed without adequate recovery may induce physiological stress, transient immunosuppression, and increase cortisol levels, potentially impairing immune function and increasing vulnerability to infection or tumour progression. This model highlights the importance of balancing exercise dose to maximise therapeutic benefit while minimising risk. Created in Biorender.com.

from preclinical and clinical research suggests that moderate-intensity exercise promotes immune function and tumour suppression (6,7), whereas excessive or prolonged high-intensity exercise may induce physiological stress, elevate cortisol levels and transiently suppress aspects of immune surveillance (8). Emerging evidence suggests that in certain contexts, particularly when not tailored to individual capacity, high-intensity exercise may inadvertently promote tumour dissemination by exacerbating physiological stress responses that enhance vascular permeability and metastatic potential, for example, by affecting platelet adhesion to tumour cells (9) or lowering the phagocytic capacity of macrophages (10,11).

Understanding how different intensities of exercise influence tumour biology, treatment tolerance and survivorship outcomes is essential for optimising exercise prescriptions in oncology. Key considerations include the identification of minimum effective doses, the potential for synergistic effects with cancer therapies, and the feasibility and safety of high-intensity protocols in clinical populations. The following sections examine how exercise intensity is defined and measured, reviewing evidence from both preclinical and clinical studies to explore mechanistic pathways, and consider how intensity-based exercise interventions may be tailored for individuals living with and beyond cancer.

6.2 Defining exercise intensity and dose

Exercise dose is a multidimensional concept, traditionally described using the FITT principle: Frequency, Intensity, Time and Type (2). While each component contributes to the physiological and clinical effects of exercise, intensity has emerged as a key determinant of biological adaptation in the context of cancer. Precise characterisation of exercise intensity is therefore essential for understanding its impact on tumour biology and for developing effective exercise prescriptions in oncology.

6.2.1 Physiological definitions of intensity

Exercise intensity can be categorised as low, moderate or high (vigorous), based on objective physiological parameters or subjective perceptions of effort (Table 6.1).

While these categories provide useful generalisations, intensity should always be interpreted relative to individual fitness levels, health status and treatment phase.

6.2.2 Distinguishing intensity from volume

Intensity refers to the effort or metabolic demand per unit of activity, whereas volume refers to the overall workload, typically calculated as

TABLE 6.1 Definitions of exercise intensities

Level	*Example activities*	*Measurements*
Low-intensity	Slow walking, stretching, light household tasks	<40% VO_2max or heart rate reserve (HRR), with a rating of perceived exertion (RPE) <3 on the Borg 6–20 scale
Moderate-intensity	Brisk walking, cycling at a steady pace, water aerobics	40–60% VO_2max or HRR, with RPE of 3–6
High-intensity	Running, high-intensity interval training (HIIT), vigorous cycling or sport	>60–70% VO_2max or HRR, with RPE >7

Abbreviations: HIIT = high-intensity interval training; HRR = heart rate reserve; RPE = rating of perceived exertion; VO2max = maximal oxygen uptake

frequency × time × intensity (2). Two exercise programmes may have the same volume but differ significantly in biological impact due to intensity variations. For example, three 10-minute sessions of high-intensity interval training may elicit distinct cellular and systemic responses compared to 30 minutes of continuous moderate-intensity activity, despite having similar energy expenditure.

6.2.3 Tools for measuring intensity

Several tools are available to assess and prescribe exercise intensity:

- Cardiopulmonary testing (e.g., VO_2max tests) provides gold-standard measurements but is not always feasible in clinical settings.
- Heart rate monitors and heart rate reserve calculations are widely used and accessible.
- Rating of perceived exertion (RPE) provides a validated, subjective tool, especially valuable for patients on medications (e.g., beta-blockers) that affect heart rate.
- Lactate threshold and ventilatory thresholds are increasingly used in performance and oncology research to individualise intensity zones.

6.2.4 Biological implications of intensity

Each intensity level elicits distinct physiological and biochemical responses. Low-intensity supports metabolic recovery, enhances fatty acid oxidation and maintains functional capacity in deconditioned patients. Moderate-intensity is associated with improved insulin sensitivity, reduced inflammation and enhanced immune surveillance—effects thought to be central to tumour suppression. High-intensity, when properly programmed, can amplify hormonal responses (e.g., catecholamine release), stimulate immune cell mobilisation and enhance vascular shear stress, potentially augmenting tumour perfusion and immune cell infiltration. However, excessive or poorly recovered high-intensity exercise may also lead to transient immunosuppression or elevated systemic stress (2). These distinctions are summarised in Table 6.2 and underscore the importance of defining not just how much exercise is performed, but the intensity at which it is performed. As research continues to refine the understanding of dose-response

TABLE 6.2 Biological effects of exercise at varying intensities

Level	*Metabolic effects*	*Hormonal responses*	*Immune modulation*	*TME effects*
Low	Fat oxidation Maintenance of metabolic function	Minimal hormonal activation	• Mild mobilisation of NK and T cells • Maintenance of immune homeostasis	May help reduce inflammation
Moderate	Improved insulin sensitivity Enhanced metabolic flexibility	IL-6 release (anti-inflammatory) Some catecholamine release	• Increased NK and CD8+ T cell mobilisation • Increased IL-10 • Decreased TNF-α	• Vascular normalisation • Improved perfusion • Immune cell infiltration
High	Glycolytic demand Increased lactate production	Significant increase in catecholamines Increased cortisol if prolonged	• Potent immune cell mobilisation • Increased NK cell cytotoxicity • Potential transient suppression post-exercise	• Increased shear stress • Activation of Hippo pathway • Suppression of Wnt/β-catenin • Potential increase in CTCs if poorly recovered

Abbreviations: CD = cluster of differentiation; CTC = circulating tumour cells; IL = interleukin; NK = natural killer; TNF = tumour necrosis factor

relationships in cancer, intensity will likely remain a focal point for both mechanistic studies and clinical translation.

6.3 Insights from preclinical studies

Animal models have been instrumental in delineating the impact of exercise intensity on tumour biology under controlled conditions (6,12–17) (see Table 6.3). These studies allow for standardisation of tumour type, exercise exposure and biological measurements, offering insights that are often difficult to obtain in human populations.

6.3.1 Voluntary versus forced exercise protocols

Preclinical studies in rodents typically compare voluntary wheel running (low-to-moderate-intensity, self-paced) with forced treadmill running (moderate-to-high-intensity, externally paced) or structured high-intensity interval training (HIIT). Some studies utilise swimming protocols in a similar vein, comparing free swimming with swimming to exhaustion. At low-to-moderate-intensity, exercise initiates several beneficial systemic responses. One of the most well-documented effects is the release of IL-6 from contracting skeletal muscle. In this context, IL-6 functions as a myokine with anti-inflammatory properties, stimulating the release of IL-10 and IL-1Ra while inhibiting TNF-α production (18–20). Moderate-intensity aerobic exercise, such as treadmill running at 60–70% VO_2max, has been shown to reduce tumour growth and enhance anti-tumour immunity, including increased CD8+ T cell infiltration and reduced regulatory T cell recruitment, when performed regularly over several weeks (12). These effects have been linked to increased cytotoxic T cell infiltration, reduced tumour hypoxia and normalisation of tumour vasculature (6,7,12,15). These experimental models simulate different aspects of human exercise behaviour and permit examination of dose-response effects on tumour development, progression and metastasis.

6.3.2 High-intensity exercise and immune modulation

While moderate intensity is generally associated with tumour-suppressive effects, high-intensity exercise appears to elicit more complex, context-dependent immune responses. Short-term high-intensity exercise protocols have shown promise in enhancing immune cell mobilisation and vascular adaptation without compromising immune function, particularly the transient redistribution of NK cells and CD8+ T lymphocytes into circulation, and potentially into the TME (21,22). These responses are largely

TABLE 6.3 Animal studies demonstrating the impact of exercise intensity on tumour biology

Study	*Exercise intensity*	*Animal model*	*Tumour outcome*
Pedersen et al., 2016 (6)	Moderate (equivalent)	1. B16F10 melanoma model, female mice 2. Male Naval Medical Research Institute (NMRI) mice 3. Lewis Lung carcinoma model (LLC), female mice 4. Tg(Grm1) EPv transgenic mice (melanoma model)	1. Reduced tumour growth by ≥60% 2. Reduced tumour incidence by ≥30% 3. Reduced tumour volume by 58% and tumour weight by 56% 4. Delayed tumour formation
Gomes-Santos et al., 2024 (12)	Low, moderate, high	FVB female syngeneic breast cancer mouse model	Only moderate-intensity exercise delayed tumour growth, reduced tumour burden, and increased CD8+ T cell infiltration with enhanced effector function.
Alves et al., 2018 (13)	High	LLC mouse model	High-intensity interval training (HIIT) group had reduced tumour mass, increased PD-L1 and VEGFA mRNA expression, and increased survival rate
Jee et al., 2022 (14)	High	CDF1 colorectal cancer mouse model	High-intensity exercise reduced tumour growth and metastases and modified the expression of genes involved in modulating immune function and suppressing cancer growth and metastasis
Voltarelli et al., 2024 (15)	Moderate	CT26 colon cancer model in Balb/c mice	Moderate-intensity exercise reduces tumour growth and hypoxia, enhances CD8+ T cell infiltration, mitochondrial density, function and IFNg production, and improves survival
Fei et al., 2020 (16)	Moderate	B16-F10 melanoma and YAC-1 lymphoma model in C57BL/6 mice	Detraining after tumour establishment increases tumour growth and reduces splenic T cell proliferation. NK cell frequency in tumours was increased in all exercised mice.

Abbreviations: CD = cluster of differentiation; IFN = interferon; NK = natural killer; NMRI = Naval Medical Research Institute; PD-L1 = programmed death ligand 1; VEGFA = vascular endothelial growth factor A

mediated by acute spikes in catecholamines, such as adrenaline and noradrenaline, which can increase NK cell cytotoxicity and support innate immune activation.

However, excessively intense or prolonged exercise may provoke physiological stress responses that lead to transient immunosuppression. Elevated glucocorticoid levels and systemic inflammation in the aftermath of intense exercise can impair NK cell activity, reduce lymphocyte proliferation and dampen immune surveillance, particularly if recovery periods are insufficient (23). This duality reflects the "J-shaped curve" hypothesis in exercise immunology, where moderate volumes of exercise enhance immune function, but excessive doses, especially when poorly adapted to the individual's condition, may suppress it (see Figure 6.1). These concerns are especially relevant for individuals with cancer or those undergoing active treatment, in whom immune function is already compromised. Further mechanistic details on immune cell mobilisation, catecholamine signalling and the impact of intensity on systemic inflammation are explored later in this chapter in Section 6.5, as well as in Chapter 3, Section 3.2.1, and Chapter 4, Section 4.9.

6.3.3 *Intensity effects on metastasis and angiogenesis*

The relationship between exercise intensity and metastatic potential has also been explored. Chronic moderate-intensity exercise appears to inhibit tumour spread by promoting vascular normalisation, reducing endothelial cell permeability and facilitating the destruction of CTCs (24–28). In a review of preclinical studies, de ten Ryen et al. (2020) caution that excessive high-intensity exercise may perturb endothelial integrity, elevate systemic stress and potentially increase the risk of tumour cell dissemination. Notably, these adverse effects may be mitigated by incorporating appropriate warm-up protocols, suggesting that exercise programming details (e.g., warm-up, recovery) are critical for maintaining safety (11).

6.3.4 *Mechanistic underpinnings*

In animal models, exercise intensity modulates several key anti-tumour pathways. For example, catecholamine signalling, primarily epinephrine (adrenaline) and norepinephrine (noradrenaline), has been shown to mobilise NK cells and enhance their cytotoxic activity, promoting their redistribution into tumour tissues (6,7). Moreover, exercise-conditioned serum can regulate the tumour suppressor Hippo pathway via catecholamines, as evidenced by phosphorylation and cytoplasmic sequestration of the downstream effector protein YAP (29). Moderate-intensity exercise in animal studies has been shown to inhibit cancer cell proliferation and induce apoptosis (30), emphasising the protective benefits of moderate-intensity exercise (31). Another candidate is irisin, a myokine released in response to high-intensity muscular contraction. Ganon et al. (2015) showed that irisin reduced the viability and invasive behaviour of breast cancer cells, while promoting apoptotic signalling (32). Moreover, it induces the release of vascular endothelial growth factor (VEGF) which leads to improved perfusion and better delivery of oxygen, immune effector cells and chemotherapeutic agents to the tumour core (7,33). Chronic moderate-intensity exercise further contributes to a reduction in systemic and local pro-inflammatory cytokines, such as IL-6 and TNF-α, which may dampen the pro-tumourigenic inflammatory TME (7,34,35).

Conversely, exercise-conditioned serum following a 9-week period of high-intensity interval training (HIIT) has been shown to suppress Wnt/β-catenin signalling (36), supporting the idea that adaptation to more extreme exercise intensities may alter the regulation of this pathway. Moreover, low-intensity exercise does not inhibit cancer cell proliferation in the same way that moderate-intensity exercise and high-intensity exercise does (3). By contrast, a study in Sprague-Dawley rats demonstrated enhanced Ki-67 expression in response to high-intensity exercise, suggesting enhanced proliferation under these conditions (37). Other animal studies corroborate these findings that strenuous exercise may show a carcinogenic effect by demonstrating increased proliferation and apoptosis in response to moderate- or high-intensity exercise (30,38). However, on balance, the majority of studies support the protective nature of moderate- and high-intensity exercise in animal models of cancer (31,39,40). Together, these mechanistic insights imply that varying levels of exercise intensity may preferentially engage distinct anti-tumour effects, with moderate-to-vigorous intensities likely providing the most robust and balanced biological benefits, provided they are appropriately dosed and are accompanied by sufficient warm-up and recovery time.

6.3.5 A threshold model for biological effect

This duality supports the concept of a threshold model of exercise oncology. While certain beneficial pathways, such as Hippo activation or NK mobilisation, are only triggered above a given intensity, excessive or cumulative stress can paradoxically induce immunosuppression, thereby promoting tumour-supportive conditions. Determining the optimal "dose" of exercise requires balancing intensity with recovery, particularly in individuals undergoing treatment or with advanced disease.

Carefully prescribed and individualised, both moderate- and high-intensity exercise can serve as potent, biologically active interventions capable of reprogramming the TME. Understanding the thresholds at which benefits outweigh risks is key to harnessing exercise as a precision oncology tool.

6.4 Clinical evidence and human trials

While preclinical models provide mechanistic insight into how exercise intensity influences tumour biology, translation into clinical practice requires robust evidence from human studies. A growing body of research has investigated the safety, feasibility and efficacy of structured exercise interventions in people with cancer, with increasing attention now being paid to the role of exercise intensity as a modifiable parameter.

6.4.1 Evidence from major clinical trials

Few clinical trials have been conducted that explicitly evaluate the impact of exercise intensity in cancer patient populations. A feasibility trial in women with recurrent ovarian cancer demonstrated that 90 minutes per week of low-to-moderate-intensity exercise was not only feasible but also significantly improved QoL, fatigue, mental health, muscular strength and balance. Participants were also able to tolerate higher doses of chemotherapy, suggesting a potential role for exercise in supporting treatment resilience (41).

The CHALLENGE trial (Canadian Cancer Trials Group CO.21) (42) investigated whether a structured physical activity programme could improve disease-free survival in individuals who had completed adjuvant chemotherapy for high-risk stage II or III colon cancer. Participants were supported to achieve approximately 150 minutes per week of predominantly moderate-intensity aerobic exercise, such as brisk walking or cycling. After a median follow-up of 8 years, the intervention group demonstrated a 28% reduction in the risk of disease recurrence or new primary cancer, and a 37% reduction in all-cause mortality compared with usual care. These findings offer some of the strongest prospective evidence to date linking moderate-intensity physical activity with improved long-term oncological outcomes.

In contrast, the INTERVAL-GAP4 trial focused on a much higher-risk population of men with metastatic castrate-resistant prostate cancer (mCRPC) (43). This international phase III study tested the effects of a high-intensity aerobic and resistance training programme, delivered under supervision, on progression-free and overall survival. While final survival outcomes are pending, interim data indicate that adherence to the high-intensity programme was feasible, with participants attending approximately 79% of scheduled sessions over the first year. Importantly, the intervention was found to be safe and well-tolerated despite the participants' advanced disease and high symptom burden.

Two trials have directly investigated the role of exercise intensity by comparing different exercise prescriptions. The Phys-Can trial (NCT02473003) enrolled patients undergoing (neo-)adjuvant therapy for breast, prostate or colorectal cancer (44), demonstrating that high-intensity exercise was safe and may confer a modest benefit in reducing physical fatigue when compared with low-to-moderate-intensity exercise. Interestingly, additional behaviour change support did not further enhance these outcomes. Similarly, Pelzer et al. (2023) conducted a four-arm randomised study in breast and prostate cancer survivors, comparing different aerobic and resistance training intensities (NCT02883699) (45). All groups showed improvements in health-related QoL and cancer-related fatigue, with no single regimen showing superiority. However, resistance training appeared to have more sustained effects over time, highlighting the importance of modality as well as intensity.

Finally, an ongoing clinical trial combining high-intensity exercise with standard treatment is investigating whether high-intensity training can mobilise and increase immune cell infiltration. The High-Intensity Aerobic exercise training and Immune cell Mobilisation (HI AIM) trial (NCT04263467) will evaluate supervised and group-based exercise training, comprising intermediate to high-intensity interval training (HIIT) three times per week over 6 weeks in combination with standard oncological treatments, checkpoint inhibitors, checkpoint inhibitors combined with chemotherapy or oncological surveillance, then measure levels of circulating NK cells, tumour immune cell infiltration, inflammatory markers and other clinical outcomes (46).

Overall, these studies suggest that both moderate- and high-intensity exercise can be delivered safely in clinical populations and may offer physiological or oncological benefits. However, the degree to which these findings can be generalised varies, with moderate-intensity interventions applicable across a broader spectrum of patients, while higher-intensity protocols often require stricter screening, closer supervision and more individualised tailoring to ensure patient safety and adherence.

6.4.2 Impact on cancer progression, recurrence and survivorship

Observational and interventional studies consistently demonstrate that greater volumes of physical activity, particularly at moderate-to-vigorous intensities, are associated with reduced cancer recurrence and improved survival (47–50). This is evident across tumour types including breast, colorectal and prostate cancer. However, while activity volume is often emphasised, exercise intensity may play a crucial role in modulating underlying biological processes such as inflammation, insulin resistance and immune function. Data from trials, such as CHALLENGE (see Section 6.4.1), support the notion that sustained, moderate-intensity aerobic exercise can reduce the risk of disease progression and improve overall survival in early-stage cancer. By contrast, high-intensity exercise protocols, though less extensively studied, appear to induce favourable changes in aerobic capacity, muscular strength and metabolic regulation—all of which may support treatment tolerance and longer-term health (95). Importantly, these benefits are not solely restricted to physical outcomes. Improvements in fatigue, psychological wellbeing, physical function and health-related QoL have also been reported across intensity levels, although high-intensity interventions are more physically demanding and require longer recovery periods.

6.4.3 *Feasibility, adherence and patient experience*

Adherence to structured exercise interventions is influenced by multiple factors, including exercise intensity, supervision, treatment side effects and patient preference. Moderate-intensity programmes tend to show higher long-term adherence and are more easily integrated into daily life, particularly when delivered in a flexible or home-based format. For example, Mizrahi et al. (2015) demonstrated that two-thirds of women with recurrent ovarian cancer were able to complete a low-to-moderate-intensity aerobic exercise programme (90 minutes per week), with no adverse events reported, supporting the feasibility of such interventions, even in advanced disease settings (41). By contrast, high-intensity exercise, while physiologically potent, is less widely implemented and may present barriers to uptake and sustainability, particularly in individuals with advanced disease, comorbidities, or treatment-related fatigue. This was reflected in findings from Scott et al. (2018), who reported that while high-intensity aerobic training was safe in patients with metastatic breast cancer, a substantial proportion of participants were unable to adhere to the programme (51). Nevertheless, in those who completed the intervention, improvements in cardiorespiratory fitness (VO_2peak) were observed, demonstrating physiological efficacy.

Other trials reinforce the feasibility of exercise during active cancer treatment. Park et al. (2023) found that patients with advanced gastrointestinal cancer undergoing palliative chemotherapy were able to comply with a moderate-intensity exercise programme (52). Those who maintained adherence preserved muscle mass and physical function over 6 weeks, with no safety concerns and QoL was maintained. Similarly, Singh et al. (2018) showed that supervised exercise in stage II and III breast cancer patients was not only feasible and safe but also led to improvements in QoL, cardiorespiratory fitness, fatigue, muscular strength, anxiety, depression, BMI and waist circumference compared to standard care (53). Breast cancer survivors who undertook 12 weeks of high-intensity interval training (HIIT) showed improvements in cardiorespiratory fitness, percentage lean mass, upper and lower muscle strength and QoL, with no adverse events reported (54). These studies suggest that while exercise intensity may influence feasibility, it is not the only determinant. When delivered with appropriate supervision, individualisation and behavioural support, both moderate- and higher-intensity interventions can be feasible and well-tolerated, as evidenced by the INTERVAL-GAP4 trial (43).

From the patient's perspective, exercise intensity is closely tied to perceived exertion, recovery needs and overall experience. While higher-intensity training may offer a sense of achievement or empowerment, it may also raise concerns about fatigue, safety or treatment interference. As such, individual preferences, goals and readiness for change should inform the design of intensity-specific exercise prescriptions. A flexible, person-centred approach is critical for optimising adherence and long-term engagement.

6.5 The concept of minimum effective dose

The idea of a minimum effective dose of exercise, which is defined as the smallest quantity required to elicit meaningful biological or clinical benefits, has become increasingly important in exercise oncology. It provides a practical benchmark for clinicians and patients, particularly in settings where time, energy or treatment side effects limit the capacity for higher volumes or intensities of activity. For instance, among colon cancer survivors, 150 minutes per week of moderate-intensity aerobic exercise produced significant reductions in IL-6 and C-reactive protein (CRP), whereas further increases to 300 minutes per week did not yield additional anti-inflammatory effects, implying a threshold above which returns diminish (55). Meta-analyses reveal 850 metabolic equivalent (MET)-minutes per week is near-optimal for QoL outcomes, with lower doses (~430 MET-minutes per week of aerobic activity) still conferring benefit (56). In resistance training contexts, guidelines often adopt a minimal prescription of two sets of 8–15 repetitions at 60–85% 1-RM (one repetition maximum), and some trials suggest that two weekly sessions may suffice to improve fitness or patient-reported outcomes (57). Finally, the exercise oncology guideline literature itself often anchors around moderate-intensity protocols of 150 minutes per week combined with two resistance training sessions per week, implicitly treating this as a working minimal therapeutic dose (58).

PATIENT VIGNETTE 6.1 "Mike"—motivation and uncertainty

Mike, 70, had prostate cancer and was deeply sceptical about exercise. "I thought it would just wear me out," he admitted. It wasn't until a clinical nurse specialist encouraged him to try light resistance bands that he gave it a go. "I was surprised how good it felt."

His confidence grew as he tracked his progress. Now he advocates for earlier exercise guidance. "If I'd had that support sooner, I might've avoided months of feeling weak and unsure."

6.5.1 The 150-minute threshold

The most widely cited recommendation is a minimum of 150 minutes per week of moderate-intensity aerobic exercise, or 75 minutes of vigorous-intensity activity, often accompanied by two to three sessions of resistance training. These guidelines, initially developed for the general population, have been endorsed for cancer survivors by organisations such as the American College of Sports Medicine (ACSM) and World Cancer Research Fund (2,59). Accumulating evidence suggests that this threshold is sufficient to improve cardiorespiratory fitness, reduce cancer-related fatigue, enhance QoL, and in some cases, lower the risk of recurrence and mortality. For example, post hoc analyses from trials such as CHALLENGE suggest that individuals who reach or exceed the 150-minute target experience superior disease-free survival compared with those who do not (60).

6.5.2 What "one size fits all" fails to capture

Despite the utility of the 150-minute guideline, growing evidence indicates that this dose may not be universally optimal. Biological responses to exercise vary across tumour types, treatment phases and individual host characteristics. For instance, people undergoing chemotherapy may experience greater fatigue or immunosuppression, altering their physiological tolerance and the biological yield of a given dose (61). Similarly, TMEs may differ in their responsiveness to exercise-induced signals, particularly across cancers with varied vascularity or immunogenicity. Indeed, the capacity of tumours to respond to exercise-induced systemic cues likely depends on their underlying vascular architecture, baseline hypoxia, immune infiltration and stromal composition (62–65). Indeed, multiple preclinical models show that not all tumours respond equally to exercise: In murine pancreatic and breast tumour xenografts, aerobic exercise induced vascular remodelling, improved perfusion and enhanced chemotherapy delivery in some models but not others (24,66,67). Similarly, Morrell et al. (2019)

demonstrated that exercise reduced endothelial permeability and improved oxygenation in a paediatric tumour model, but the magnitude of effect likely depends on tumour-specific traits (26).

This accumulating evidence reinforces the need to move beyond generic exercise prescriptions in oncology. In their seminal paper, Jones et al. (2017) challenged the prevailing assumption that a uniform exercise dose can elicit consistent physiological or tumour-modifying effects across diverse populations (68). Drawing on mechanistic insights from exercise physiology, they argued that distinct physiological systems respond to specific combinations of intensity, duration and frequency. For example, in healthy participants, high-intensity exercise sessions of shorter duration (approximately 30 minutes) activate mitochondrial biogenesis and angiogenesis within skeletal muscle, effects which do not occur in response to low-to-moderate-intensity sessions of longer duration (≥60 minutes) (69,70). Importantly, exercise-induced benefits may differ across tumour subtypes or molecular profiles. For instance, in the context of breast cancer, oestrogen receptor (ER)-positive tumours are particularly responsive to exercise (71), supporting the idea that exercise prescriptions should be based on a rational hypothesis designed to optimise ER inhibition, or that of its 74 ligands or coactivators. This perspective aligns with the broader recognition that host- and tumour-specific factors, including vascularity, immunogenicity and treatment phase, modulate the biological response to exercise. This movement towards precision exercise oncology in which prescriptions are rationally designed and matched to individual and disease-specific variables holds promise for enhancing therapeutic efficacy and clinical relevance.

6.5.3 Heterogeneity in response

Individual differences in exercise response are influenced by multiple factors, including treatment status (e.g., ongoing chemotherapy versus post-treatment), comorbidities and functional status, age and sex, genetic and epigenetic modifiers of trainability, and baseline inflammatory and metabolic profiles (72) (see Section 6.6). For some individuals, lower doses of exercise may still elicit measurable benefit, while others may require a higher volume or intensity to achieve similar outcomes. Notably, even small increases in physical activity above a sedentary baseline appear to improve health and QoL, and may provide partial protection against cancer progression, particularly in physically deconditioned or frail populations (73,74).

6.6 Towards precision exercise prescription

The concept of precision exercise prescription draws from the broader movement towards personalised medicine and aims to match exercise parameters to the unique biological, clinical and psychosocial profile of each patient.

6.6.1 Personalising exercise: key determinants

Multiple factors influence the optimal type, intensity and timing of exercise for individual living with and beyond cancer (Figure 6.2) and are briefly mentioned below but are discussed in more detail in Chapter 7. These factors include:

Cancer type and stage: Exercise may interact differently with tumours depending on their vascularity, immunogenicity and metastatic potential. For instance, vascular normalisation may be particularly beneficial in solid tumours with hypoxic cores, while immune mobilisation may be more relevant in immunogenic cancers such as melanoma (68,75).

Treatment status and modality: Individuals undergoing chemotherapy, immunotherapy, radiation or targeted therapy present distinct physiological challenges. Exercise must be adapted to mitigate treatment-related side effects without exacerbating fatigue or immunosuppression (76).

Baseline fitness and comorbidities: Functional capacity, cardiorespiratory fitness and the presence of comorbid conditions (e.g., CVD, diabetes) determine both the safety and efficacy of different exercise intensities (77).

Age, sex and body composition: Hormonal status, sarcopenia risk and metabolic differences may shape both responsiveness and recovery from exercise (72).

Biological markers of response: Emerging evidence suggests that individual variability in inflammatory markers, stress hormones, mitochondrial function and even tumour genomics may predict exercise responsiveness, opening the door for biomarker-guided prescription (78).

6.6.2 From population guidelines to precision interventions

Current public health guidelines provide a valuable baseline for exercise promotion in cancer care. However, a key challenge ahead lies in transitioning from these broad recommendations to individualised regimens, guided by ongoing assessment, patient goals and adaptive programming. This approach echoes the principles of precision oncology, in which treatments are matched to tumour biology. Similarly, exercise prescriptions could potentially be stratified by molecular subtype, treatment trajectory and host factors, using tools such as cardiopulmonary exercise testing (CPET), wearable technology (e.g., smart w atches) and blood-based biomarkers to refine dose and monitor efficacy. As more trials begin to account for baseline fitness, tumour phenotype and treatment status, there

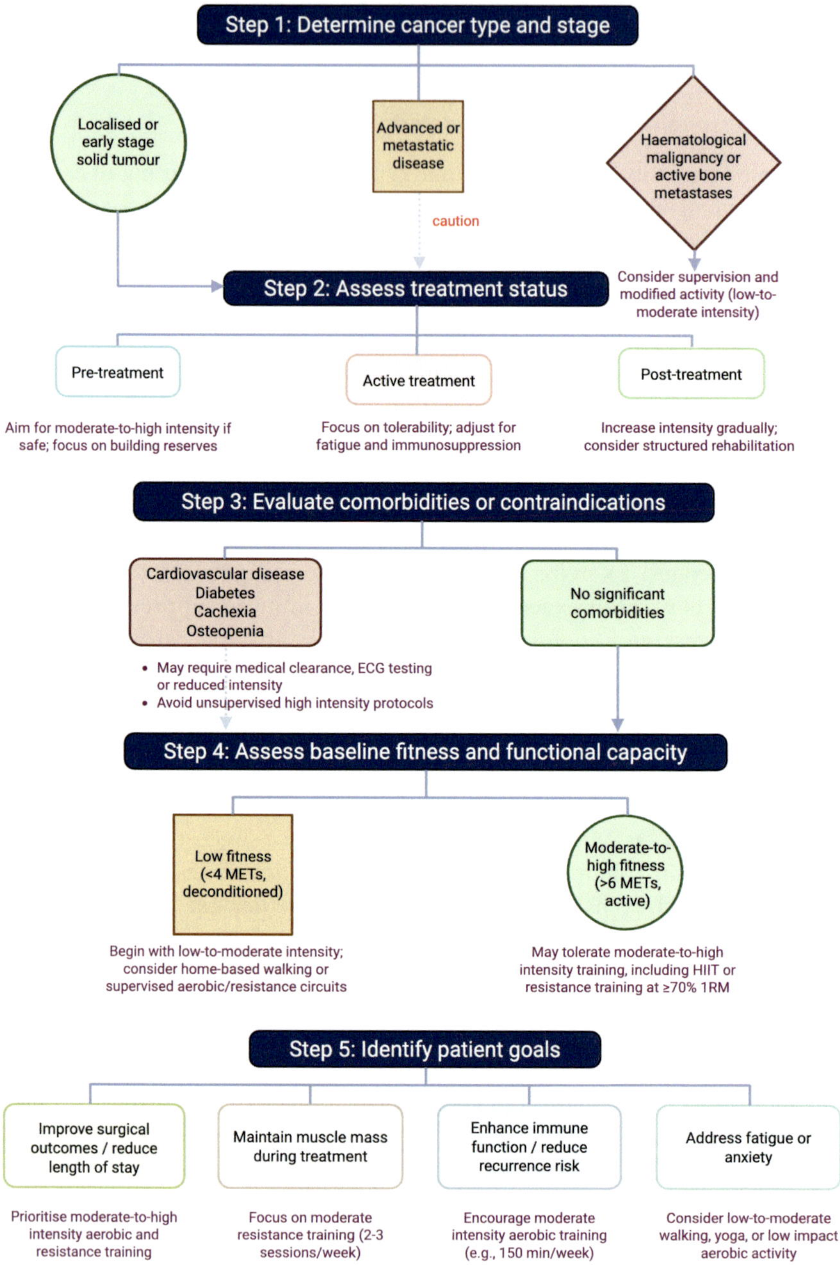

FIGURE 6.2 Clinical decision-making framework for tailoring exercise intensity in cancer care. This flowchart outlines a stepwise approach for determining appropriate exercise intensity in individuals living with and beyond cancer. Starting with cancer type and stage (Step 1),

(*Continued*)

FIGURE 6.2 (Continued) the framework incorporates treatment status (Step 2), comorbidities (Step 3), baseline functional capacity (Step 4), and patient-specific goals (Step 5) to inform safe and effective exercise prescription. Recommendations consider common clinical scenarios, such as prehabilitation, active treatment, and survivorship, as well as common goals including immune enhancement, fatigue reduction, and surgical optimisation. Caution is advised for individuals with advanced disease, haematological malignancies, or significant comorbidities, with emphasis on supervision, gradual progression, and individualisation of intensity. This framework supports the delivery of precision exercise intervention in oncology, balancing efficacy with feasibility and patient safety. Created in Biorender.com.

is growing interest in "exercise phenotyping" as a potential foundation for safer, more effective and personalised interventions across the cancer continuum (75).

6.7 Practical considerations for clinicians

Translating evidence on exercise intensity into clinical care requires consideration of both benefit and risk, along with a flexible, patient-centred approach to prescription.

6.7.1 Balancing benefit and risk by intensity

Moderate-intensity exercise is the most widely supported and feasible option in oncology care. It is consistently associated with improvements in fatigue, fitness, QoL, and in some contexts, disease-free survival (60,79). High-intensity exercise may offer added physiological or immunological benefits, particularly for patients with good baseline fitness or metabolic dysfunction, but requires more cautious implementation. Screening, supervision and structured progression are essential to mitigate risks such as transient immunosuppression or overtraining (80–82). Low-intensity activity, while less likely to trigger tumour-suppressive mechanisms, remains important for maintaining mobility, reducing sedentary behaviour and supporting mental wellbeing, especially in frail or treatment-restricted individuals (81,83). Evidence also supports the inclusion of presurgical aerobic and resistance training for patients preparing for cancer surgery. Structured prehabilitation programmes have been shown to improve cardiovascular fitness, muscle strength and QoL, and may reduce the length of hospital stay (80,84,85). Effective interventions have ranged from high-intensity interval training (e.g., cycling five days per week for 30 minutes at 50–100% of VO_2max) to combined moderate aerobic and resistance training (3 hours per week of moderate aerobic exercise plus 40 minutes of strength training) (86,87). Current guidelines recommend a pre-surgical protocol that includes endurance exercise (60–90% of VO_2max) for 20–35 minutes and strength training involving whole-body movements using bodyweight or light resistance (0–40% of 1RM), typically performed in two sets of ten repetitions, alongside stretching exercises for major muscle groups (58,88–92). These structured programmes reflect a growing clinical consensus that exercise intensity can, and should, be safely prescribed even in pre-operative oncology settings to optimise outcomes.

6.7.2 *The role of warm-up, recovery and monitoring*

Warm-up prior to exercise is especially critical before higher-intensity sessions. A progressive warm-up enhances vascular function, reduces endothelial shear stress and may prevent acute spikes in blood pressure that could promote tumour cell dissemination (93,96). Adequate recovery between sessions is essential to prevent chronic inflammation, immune suppression and fatigue accumulation (94,97). Clinicians should monitor for signs of over-reaching and adjust accordingly. Use of heart rate, perceived exertion (e.g., Borg RPE scale) and symptom checklists can help titrate intensity safely. For selected patients, objective measures such as heart rate variability (HRV), CPET or wearable data may provide further insight (2).

6.7.3 *Communication and collaboration*

Clinicians play a key role in educating patients, setting realistic goals and referring to qualified exercise professionals where available. Integrating exercise into survivorship care plans requires interdisciplinary collaboration and recognition of exercise as a biological therapy with dose, side effects and response variation, not merely a lifestyle adjunct. Greater consideration of the role of the multidisciplinary treatment team is provided in Chapter 8.

6.8 Summary and key takeaways

Exercise intensity is a critical variable in the context of cancer biology and survivorship. This chapter has explored how different levels of intensity, from low to high, elicit distinct systemic and molecular responses, each with implications for tumour progression, immune function and treatment tolerance. Preclinical studies demonstrate that moderate-intensity aerobic exercise exerts robust anti-tumour effects, including enhanced immune surveillance, improved vascular function and reduced metastatic spread. By contrast, high-intensity exercise may amplify certain beneficial responses such as NK cell mobilisation and angiogenesis, but also carries the risk of transient immunosuppression or stress-induced dissemination if not properly dosed or recovered.

Clinical trials, including CHALLENGE and INTERVAL-GAP4, confirm that both moderate and vigorous exercise can be delivered safely in oncology populations, with emerging evidence suggesting potential survival benefits. However, adherence, feasibility and patient experience vary by intensity, emphasising the need for flexible, individualised programming. As such, the concept of a minimum effective dose provides a pragmatic starting point for many: typically, 150 minutes per week of moderate-intensity activity. However, individual variability, tumour biology, treatment context and patient goals all necessitate more personalised approaches. Precision exercise prescription, guided by host, tumour and treatment characteristics, is likely to represent the future of exercise oncology.

Ultimately, the challenge lies in balancing biological efficacy with clinical feasibility. Exercise should be recognised as a scalable, dose-dependent intervention capable of reprogramming the TME. When intensity is individualised, it becomes a powerful tool in cancer care, enhancing resilience, improving outcomes and supporting survivorship across the cancer continuum.

Chapter 6 Test your understanding question bank

1. Which physiological parameter is considered the most accurate objective measure of exercise intensity?
2. Explain the difference between exercise volume and intensity.
3. Which type of immune cell is most acutely mobilised in response to high-intensity exercise?
4. What is the "J-shaped curve" in exercise immunology, and how does it apply to exercise oncology?
5. List two biological pathways activated by high-intensity exercise that may influence tumour biology.
6. Name one potential risk associated with poorly recovered high-intensity exercise in cancer patients.

7. Describe one benefit and one limitation of using RPE (rating of perceived exertion) to measure exercise intensity in cancer patients.
8. What does the term "minimum effective dose" mean in the context of exercise oncology?
9. What is meant by "precision exercise prescription"?
10. What are some recommended features of a prehabilitation programme for cancer surgery?
11. Why is warm-up considered essential before high-intensity exercise, particularly in cancer populations?
12. Summarise one mechanistic reason by moderate-intensity exercise is beneficial in suppressing tumour growth?
13. What are some of the individual factors that may influence exercise response in cancer patients?
14. A patient undergoing chemotherapy reports severe fatigue. What intensity of exercise might be appropriate to recommend and why?
15. How might future exercise oncology trials integrate the concept of phenotyping?

References

1. MacIntosh BR, Murias JM, Keir DA, Weir JM. What is moderate to vigorous exercise intensity? Front Physiol [Internet]. 2021 Sep 22 [cited 2025 Nov 22];12:682233. Available from: https://pmc.ncbi.nlm.nih.gov/articles/PMC8493117/
2. American College of Sports Medicine. ACSM's guidelines for exercise testing and prescription / [Internet]. Wolters Kluwer. 2022 [cited 2025 Nov 14]. Available from: https://books.google.com/books/about/ACSM_s_Guidelines_for_Exercise_Testing_a.html?hl=sl&id=hTKvzgEACAAJ
3. Wang Q, Zhou W. Roles and molecular mechanisms of physical exercise in cancer prevention and treatment. J Sport Health Sci [Internet]. 2020 Mar 1 [cited 2025 Nov 22];10(2):201. Available from: https://pmc.ncbi.nlm.nih.gov/articles/PMC7987556/
4. Nieman DC. Risk of upper respiratory tract infection in athletes: An epidemiologic and immunologic perspective. J Athl Train [Internet]. 1997 Oct [cited 2025 Nov 22];32(4):344. Available from: https://pmc.ncbi.nlm.nih.gov/articles/PMC1320353/
5. Chamorro-Viña C, Fernandez-Del-Valle M, Tacón AM. Excessive exercise and immunity: The J-shaped curve. The Active Female [Internet]. 2013 Jan 1 [cited 2025 Nov 22];357. Available from: https://pmc.ncbi.nlm.nih.gov/articles/PMC7176256/
6. Pedersen L, Idorn M, Olofsson GH, Lauenborg B, Nookaew I, Hansen RH, et al. Voluntary running suppresses tumor growth through epinephrine- and IL-6-dependent NK cell mobilization and redistribution. Cell Metab. 2016 Mar 8;23(3):554–62.
7. Idorn M, thor Straten P. Exercise and cancer: From "healthy" to "therapeutic"? Cancer Immunol Immunother [Internet]. 2017 May 1 [cited 2025 Nov 16];66(5):667–71. Available from: https://pubmed.ncbi.nlm.nih.gov/28324125/

8. Luu TV, Fleischer Hach L, Seremet T, Leuchte K, thor Straten P, Holmen Olofsson G. Exercise duration modulates cortisol release and chronic cortisol exposure jeopardises T cell effector functions. Immunology [Internet]. 2025 [cited 2025 Nov 22]. Available from: https://pubmed.ncbi.nlm.nih.gov/40796353/
9. Wang JS, Chang CY, Chow SE, Chen YW, Yang CM. Exercise modulates platelet-nasopharyngeal carcinoma cell aggregation and subsequent tissue factor and matrix metalloproteinase activities. J Appl Physiol [Internet]. 2007 Sep [cited 2025 Nov 22];103(3):763–70. Available from: https://journals.physiology.org/doi/10.1152/japplphysiol.00165.2007
10. Woods JA, Davis JM, Mayer EP, Ghaffar A, Pate RR. Effects of exercise on macrophage activation for antitumor cytotoxicity. J Appl Physiol (1985) [Internet]. 1994 [cited 2025 Nov 22];76(5):2177–85. Available from: https://pubmed.ncbi.nlm.nih.gov/8063684/
11. de ten Ryen S van D, Deldicque L. The regulation of the metastatic cascade by physical activity: A narrative review. Cancers (Basel) [Internet]. 2020 [cited 2025 Nov 14];12(1):153. Available from: https://pmc.ncbi.nlm.nih.gov/articles/PMC7017263/
12. Gomes-Santos IL, Kumar AS, Hausmann F, Meyer MN, Shiferaw SZ, Amoozgar Z, et al. Exercise intensity governs tumor control in mice with breast cancer. Front Immunol. 2024 Mar 1;15:1339232.
13. Alves CRR, Neves W das, Tobias GC, Almeida NR de, Barreto RF, Melo CM, et al. High-intensity interval training slows down tumor progression in mice bearing Lewis lung carcinoma. JCSM Rapid Commun [Internet]. 2018 Jul 1 [cited 2025 Nov 22];1(2):1–10. Available from: https://onlinelibrary.wiley.com/doi/full/10.1002/j.2617-1619.2018.tb00008.x
14. Jee H, Park E, Hur K, Kang M, Kim Y. High-intensity aerobic exercise suppresses cancer growth by regulating skeletal muscle-derived oncogenes and tumor suppressors. Front Mol Biosci [Internet]. 2022 Jun 21 [cited 2025 Nov 22];9:818470. Available from: www.frontiersin.org
15. Voltarelli VA, Amano MT, Tobias GC, Borges GS, Oliveira da Paixão A, Pereira MG, et al. Moderate-intensity aerobic exercise training improves CD8+ tumor-infiltrating lymphocytes effector function by reducing mitochondrial loss. iScience. 2024 Jun 21;27(6):110121.
16. Fei Z, Li D, Li K, Zhou M, Li Y, Li Y, et al. Detraining after tumor-bearing accelerates tumor growth while continuous training decreases tumor growth in mice. J Tradit Chin Med Sci. 2020 Mar 1;7(1):75–81.
17. Eschke RCKR, Lampit A, Schenk A, Javelle F, Steindorf K, Diel P, et al. Impact of physical exercise on growth and progression of cancer in rodents—A systematic review and meta-analysis. Front Oncol [Internet]. 2019 Feb [cited 2025 Nov 22];9:35. Available from: https://pmc.ncbi.nlm.nih.gov/articles/PMC6370688/
18. Campbell JP, Riddell NE, Burns VE, Turner M, van Zanten JJCSV, Drayson MT, et al. Acute exercise mobilises CD8+ T lymphocytes exhibiting an effector-memory phenotype. Brain Behav Immun [Internet]. 2009 Aug [cited 2025 Nov 22];23(6):767–75. Available from: https://pubmed.ncbi.nlm.nih.gov/19254756/
19. Djurhuus SS, Simonsen C, Toft BG, Thomsen SN, Wielsøe S, Røder MA, et al. Exercise training to increase tumour natural killer-cell infiltration in men with localised prostate cancer: A randomised controlled trial. BJU Int [Internet]. 2023 Jan 1 [cited 2025 Nov 22];131(1):116–24. Available from: https://pubmed.ncbi.nlm.nih.gov/35753072/

20. Muscari I, Fierabracci A, Adorisio S, Moretti M, Cannarile L, Thi Minh Hong V, et al. Glucocorticoids and natural killer cells: A suppressive relationship. Biochem Pharmacol. 2022 Apr 1;198:114930.
21. Schadler KL, Thomas NJ, Galie PA, Bhang DH, Roby KC, Addai P, et al. Tumor vessel normalization after aerobic exercise enhances chemotherapeutic efficacy. Oncotarget [Internet]. 2016 [cited 2025 Nov 14];7(40):65429. Available from: https://pmc.ncbi.nlm.nih.gov/articles/PMC5323166/
22. Regmi S, Fu A, Luo KQ. High shear stresses under exercise condition destroy circulating tumor cells in a microfluidic system. Sci Rep [Internet]. 2017 Jan 5 [cited 2025 Nov 18];7. Available from: https://pubmed.ncbi.nlm.nih.gov/28054593/
23. Morrell MBG, Alvarez-Florez C, Zhang A, Kleinerman ES, Savage H, Marmonti E, et al. Vascular modulation through exercise improves chemotherapy efficacy in Ewing sarcoma. Pediatr Blood Cancer [Internet]. 2019 Sep 1 [cited 2025 Nov 22];66(9):e27835. Available from: https://onlinelibrary.wiley.com/doi/full/10.1002/pbc.27835
24. Magnussen AL, Mills IG. Vascular normalisation as the stepping stone into tumour microenvironment transformation. Br J Cancer [Internet]. 2021 Apr 7 [cited 2025 Nov 22];125(3):324–36. Available from: https://www.nature.com/articles/s41416-021-01330-z
25. Brown JC, Rhim AD, Manning SL, Brennan L, Mansour AI, Rustgi AK, et al. Effects of exercise on circulating tumor cells among patients with resected stage I-III colon cancer. PLoS One [Internet]. 2018 Oct 1 [cited 2025 Nov 22];13(10):e0204875. Available from: https://journals.plos.org/plosone/article?id=10.1371/journal.pone.0204875
26. Dethlefsen C, Hansen LS, Lillelund C, Andersen C, Gehl J, Christensen JF, et al. Exercise-induced catecholamines activate the hippo tumor suppressor pathway to reduce risks of breast cancer development. Cancer Res [Internet]. 2017 Sep 15 [cited 2019 Dec 6];77(18):4894–904. Available from: http://cancerres.aacrjournals.org/lookup/doi/10.1158/0008-5472.CAN-16-3125
27. Westerlind KC, Mccarty HL, Gibson KJ, Strange R. Effect of exercise on the rat mammary gland: Implications for carcinogenesis. Acta Physiol Scand [Internet]. 2002 [cited 2025 Nov 22];175(2):147–56. Available from: https://pubmed.ncbi.nlm.nih.gov/12028135/
28. Cohen LA, Boylan E, Epstein M, Zang E. Voluntary exercise and experimental mammary cancer. Adv Exp Med Biol [Internet]. 1992 [cited 2025 Nov 22];322:41–59. Available from: https://pubmed.ncbi.nlm.nih.gov/1442300/
29. Zheng A, Zhang L, Yang J, Yin X, Zhang T, Wu X, et al. Physical activity prevents tumor metastasis through modulation of immune function. Front Pharmacol. 2022 Oct 12;13:1034129.
30. Nash D, Hughes MG, Butcher L, Aicheler R, Smith P, Cullen T, et al. IL-6 signaling in acute exercise and chronic training: Potential consequences for health and athletic performance. Scand J Med Sci Sports [Internet]. 2022 Jan 1 [cited 2025 Nov 22];33(1):4. Available from: https://pmc.ncbi.nlm.nih.gov/articles/PMC10092579/
31. Jiménez-Maldonado A, Montero S, Lemus M, Cerna-Cortés J, Rodríguez-Hernández A, Mendoza MA, et al. Moderate and high intensity chronic exercise reduces plasma tumor necrosis factor alpha and increases the Langerhans islet area in healthy rats. J Musculoskelet Neuronal Interact [Internet]. 2019 Sep 1 [cited 2025 Nov 22];19(3):354. Available from: https://pmc.ncbi.nlm.nih.gov/articles/PMC6737555/
32. Baldelli G, De Santi M, Gervasi M, Annibalini G, Sisti D, Højman P, et al. The effects of human sera conditioned by high-intensity exercise sessions and

training on the tumorigenic potential of cancer cells. Clin Transl Oncol [Internet]. 2021 Jan 1 [cited 2025 Nov 16];23(1):22–34. Available from: https://pubmed.ncbi.nlm.nih.gov/32447643/

33. Siewierska K, Malicka I, Kobierzycki C, Paslawska U, Cegielski M, Grzegrzolka J, et al. The impact of exercise training on breast cancer. In Vivo [Internet]. 2018 [cited 2025 Nov 22];32(2):249–54. Available from: https://pubmed.ncbi.nlm.nih.gov/29475906/
34. Sáez M del C, Barriga C, García JJ, Rodríguez AB, Ortega E. Exercise-induced stress enhances mammary tumor growth in rats: Beneficial effect of the hormone melatonin. Mol Cell Biochem [Internet]. 2007 Jan [cited 2025 Nov 22];294(1–2):19–24. Available from: https://pubmed.ncbi.nlm.nih.gov/17136443/
35. Thompson HJ, Westerlind KC, Snedden J, Singh M. Exercise intensity dependent inhibition of 1-methyl-1-nitrosourea induced mammary carcinogenesis in female F-344 rats. Carcinogenesis [Internet]. 1995 Aug [cited 2025 Nov 22];16(8):1783–6. Available from: https://pubmed.ncbi.nlm.nih.gov/7634404/
36. Thompson HJ. Effects of physical activity and exercise on experimentally-induced mammary carcinogenesis. Breast Cancer Res Treat. 1997;46(2–3):135–41.
37. Mizrahi D, Broderick C, Friedlander M, Ryan M, Harrison M, Pumpa K, et al. An exercise intervention during chemotherapy for women with recurrent ovarian cancer: A feasibility study. Int J Gynecol Cancer. 2015 Jul 1;25(6):985–92.
38. Booth CM, Vardy JL, O'Callaghan CJ, Gill S, Friedenreich C, Wong RK, et al. A randomized phase III trial of the impact of a structured exercise program on Disease-Free Survival (DFS) in stage 3 or high-risk stage 2 colon cancer: Canadian Cancer Trials Group (CCTG) CO.21 (Challenge). J Clin Oncol [Internet]. 2025 Jun 10 [cited 2025 Nov 22];43(17_suppl). Available from: https://ascopubs.org/doi/10.1200/JCO.2025.43.17_suppl.LBA3510
39. Newton RU, Lopez P, Hart NH, Galvao DA, Taaffe DR, Clay TD, et al. Intense exercise for survival among men with metastatic prostate cancer: 12 months feasibility results from the INTERVAL-GAP4 trial. JCO Glob Oncol [Internet]. 2023 Aug [cited 2025 Nov 22];9(Supplement_1):81. Available from: https://ascopubs.org/doi/10.1200/GO.2023.9.Supplement_1.81
40. Demmelmaier I, Brooke HL, Henriksson A, Mazzoni AS, Bjørke ACH, Igelström H, et al. Does exercise intensity matter for fatigue during (neo-)adjuvant cancer treatment? The Phys-Can randomized clinical trial. Scand J Med Sci Sports [Internet]. 2021 May 1 [cited 2025 Nov 22];31(5):1144–59. Available from: https://pubmed.ncbi.nlm.nih.gov/33527488/
41. Pelzer F, Leisge K, Schlüter K, Schneider J, Wiskemann J, Rosenberger F. Effects of exercise mode and intensity on patient-reported outcomes in cancer survivors: A four-arm intervention trial. Supportive Care in Cancer [Internet]. 2023 May 1 [cited 2025 Nov 22];31(5):315. Available from: https://pmc.ncbi.nlm.nih.gov/articles/PMC10154283/
42. Holmen Olofsson G, Mikkelsen MK, Ragle AM, Christiansen AB, Olsen AP, Heide-Ottosen L, et al. High intensity aerobic exercise training and Immune cell mobilization in patients with lung cancer (HI AIM)—A randomized controlled trial. BMC Cancer [Internet]. 2022 Dec 1 [cited 2025 Nov 22];22(1):246. Available from: https://bmccancer.biomedcentral.com/articles/10.1186/s12885-022-09349-y
43. Mctiernan A, Friedenreich CM, Katzmarzyk PT, Powell KE, Macko R, Buchner D, et al. Physical activity in cancer prevention and survival: A systematic review. Med Sci Sports Exerc [Internet]. 2019 Jun [cited 2024 Nov 8];51(6):1252–61. Available from: https://journals.lww.com/00005768-201906000-00020
44. Schmid D, Leitzmann MF. Association between physical activity and mortality among breast cancer and colorectal cancer survivors: A systematic review and

meta-analysis. Ann Oncol [Internet]. 2014 [cited 2025 Nov 22];25(7):1293–311. Available from: https://pubmed.ncbi.nlm.nih.gov/24644304/
45. Friedenreich CM, Neilson HK, Farris MS, Courneya KS. Physical activity and cancer outcomes: A precision medicine approach. Clin Cancer Res [Internet]. 2016 Oct 1 [cited 2025 Nov 22];22(19):4766–75. Available from: https://pubmed.ncbi.nlm.nih.gov/27407093/
46. Takemura N, Chan SL, Smith R, Cheung DST, Lin CC. The effects of physical activity on overall survival among advanced cancer patients: A systematic review and meta-analysis. BMC Cancer [Internet]. 2021 Dec 1 [cited 2025 Nov 22];21(1):242. Available from: https://bmccancer.biomedcentral.com/articles/10.1186/s12885-021-07988-1
47. Scott JM, Iyengar NM, Nilsen TS, Michalski M, Thomas SM, Herndon J, et al. Feasibility, safety, and efficacy of aerobic training in pretreated patients with metastatic breast cancer: A randomized controlled trial. Cancer [Internet]. 2018 Jun 15 [cited 2025 Nov 22];124(12):2552–60. Available from: https://onlinelibrary.wiley.com/doi/full/10.1002/cncr.31368
48. Park SE, Kim DH, Kim DK, Ha JY, Jang JS, Choi JH, et al. Feasibility and safety of exercise during chemotherapy in people with gastrointestinal cancers: A pilot study. Supportive Care in Cancer [Internet]. 2023 Oct 1 [cited 2025 Nov 22];31(10):561. Available from: https://pmc.ncbi.nlm.nih.gov/articles/PMC10480261/
49. Singh B, Spence RR, Steele ML, Sandler CX, Peake JM, Hayes SC. A systematic review and meta-analysis of the safety, feasibility, and effect of exercise in women with stage II+ breast cancer. Arch Phys Med Rehabil [Internet]. 2018 Dec 1 [cited 2025 Nov 22];99(12):2621–36. Available from: https://www.archives-pmr.org/action/showFullText?pii=S0003999318302806
50. Bettariga F, Taaffe DR, Crespo-Garcia C, Clay TD, Galvão DA, Newton RU. Effects of resistance training vs high intensity interval training on body composition, muscle strength, cardiorespiratory fitness, and quality of life in survivors of breast cancer: A randomized trial. Breast Cancer Res Treat [Internet]. 2025 Apr 1 [cited 2025 Nov 22];210(2):261–70. Available from: https://pubmed.ncbi.nlm.nih.gov/39557768/
51. Pedersen BK, Febbraio MA. Muscle as an endocrine organ: Focus on muscle-derived interleukin-6. Physiol Rev [Internet]. 2008 Oct [cited 2025 Nov 22];88(4):1379–406. Available from: https://pubmed.ncbi.nlm.nih.gov/18923185/
52. Benatti FB, Pedersen BK. Exercise as an anti-inflammatory therapy for rheumatic diseases-myokine regulation. Nat Rev Rheumatol [Internet]. 2015 Feb 17 [cited 2025 Nov 22];11(2):86–97. Available from: https://pubmed.ncbi.nlm.nih.gov/25422002/
53. Docherty S, Harley R, McAuley JJ, Crowe LAN, Pedret C, Kirwan PD, et al. The effect of exercise on cytokines: implications for musculoskeletal health: A narrative review. BMC Sports Sci Med Rehabil [Internet]. 2022 Dec 1 [cited 2025 Nov 16];14(1):5. Available from: https://pmc.ncbi.nlm.nih.gov/articles/PMC8740100/
54. Timper K, Denson JL, Steculorum SM, Heilinger C, Engström-Ruud L, Wunderlich CM, et al. IL-6 improves energy and glucose homeostasis in obesity via enhanced central IL-6 trans-signaling. Cell Rep. 2017 Apr 11;19(2):267–80.
55. Carey AL, Steinberg GR, Macaulay SL, Thomas WG, Holmes AG, Ramm G, et al. Interleukin-6 increases insulin-stimulated glucose disposal in humans and glucose uptake and fatty acid oxidation in vitro via AMP-activated protein kinase. Diabetes [Internet]. 2006 Oct [cited 2025 Nov 22];55(10):2688–97. Available from: https://pubmed.ncbi.nlm.nih.gov/17003332/

56. Idorn M, Hojman P. Exercise-dependent regulation of NK cells in cancer protection. Trends Mol Med [Internet]. 2016 Jul 1 [cited 2025 Nov 22];22(7):565–77. Available from: https://www.cell.com/action/showFullText?pii=S1471491416300417
57. Gannon NP, Vaughan RA, Garcia-Smith R, Bisoffi M, Trujillo KA. Effects of the exercise-inducible myokine irisin on malignant and non-malignant breast epithelial cell behavior in vitro. Int J Cancer [Internet]. 2015 Feb 15 [cited 2025 Nov 16];136(4):E197–202. Available from: https://pubmed.ncbi.nlm.nih.gov/25124080/
58. Brown JC, Compton SLE, Meyerhardt JA, Spielmann G, Yang S. The dose-response effect of aerobic exercise on inflammation in colon cancer survivors. Front Oncol. 2023 Dec 12;13:1257767.
59. Xiong Z, Yuan Y, Yang Y, Qiu B, Bai Y, Wang T, et al. Optimal exercise dose-response improves health-related quality of life in cancer survivors: A systematic review and Bayesian network meta-analysis of RCTs. Front Oncol [Internet]. 2024 [cited 2025 Nov 22];14. Available from: https://pubmed.ncbi.nlm.nih.gov/39737404/
60. Lopez P, Taaffe DR, Newton RU, Buffart LM, Galvão DA. What is the minimal dose for resistance exercise effectiveness in prostate cancer patients? Systematic review and meta-analysis on patient-reported outcomes. Prostate Cancer Prostatic Dis [Internet]. 2020 Jun 1 [cited 2025 Nov 22];24(2):465. Available from: https://pmc.ncbi.nlm.nih.gov/articles/PMC8134054/
61. Campbell KL, Winters-Stone KM, Wiskemann J, May AM, Schwartz AL, Courneya KS, et al. Exercise guidelines for cancer survivors. Med Sci Sports Exerc [Internet]. 2019 Nov [cited 2019 Dec 6];51(11):2375–90. Available from: http://www.ncbi.nlm.nih.gov/pubmed/31626055
62. Aicr WCRF. Diet, nutrition, physical activity and cancer: A global perspective A summary of the third expert report. [cited 2025 Nov 14]. Available from: http://gco.iarc.fr/today
63. Booth CM, Vardy JL, O'Callaghan CJ, Gill S, Friedenreich C, Wong RK, et al. A randomized phase III trial of the impact of a structured exercise program on Disease-Free Survival (DFS) in stage 3 or high-risk stage 2 colon cancer: Canadian Cancer Trials Group (CCTG) CO.21 (CHALLENGE). J Clin Oncol [Internet]. 2025 Jun 10 [cited 2025 Nov 22];43(17_suppl). Available from: https://ascopubs.org/doi/10.1200/JCO.2025.43.17_suppl.LBA3510
64. De Hoop AMS, Valkenet K, Dronkers JJ, Krul CAM, Ruurda JP, Veenhof C, et al. Effects of exercise during chemo- or radiotherapy on immune markers: A systematic review. Oncology [Internet]. 2024 May 6 [cited 2025 Nov 22];102(5):425–40. Available from: https://dx.doi.org/10.1159/000534390
65. Buss LA, Dachs GU. Effects of exercise on the tumour microenvironment. Adv Exp Med Biol [Internet]. 2020 [cited 2025 Nov 22];1225:31–51. Available from: https://pubmed.ncbi.nlm.nih.gov/32030646/
66. Koelwyn GJ, Quail DF, Zhang X, White RM, Jones LW. Exercise-dependent regulation of the tumour microenvironment. Nat Rev Cancer [Internet]. 2017 Oct 25 [cited 2019 Dec 6];17(10):620–32. Available from: http://www.nature.com/articles/nrc.2017.78
67. Feng Y, Feng X, Wan R, Luo Z, Qu L, Wang Q. Impact of exercise on cancer: Mechanistic perspectives and new insights. Front Immunol [Internet]. 2024 [cited 2025 Nov 22];15. Available from: https://pubmed.ncbi.nlm.nih.gov/39346906/
68. Jones LW, Eves ND, Scott JM. Bench-to-bedside approaches for personalized exercise therapy in cancer. Am Soc Clin Oncol Educ Book [Internet]. 2017 May [cited 2025 Nov 22];37(37):684–94. Available from: https://pubmed.ncbi.nlm.nih.gov/28561646/

69. Jia N, Zhou Y, Dong X, Ding M. The antitumor mechanisms of aerobic exercise: A review of recent preclinical studies. Cancer Med [Internet]. 2021 Sep 1 [cited 2025 Nov 22];10(18):6365–73. Available from: https://onlinelibrary.wiley.com/doi/full/10.1002/cam4.4169
70. Florez Bedoya CA, Cardoso ACF, Parker N, Ngo-Huang A, Petzel MQ, Kim MP, et al. Exercise during preoperative therapy increases tumor vascularity in pancreatic tumor patients. Sci Rep [Internet]. 2019 Sep 27 [cited 2025 Nov 22];9(1):13966. Available from: https://www.nature.com/articles/s41598-019-49582-3
71. Wakefield ZR, Tanaka M, Pampo C, Lepler S, Rice L, Guingab-Cagmat J, et al. Normal tissue and tumor microenvironment adaptations to aerobic exercise enhance doxorubicin anti-tumor efficacy and ameliorate its cardiotoxicity in retired breeder mice. Oncotarget [Internet]. 2021 Aug 31 [cited 2025 Nov 22];12(18):1737–48. Available from: https://www.oncotarget.com/article/28057/text/
72. MacInnis MJ, Gibala MJ. Physiological adaptations to interval training and the role of exercise intensity. J Physiol [Internet]. 2017 May 1 [cited 2025 Nov 22];595(9):2915–30. Available from: https://pubmed.ncbi.nlm.nih.gov/27748956/
73. MacInnis MJ, Zacharewicz E, Martin BJ, Haikalis ME, Skelly LE, Tarnopolsky MA, et al. Superior mitochondrial adaptations in human skeletal muscle after interval compared to continuous single-leg cycling matched for total work. J Physiol [Internet]. 2017 May 1 [cited 2025 Nov 22];595(9):2955–68. Available from: https://pubmed.ncbi.nlm.nih.gov/27396440/
74. Jones LW, Kwan ML, Weltzien E, Chandarlapaty S, Sternfeld B, Sweeney C, et al. Exercise and prognosis on the basis of clinicopathologic and molecular features in early-stage breast cancer: The LACE and pathways studies. Cancer Res [Internet]. 2016 Sep 15 [cited 2025 Nov 22];76(18):5415–22. Available from: https://pubmed.ncbi.nlm.nih.gov/27488523/
75. Cao C, Friedenreich CM, Yang L. Association of daily sitting time and leisure-time physical activity with survival among US cancer survivors. JAMA Oncol [Internet]. 2022 Mar 1 [cited 2025 Nov 22];8(3):395–403. Available from: https://jamanetwork.com/journals/jamaoncology/fullarticle/2787951
76. Misiąg W, Piszczyk A, Szymańska-Chabowska A, Chabowski M. Physical activity and cancer care—A review. Cancers (Basel) [Internet]. 2022 Sep 1 [cited 2025 Nov 22];14(17):4154. Available from: https://pmc.ncbi.nlm.nih.gov/articles/PMC9454950/
77. Schumacher O, Galvão DA, Taaffe DR, Chee R, Spry N, Newton RU. Exercise modulation of tumour perfusion and hypoxia to improve radiotherapy response in prostate cancer. Prostate Cancer Prostatic Dis [Internet]. 2020 Mar 1 [cited 2025 Nov 22];24(1):1. Available from: https://pmc.ncbi.nlm.nih.gov/articles/PMC8012204/
78. Buffart LM, Kenkhuis MF, Newton RU, May AM, Galvão DA, Courneya KS. Accelerating precision exercise medicine in cancer patients using pooled individual patient data: POLARIS experience. JNCI Cancer Spectr [Internet]. 2025 Sep 1 [cited 2025 Nov 22];9(5). Available from: https://dx.doi.org/10.1093/jncics/pkaf078
79. Azevedo MJ, Viamonte S, Castro A. Exercise prescription in oncology patients: General principles. Rehabilitacion (Madr). 2013 Jul 1;47(3):170–8.
80. Sasso JP, Eves ND, Christensen JF, Koelwyn GJ, Scott J, Jones LW. A framework for prescription in exercise-oncology research. J Cachexia Sarcopenia Muscle [Internet]. 2015 [cited 2025 Nov 22];6(2):115. Available from: https://pmc.ncbi.nlm.nih.gov/articles/PMC4458077/

81. Wang J, He Y, Wang Z, Miao Y, Choi JY. Effects of different exercise prescription parameters on metabolic and inflammatory biomarkers in cancer patients: A systematic review, meta-analysis, and meta-regression. Front Immunol [Internet]. 2025 [cited 2025 Nov 22];16:1663560. Available from: https://pmc.ncbi.nlm.nih.gov/articles/PMC12390815/
82. Mulero Portela AL, Colón Santaella CL, Rogers LQ, Missaghian Vissepo M. Effect of low- and moderate-intensity endurance exercise on physical functioning among breast cancer survivors: A randomized controlled trial. Support Care Cancer [Internet]. 2024 Jan 1 [cited 2025 Nov 22];33(1):49. Available from: https://pmc.ncbi.nlm.nih.gov/articles/PMC11806920/
83. Clemente-Suárez VJ, Martín-Rodríguez A, Redondo-Flórez L, Ruisoto P, Navarro-Jiménez E, Ramos-Campo DJ, et al. Metabolic health, mitochondrial fitness, physical activity, and cancer. Cancers (Basel) [Internet]. 2023 Feb 1 [cited 2025 Nov 22];15(3):814. Available from: https://pmc.ncbi.nlm.nih.gov/articles/PMC9913323/
84. Van Waart H, Stuiver MM, Van Harten WH, Geleijn E, Kieffer JM, Buffart LM, et al. Effect of low-intensity physical activity and moderate- to high-intensity physical exercise during adjuvant chemotherapy on physical fitness, fatigue, and chemotherapy completion rates: Results of the PACES randomized clinical trial. J Clin Oncol [Internet]. 2015 Jun 10 [cited 2025 Nov 22];33(17):1918–27. Available from: https://ascopubs.org/doi/10.1200/JCO.2014.59.1081
85. Hofmann P. Cancer and exercise: Warburg hypothesis, tumour metabolism and high-intensity anaerobic exercise. Sports [Internet]. 2018 Mar 1 [cited 2025 Nov 22];6(1):10. Available from: https://pmc.ncbi.nlm.nih.gov/articles/PMC5969185/
86. Siewierska K, Malicka I, Kobierzycki C, Paslawska U, Cegielski M, Grzegrzolka J, et al. The impact of exercise training on breast cancer. In Vivo [Internet]. 2018 [cited 2025 Nov 22];32(2):249–54. Available from: https://pubmed.ncbi.nlm.nih.gov/29475906/
87. Singh F, Newton RU, Galvão DA, Spry N, Baker MK. A systematic review of pre-surgical exercise intervention studies with cancer patients. Surg Oncol [Internet]. 2013 Jun [cited 2025 Nov 14];22(2):92–104. Available from: https://pubmed.ncbi.nlm.nih.gov/23434347/
88. Liu L, Shi Y, Li T, Qin Q, Yin J, Pang S, et al. Leisure time physical activity and cancer risk: Evaluation of the WHO's recommendation based on 126 high-quality epidemiological studies. Br J Sports Med [Internet]. 2016 Mar 1 [cited 2025 Nov 22];50(6):372–8. Available from: https://pubmed.ncbi.nlm.nih.gov/26500336/
89. Jones LW, Eves ND, Peddle CJ, Courneya KS, Haykowsky M, Kumar V, et al. Effects of presurgical exercise training on systemic inflammatory markers among patients with malignant lung lesions. Appl Physiol Nutr Metab [Internet]. 2009 Apr [cited 2025 Nov 22];34(2):197–202. Available from: https://pubmed.ncbi.nlm.nih.gov/19370050/
90. Ligibel J, Irwin M, Dillon D, Barry W, Giobbie-Hurder A, Frank E, et al. Abstract S5–05: Impact of pre-operative exercise on breast cancer gene expression. Cancer Res [Internet]. 2017 Feb 15 [cited 2025 Nov 22];77(4_Supplement):S5–05. Available from: /cancerres/article/77/4_Supplement/S5-05/624551/Abstract-S5-05-Impact-of-pre-operative-exercise-on
91. Gil-Rey E, Quevedo-Jerez K, Maldonado-Martin S, Herrero-Román F. Exercise intensity guidelines for cancer survivors: A comparison with reference values. Int J Sports Med [Internet]. 2014 Dec [cited 2025 Nov 22];35(14):e1–9. Available from: https://pubmed.ncbi.nlm.nih.gov/25429545/

92. Schmid D, Leitzmann MF. Cardiorespiratory fitness as predictor of cancer mortality: A systematic review and meta-analysis. Ann Oncol [Internet]. 2015 Feb 1 [cited 2025 Nov 22];26(2):272–8. Available from: https://pubmed.ncbi.nlm.nih.gov/25009011/
93. Fuller JT, Hartland MC, Maloney LT, Davison K. Therapeutic effects of aerobic and resistance exercises for cancer survivors: A systematic review of meta-analyses of clinical trials. Br J Sports Med [Internet]. 2018 Oct 1 [cited 2025 Nov 22];52(20):1311. Available from: https://pubmed.ncbi.nlm.nih.gov/29549149/
94. Zhuang C Le, Zhang FM, Li W, Wang KH, Xu HX, Song CH, et al. Associations of low handgrip strength with cancer mortality: A multicentre observational study. J Cachexia Sarcopenia Muscle [Internet]. 2020 Dec 1 [cited 2025 Nov 22];11(6):1476–86. Available from: https://pubmed.ncbi.nlm.nih.gov/32910535/
95. Ruiz JR, Sui X, Lobelo F, Lee DC, Morrow JR, Jackson AW, et al. Muscular strength and adiposity as predictors of adulthood cancer mortality in men. Cancer Epidemiol Biomarkers Prev [Internet]. 2009 May [cited 2025 Nov 22];18(5):1468–76. Available from: https://pubmed.ncbi.nlm.nih.gov/19366909/
96. Padilla J, Simmons GH, Bender SB, Arce-Esquivel AA, Whyte JJ, Laughlin MH. Vascular effects of exercise: Endothelial adaptations beyond active muscle beds. Physiology (Bethesda) [Internet]. 2011 [cited 2025 Nov 22];26(3):132. Available from: https://pmc.ncbi.nlm.nih.gov/articles/PMC3286126/
97. Dupuy O, Douzi W, Theurot D, Bosquet L, Dugué B. An evidence-based approach for choosing post-exercise recovery techniques to reduce markers of muscle damage, soreness, fatigue, and inflammation: A systematic review with meta-analysis. Front Physiol [Internet]. 2018 Apr 26 [cited 2025 Nov 22];9:403. Available from: https://pmc.ncbi.nlm.nih.gov/articles/PMC5932411/

7

FREQUENCY AND LENGTH OF EXERCISE BOUTS

7.1 Introduction

Building on the FITT principle introduced in earlier chapters, this chapter shifts its focus to two often overlooked but essential components of exercise prescription: Frequency (how often) and time (how long). While the type and intensity of exercise, explored in Chapters 5 and 6, have received substantial attention in the cancer and exercise literature, the dose of exercise—comprising frequency and duration—plays a critical role in determining its biological and clinical effects. This chapter focuses on how the dimensions of frequency and time shape outcomes such as tumour biology, immune modulation, treatment tolerance, fatigue and adherence.

From a biological perspective, the frequency and duration of exercise can influence the magnitude and sustainability of molecular and cellular responses. Acute sessions may trigger transient but powerful systemic changes, such as cytokine release, immune mobilisation and metabolic alterations, while regular, repeated bouts are required to induce longer-term adaptations, including changes in gene expression, angiogenesis and tissue remodelling (1–3). Physiologically, adequate frequency and time are needed to achieve training effects on cardiorespiratory fitness, muscular strength and metabolic health, which are all factors known to influence cancer outcomes. Meanwhile, from a behavioural standpoint, the feasibility and acceptability of different exercise schedules affect adherence, which is itself a major determinant of benefit (4,5).

DOI: 10.4324/9781003511519-9

This chapter therefore tackles three central questions in exercise oncology:

1. How often should individuals who are living with or beyond cancer exercise?
2. How long should each exercise session last?
3. For whom are particular exercise doses appropriate?

By integrating current evidence from both laboratory and clinical studies, this chapter aims to provide a nuanced understanding of how frequency and time interact with individual, tumour-related and treatment-specific factors to influence cancer progression, symptom control and survivorship outcomes.

BOX-OUT 7.1 THE FITT PRINCIPLE: A RECAP

The FITT principle is a foundational concept in exercise prescription, used to structure and personalise physical activity interventions. It consists of four key variables:

1. Frequency: How often exercise is performed (e.g., sessions per week)
2. Intensity: How hard the exercise is (e.g., low, moderate, vigorous, % HR_{max} or RPE)
3. Time: The duration of each session (e.g., minutes per bout)
4. Type: The modality of activity (e.g., aerobic, resistance, flexibility)

In the context of exercise oncology, each component of the FITT framework influences the physiological and psychosocial responses to exercise, as well as its safety and efficacy at different stages of the cancer continuum.

7.2 Biological basis for exercise dosing

7.2.1 Acute versus chronic effects

The distinction between acute and chronic exercise is central to understanding how the dose of exercise, particularly frequency and duration, affects cancer biology (6). Acute bouts of exercise trigger immediate, transient physiological responses, while chronic training induces longer-term adaptations across multiple organ systems (7). These two modes of response are not mutually exclusive; rather, they interact dynamically to shape the TME, anti-tumour immune surveillance and systemic homeostasis (8).

Acute exercise, even as a single session, can generate significant systemic perturbations (9). For instance, a single bout of resistance training or high-intensity interval training (HIIT) in breast cancer survivors significantly elevated anti-cancer myokines, such as IL-6, SPARC and decorin, and suppressed the growth of breast cancer cell lines in vitro (10). Similarly, high-intensity endurance cycling has been shown to elevate circulating levels of catecholamines and IL-6, which in turn activate pathways involved in tumour suppression (11). In both murine and in vitro models, these acute hormonal and cytokine surges have been linked to increased mobilisation and redistribution of NK cells, enhanced tumour cell apoptosis and reduced tumour proliferation (11,12). Dethlefsen and colleagues notably demonstrated that catecholamines released during intense exercise activated the Hippo tumour suppressor pathway, reducing breast cancer cell viability via YAP inhibition (11). These rapid-onset changes highlight how single sessions of intense physical activity can act as biological "pulses" that disrupt tumour-supportive signalling.

In contrast, chronic exercise training, defined as regular, repeated bouts over weeks or months, leads to adaptive physiological changes that are stabilising and cumulative (Figure 7.1). These include improvements in mitochondrial biogenesis, systemic insulin sensitivity, enhanced antioxidant capacity and immune reprogramming (13). Such adaptations contribute to a more hostile internal environment for tumour growth and are often associated with a shift towards anti-inflammatory and anti-tumour immune phenotypes (7,8). For example, sustained exercise has been shown to increase CD8+ T cell infiltration into tumours, enhance antigen presentation and downregulate tumour-promoting MDSCs (14). Together, these insights underscore the need to consider both the immediate and cumulative biological effects of exercise when designing dosing strategies. The remainder of this chapter will examine how frequency and time influence these responses and how they can be tailored to individual needs.

7.2.2 Insights from serum studies

One of the most direct ways to explore how exercise modulates cancer biology is through serum transfer studies, in which blood serum collected from individuals before and after exercise is applied to cancer cell cultures. These *in vitro* experiments offer powerful insights into the acute molecular signals mobilised by exercise and the extent to which they alter tumour cell behaviour. A prime example comes from Baldelli et al. (2021), who investigated the effects of serum collected from sedentary individuals

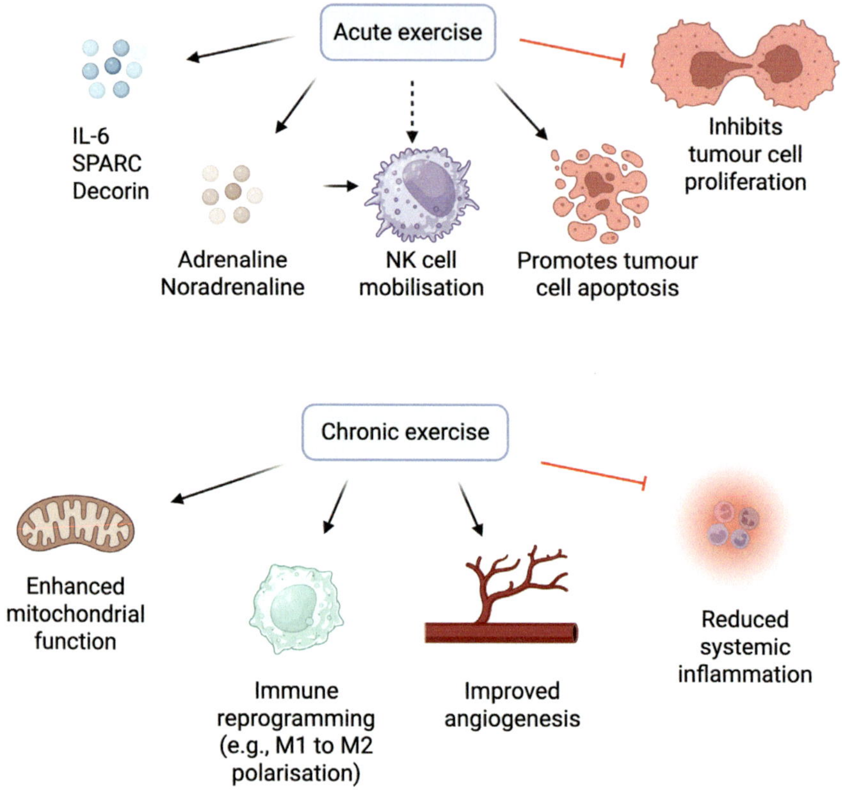

FIGURE 7.1 Acute and chronic exercise exert distinct but complementary anticancer effects. Acute exercise triggers rapid, transient systemic responses, including elevations in catecholamines, IL-6 and other myokines, which mobilise cytotoxic immune cells (e.g., NK cells) and transiently suppress tumour cell proliferation. These acute biological "pulses" can inhibit tumour-promoting signalling pathways within minutes to hours after a single exercise session. By contrast, chronic exercise training induces longer-term physiological adaptations such as increased mitochondrial function, enhanced immune competence, improved metabolic regulation and more ordered vascular remodelling. These cumulative changes contribute to a less inflamed, less tumour-promoting microenvironment, improving tissue oxygenation and limiting tumour growth over time, highlighting how both the frequency and duration of exercise influence pathways that govern tumour growth and development through distinct acute and chronic adaptations. Created in Biorender.com.

undergoing high-intensity endurance cycling (HIEC), both before and after a 9-week high-intensity interval training programme (HIIT) (15). The authors found that serum collected immediately after a single HIEC session significantly reduced the proliferative and tumourigenic potential of both TNBC and prostate cancer cell lines. Crucially, no additional tumour-suppressive benefit was observed after the training period, indicating that it was the acute session, rather than accumulated training, that triggered the most biologically active systemic responses. Further supporting this conclusion, the authors reported no significant change in participants' body weight across the study period, suggesting that the anti-tumour effects were independent of weight loss, which has previously been proposed as a mediator of cancer risk reduction through exercise (15). This points to the importance of exercise-induced molecular signalling rather than indirect metabolic changes as a primary driver of the observed effects.

These findings echo earlier work by Dethlefsen et al. (2017), who demonstrated that catecholamines released during acute exercise act via the β-adrenergic receptor to activate the Hippo signalling pathway, a well-known tumour suppressor cascade. The activation of this pathway led to phosphorylation and cytoplasmic retention of YAP, a transcriptional co-activator that promotes tumour proliferation when active (see Chapter 4, Section 4.3.3). Serum from exercised individuals inhibited YAP activity and reduced downstream gene expression associated with tumour growth, providing a mechanistic link between the neuroendocrine response to exercise and its anti-cancer potential (11).

Many other in vitro studies corroborate the tumour-suppressive effects of exercise-conditioned serum across diverse cancer types. In prostate cancer, serum collected immediately after acute endurance exercise inhibited LNCaP prostate cancer cell proliferation by 31%, potentially due to increased IGFBP-1 and reduced EGF levels (16). In colon cancer, serum collected post-exercise significantly suppressed LoVo cell proliferation and DNA damage, an effect that was mediated via IL-6-induced reductions in γ-H2AX expression (17). Similarly, Kurgan et al. (2017) demonstrated that serum obtained after a single bout of high-intensity interval training reduced proliferation and survival of non-small cell lung cancer cells, alongside decreased activation of key pro-survival signalling pathways, including Akt, mTOR and ERK1/2 (18). In breast cancer, both resistance and high-intensity interval training elevated anti-cancer myokines and suppressed breast cancer cell growth, with HIIT producing slightly greater effects (10). Together, these studies demonstrate that even short bouts of exercise can transiently reprogramme the systemic environment in ways that directly impact tumour cell behaviour, detectable across multiple cell types. This has important implications for frequency and duration, suggesting that regular exposure to these acute biochemical shifts, rather than sustained physical training alone, may be key to achieving meaningful tumour control.

7.3 Preclinical and clinical evidence for frequency and duration

7.3.1 Frequency: How often should patients exercise?

How often exercise should be performed remains a central question in exercise oncology. While guidelines for the general population are well established, tailoring frequency to individual cancer patients, accounting for treatment status, symptom burden and comorbidities, requires a more nuanced approach (19). The ACSM and other expert panels recommend that cancer survivors engage in at least three sessions of moderate-intensity aerobic exercise per week, ideally accumulating 150 minutes per week, and include resistance training two to three times per week (19,20). This mirrors public health recommendations for healthy adults, reflecting a default "one-size-fits-all" model that, while practical, may not be optimal across diverse cancer populations.

From a preclinical standpoint, while very few studies in murine models have evaluated frequency, per se, a comprehensive systematic review and meta-analysis of the impact of exercise on cancer growth in rodents has demonstrated differential effects depending on exercise frequency and length (21). Synthesising data from 19 preclinical studies in models encompassing a range of tumour types, including breast, lung, liver and skin cancer, with a variety of exercise modalities (swimming, running and aquatic jumping), this meta-analysis demonstrated consistent findings that tumour growth is abrogated in response to exercise. Across the studies, training programmes typically involved between four and seven sessions a week, lasting from 5 to 180 minutes per day. Despite this heterogeneity, the magnitude of reduction in tumour weight or volume (compared with sedentary controls) appeared to be influenced by training frequency and duration since more regular and sustained exercise regimens, typically ≥5 sessions per week for ≥6 weeks, was associated with greater tumour suppression (21). Both forced and voluntary exercise paradigms were effective, although voluntary running produced more variable results, likely reflecting differences in exercise dose and individual variability in activity levels. A minority of studies observed neutral or even adverse effects (22–25). It is interesting to note that these four studies that demonstrated neutral or adverse effects of exercise used either female Sprague-Dawley mice or

C57BL/6 mice, suggesting that the tumour response may depend on specific model characteristics. For instance, Sprague-Dawley rats are outbred and genetically diverse, which may introduce variability in immune surveillance, tumour recognition and inflammatory responses. They also tend to have higher baseline adiposity and may be more prone to metabolic disturbances induced by exercise, underscoring the importance of considering host-tumour-exercise interactions in preclinical studies. Overall, this meta-analysis supports the conclusion that regular, moderate-to-high frequency exercise exerts tumour-suppressive effects in animal models, with evidence that both the duration of the training and the number of weekly sessions (frequency) are critical determinants of biological efficacy.

In clinical settings, frequency must be balanced against real-world considerations such as fatigue, pain, treatment-related side effects and psychological burden. Adherence to high-frequency protocols can be particularly challenging during chemotherapy or radiotherapy. Studies show that even patients who are motivated may struggle to meet minimum frequency recommendations due to fluctuating energy levels or symptom flares (8,26). A meta-analysis found that interventions lasting less than 12 weeks and performed three times a week produced the greatest reductions in cancer-related fatigue and improvements in QoL (27). Indeed, the consensus statement from the ACSM for cancer survivors indicates that aerobic programmes of moderate intensity undertaken three times a week over 8–12 weeks or more are associated with meaningful improvements in fatigue, QoL and physical function (28). In this context, individualised exercise prescriptions that adapt frequency to the patient's capacity and treatment phase are essential. Some trials have explored the utility of "exercise snacking" (i.e., multiple short bouts spread across the day) or low-volume, high-frequency walking programmes, both of which show promising adherence and efficacy, particularly in deconditioned patients or older adults (29). Ultimately, the evidence supports a minimum effective frequency of ≥3 sessions per week. However, how long each session lasts adds another critical layer to this prescription.

7.3.2 Duration: How long is enough?

Just as frequency shapes the regularity of biological exposure to exercise-induced signalling, duration determines the dose per session—a key variable influencing both the mechanistic effects and patient adherence. Emerging evidence suggests that even short bouts of exercise (as little as 10–30 minutes) may be sufficient to activate key anti-cancer immune cells (30) (Table 7.1). For instance, acute sessions of high-intensity cycling lasting 20–30 minutes have been shown to induce significant

TABLE 7.1 Summary of exercise frequency and time in human studies

Study	*Cancer type*	*Frequency (sessions per week)*	*Session duration (min)*	*Duration (weeks)*	*Major outcomes*
Mustian et al., 2017 (43)	Mixed (meta-analysis)	3–5	20–60	≥12	Reduced fatigue, improved QoL
Cormie et al., 2015 (44)	Prostate	2–3	60	12	Improved strength, body composition
Mishra et al., 2012 (39)	Mixed (review)	3	30–60	8–12	QoL and fatigue improvements peak with 3 x weekly sessions
Pelzer et al., 2023 (45)	Breast & prostate	2	30–38	12	HRQoL, fatigue, sustained RT benefits
Phys-Can trial (van Waart et al., 2021) (46)	Breast, colorectal	5	20–30	24	Less decline in cardiorespiratory fitness, better physical function, less nausea, vomiting and pain
CHALLENGE trial (Booth et al., 2025) (47)	Colon	≥3	45–60	156 (3 yrs)	Lower recurrence, better DFS, OS, improved physical function
INTERVAL-GAP4 trial (Newton et al., 2023) (48)	Prostate (mCRPC)	3	60–75	52 (12 months)	Feasible, safe in advanced cancer, adherence 79%
HI AIM trial (Olofsson et al., 2022) (49)	Various (checkpoint inhibitors)	3	40–60	6	Testing immune mobilisation and clinical endpoints

Abbreviations: CRF = cancer-related fatigue; DFS = disease-free survival; HRQoL = health-related quality of life; mCRPC = metastatic castrate-resistant prostate cancer; OS = overall survival; QoL = quality of life; RT = resistance training

systemic changes, including catecholamine release, IL-6 elevation and NK cell mobilisation, all of which contribute to transient suppression of tumour proliferation when assessed via serum transfer studies (11,12). These findings yet again point to a "minimum effective dose" for triggering molecular events relevant to tumour control. Preclinical studies support this whereby repeated short-duration exercise bouts in rodent models, whether via treadmill or wheel running, can reduce tumour growth and improve immune function without requiring prolonged sessions (31,32). Similarly, clinical observations suggest that short, structured exercise sessions and self-paced, home-based interventions are more achievable for individuals undergoing treatment, who often face fatigue, nausea and time constraints as barriers to longer workouts (33,34).

By contrast, longer-duration sessions (≥60 minutes) may provide additional physiological benefits (e.g., cardiovascular fitness, body composition changes), but these come with diminishing returns in terms of molecular or immune activation and may increase the risk of overtraining, injury or non-adherence, particularly in vulnerable or deconditioned patients (3,35,36) (see Chapter 4, Section 4.10). Moreover, as previously discussed, prolonged bouts of exercise can elevate circulating cortisol levels and transiently suppress some aspects of immune surveillance, which are likely counterproductive in terms of reducing cancer growth and development where maintaining a vigilant anti-tumour immune response is critical (37,38). It is also worth noting that consistent engagement in shorter exercise sessions may be more achievable for many individuals undergoing cancer treatment and in some cases correlate with greater improvements in patient-reported outcomes than less frequent, longer sessions. While direct comparisons are limited, evidence suggests that feasibility and regularity often outweigh duration alone in driving psychological and physical benefits (39–41). A patient who completes 5 × 20-minute walks per week may derive greater benefit, both physically and psychologically, than one who manages a single 90-minute session but struggles to recover. Broader behavioural science findings show that habit formation and sustainable adherence are more likely with shorter, more frequent routines. Moreover, such patterns better support recovery and minimise symptom exacerbation during treatment, contributing to greater long-term engagement and cumulative benefit (42). In practice, this means that while 30 minutes per session remains a widely recommended benchmark, shorter sessions should not be discounted, especially if performed frequently and consistently. For some individuals, accumulating activity in brief intervals throughout the day may offer a more accessible and sustainable model of care.

7.3.3 Timing across the cancer continuum

The timing of exercise relative to a patient's position along the cancer continuum, be it before, during or after treatment, strongly influences the safety, tolerability and effectiveness of both frequency and duration.

As outlined in Jones and Alfano (2013) in their adaptation to the Physical Exercise Across the Cancer Experience (PEACE) framework (50), patients' physiological and psychosocial responses to exercise vary substantially depending on whether they are in the pre-treatment (prehabilitation), active treatment or post-treatment (survivorship or palliative care) phases. Each stage presents unique challenges and opportunities for optimising exercise dose (51). Building on this foundation, the 2024 review by An et al. (2024) elaborates a refined phase-based approach across four discrete survivorship periods: 1) post-diagnosis before surgery; 2) after surgery and before adjuvant treatment; 3) during non-surgical treatment (neoadjuvant/adjuvant); and 4) extended survival/long-term survivorship (52). This analysis emphasises that exercise prescription must align not only with treatment status and timing but also with the evolving biological, functional and psychosocial needs of the individual at each stage. Tailoring variables such as frequency, intensity, modality and progression according to these phases is essential for maximising benefit, maintaining safety and supporting long-term health outcomes. A summary of the benefits of exercise across the cancer continuum is given in Figure 7.2.

7.3.3.1 Before treatment (prehabilitation)

In the pre-treatment window, patients are typically more robust, making it an ideal time to establish baseline fitness and physiological reserve. Some studies have shown that moderate-to-high frequency exercise programmes (e.g., four to five sessions per week) of 20–60 minutes can enhance cardiorespiratory fitness, reduce surgical complication risk and improve mental preparedness (53–55). A systematic review and meta-analysis reported that cancer patients who already had higher levels of physical activity before surgical resection of their tumour had shorter post-operative hospital stays and enhanced QoL (56). In obese or overweight patients, pre-operative exercise benefits weight loss and lowers the risk of adverse effects related to surgery (57–59). In oesophageal cancer patients, early exercise can preserve muscle mass during pre-operative neoadjuvant chemotherapy treatment (60). Moreover, exercise prehabilitation can enhance cardiopulmonary function and muscle strength in lung cancer patients (61). Even brief interventions in this phase have shown benefit in improving post-treatment recovery trajectories.

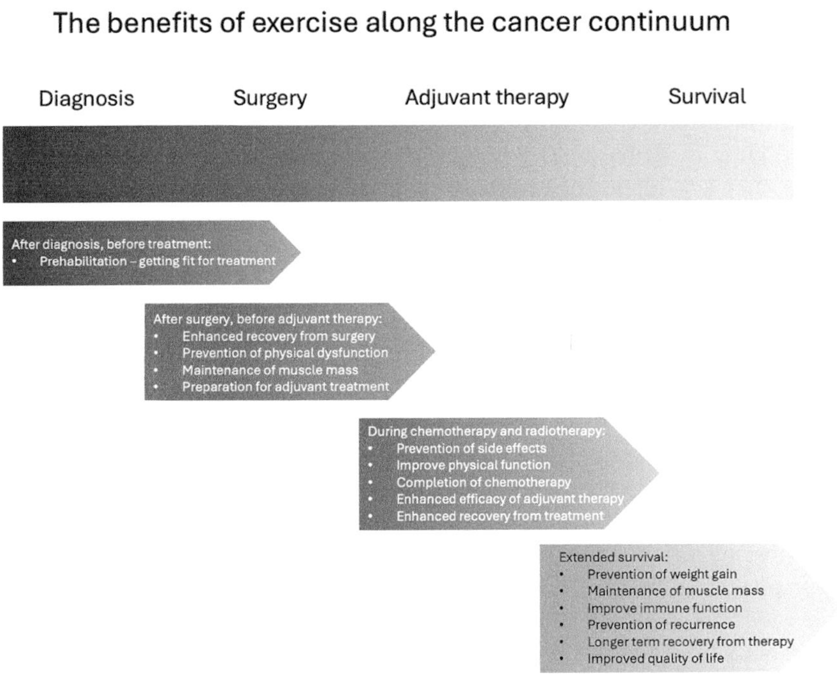
The benefits of exercise along the cancer continuum
Diagnosis
Surgery
Adjuvant therapy
Survival
After diagnosis, before treatment:
• Prehabilitation – getting fit for treatment
After surgery, before adjuvant therapy:
• Enhanced recovery from surgery
• Prevention of physical dysfunction
• Maintenance of muscle mass
• Preparation for adjuvant treatment
During chemotherapy and radiotherapy:
• Prevention of side effects
• Improve physical function
• Completion of chemotherapy
• Enhanced efficacy of adjuvant therapy
• Enhanced recovery from treatment
Extended survival:
• Prevention of weight gain
• Maintenance of muscle mass
• Improve immune function
• Prevention of recurrence
• Longer term recovery from therapy
• Improved quality of life

FIGURE 7.2 The benefits of exercise along the cancer continuum. This schematic illustrates the role and potential benefits of exercise at different stages of the cancer care continuum, from diagnosis and surgery through to adjuvant therapy and long-term survivorship. At each phase, tailored exercise interventions can help mitigate treatment-related side effects, preserve or restore physical function, and support psychological and physiological resilience. In the pre-treatment phase, prehabilitation can improve readiness for surgery or therapy. During and between treatments, exercise contributes to recovery, treatment tolerance and enhanced therapeutic efficacy. In survivorship, it supports long-term health, reduces recurrence risk and improves quality of life. Adapted from (52).

7.3.3.2 During treatment

During chemotherapy, radiotherapy or targeted therapies, patients often experience fatigue, nausea, myelosuppression and general deconditioning. The most common outcome measured in many systematic reviews and meta-analyses investigating the impact of exercise in cancer patients was fatigue, with many consistently reporting a reduction in fatigue with exercise during treatment in breast cancer (62–65) and colorectal cancer

(66,67). Other outcome measures include improvements in physical fitness measures, such as cardiorespiratory fitness (64), muscular strength (64,68) and lean mass (68). Moreover, in breast cancer, additional benefits include improved shoulder mobility, upper body function, arm mobility and reduced lymphoedema (64).

Another key benefit of exercise during treatment is improving treatment-related outcomes, such as improved treatment tolerance, positive indicators of cancer-related biomarkers and potentially reducing cancer recurrence. In a review of eight RCTs, only two reported significant beneficial effects of exercise on chemotherapy completion (69). These were the START trial by Courneya et al. (2014), which compared aerobic and resistance exercise to usual care and demonstrated that resistance exercise significantly improved chemotherapy completion rates (70), and the PACES trial by van Waart et al. (2015), which compared a home-based low-intensity exercise programme to a supervised moderate-to-high-intensity combined aerobic and resistance programme to usual care and found that those who participated in the supervised moderate-to-high-intensity exercise trial required four times fewer dose adjustments in their prescribed chemotherapy regimen compared to the usual care and low intensity groups (46). Other studies have demonstrated enhanced treatment tolerability and higher complete response rates with exercise. For example, in colorectal cancer patients, relative dose intensity was higher in the exercise intervention group compared with the usual care group (63), and in the phase II EXERT trial, the number of patients who achieved a complete response was significantly higher than in the exercise group (71). Furthermore, in a pooled analysis of two multicentre trials, higher baseline cardiovascular fitness and muscular strength were found to be the strongest predictors of chemotherapy completion, supporting the idea that exercise that increases physical fitness may improve treatment tolerance (72). Finally, a systematic review reported improved biomarker levels, including insulin-like growth factor (IGF)-I, IGF-II, CD4+ cells, immune function and decreased inflammatory markers (73).

During active treatment, exercise may need to be gentler, shorter and more flexible, with some studies showing that as little as 10–20 minutes per day, even at low intensity, can help maintain function and reduce treatment-related side effects (74,75). High-frequency, low-duration models may be most effective here, prioritising consistency over intensity or volume. Monitoring for overtraining and immune suppression is essential during this phase.

7.3.3.3 After treatment (survivorship and beyond)

Post-treatment, the physiological context shifts again. Here, the goals often include restoring physical capacity, managing late effects, preventing recurrence and improving QoL (51). This is the phase in which traditional public health guidelines (e.g., 150 minutes per week of moderate-intensity exercise) are most often achievable and appropriate. Both frequency and duration can be gradually increased, depending on individual recovery, comorbidities and motivation. For some, particularly those with metastatic or advanced disease, the focus of exercise in the post-treatment phase shifts towards function preservation and symptom relief rather than tumour suppression. Here, low-impact, frequent movement may provide better outcomes than conventional training structures.

Exercise following cancer treatment offers significant physical and psychological benefits, both in the immediate rehabilitation phase and throughout long-term survivorship. Clinical trials, particularly in breast and colorectal cancer populations, have shown that structured aerobic and resistance training improves physical functioning, fatigue, QoL and biomarkers such as immune function and insulin resistance (73,76,77). While evidence for other tumour types remains limited, exercise is generally safe and feasible across populations (78). Long-term observational studies further support these findings, linking higher post-diagnosis physical activity with substantial reductions in cancer-specific and all-cause mortality, particularly in breast, colorectal and prostate cancers (79). These data have informed current guidelines from the American Cancer Society, which recommend ongoing physical activity to enhance survivorship outcomes and reduce recurrence risk (80).

Overall, timing matters: Not only in terms of when exercise is introduced but also how its frequency and duration are adjusted to match an individual patient's physiological capacity. A personalised, continuum-based approach is critical to ensure that exercise remains safe, meaningful and beneficial throughout the cancer journey.

7.4 Patient-specific modifiers

No two individuals with cancer experience the disease, or respond to exercise, in the same way. As such, exercise prescriptions must be tailored, not just by tumour type or treatment modality, but by individual physiological, clinical and behavioural characteristics. Two of the most important modifiers of frequency and duration are the treatment phase and the patient's baseline fitness and comorbidity profile.

7.4.1 Treatment phase

Each treatment modality imposes unique demands on the body, which influence the appropriateness of different exercise doses.

7.4.1.1 Chemotherapy

Fatigue, neutropenia, anaemia and nausea are common barriers to sustained or prolonged activity (81). While frequent movement is beneficial for fatigue mitigation (82), sessions often need to be shorter (10–20 minutes) and adapted to daily fluctuations in energy. Resistance training has been shown to improve lower-body strength in patients undergoing chemotherapy but may need to be scaled back during periods of immune suppression (83). However, low-intensity aerobic exercise is generally safe and effective for most patients.

7.4.1.2 Immunotherapy

As a newer and rapidly evolving treatment class, the interaction between exercise and immune checkpoint inhibitors is still under investigation. Not all tumour types respond to checkpoint inhibition; however, given that exercise can mediate changes in intratumoural immune cell composition, it stands to reason that exercise may boost the efficacy of checkpoint inhibitor therapy. Indeed, both preclinical and clinical data support this paradigm. In preclinical mouse models, exercise has shown promising effects on the TME and response to immunotherapy. In B16 melanoma-bearing mice, voluntary wheel running for four weeks before tumour inoculation skewed the TME towards an anti-tumour phenotype and upregulated immune checkpoint expression (PD-1 and PD-L1, among others) and wheel running alone reduced tumour growth by 72% (84). Interestingly, combining wheel running with anti-PD-1 or anti-PD-L1 therapy did not further inhibit tumour growth, likely because the effect of exercise was already significant. However, in a pancreatic adenocarcinoma model, exercise post-transplant sensitised tumours to anti-PD-1 therapy, yielding significant tumour growth inhibition (85). Similarly, in a hepatocellular carcinoma (HCC) model, exercise prevented the emergence of an immunosuppressive TME, marked by Treg infiltration and checkpoint upregulation, that was observed in mice treated long-term with anti-PD-1 plus Lenvatinib (86). Additionally, breast cancer models showed enhanced responses to combined immune checkpoint inhibition with exercise or checkpoint inhibition with radiation plus exercise when compared to checkpoint inhibition alone (87,88). However, not all studies found positive synergies: Buss et al. (2021) observed no beneficial effect of voluntary exercise on immune checkpoint responses in B16-F10 melanoma or E0771 breast cancer-bearing mice, underscoring the importance of exercise dose and model selection (89).

In clinical studies, patients with unresectable HCC receiving first-line Lenvatinib alongside anti-PD-1 were trained unsupervised (five times per week, moderate aerobic activity or three times per week, vigorous activity for more than 30 minutes per session) before or soon after therapy and displayed improved overall survival (OS), progression-free survival (PFS) and overall response rate (ORR) (86). The SPORTIVUMAB study in melanoma patients on immune checkpoint inhibitors undertaking twice-weekly supervised sessions of 60 minutes duration will be the first trial to evaluate the safety, feasibility and effectiveness of a 12-week combined resistance and endurance exercise intervention programme during checkpoint inhibitor treatment (90). At the time of writing, the study is complete but the results are yet to be published. Upcoming RCTs include ERICA, which will evaluate the acute effects of an hour of exercise prior to treatment with the checkpoint inhibitor, pembrolizumab, plus platinum-based chemotherapy in 30 non-small cell lung carcinoma (NSCLC) patients (91) and HI AIM, which will investigate the impact of exercise on immune cells in 70 NSCLC patients undergoing checkpoint inhibition or combined checkpoint inhibitor plus chemotherapy (49). Other RCTs in skin cancer include EDEN, which explored the impact of diet and exercise on immunotherapy and the microbiome (90), and Moffitt Cancer Center's randomised arm-ergometer/treadmill intervention before each checkpoint inhibitor infusion on various skin cancers (90). Although final results are pending, these studies may clarify how exercise can modulate immune responses to immunotherapy. Given the capacity of exercise to influence immune cell trafficking, cytokine release and overall immune tone, it is important to avoid excessive or poorly timed training during active immunotherapy. Until more definitive data emerge, a moderate approach of three to four sessions per week of 20–40 minutes in duration at a light-to-moderate intensity appears safest and most likely to support, rather than compete with, therapeutic immune activation.

7.4.1.3 Surgery

In the surgical context, exercise dose must be carefully tailored to the physiological disturbances and recovery demands imposed by surgery. In the perioperative period, when time permits between diagnosis and surgery, prehabilitation efforts may allow for higher training loads. Emerging evidence indicates that preoperative exercise interventions significantly improve functional capacity (e.g., the 6-minute walk test) and may reduce postoperative complications and length of hospital stay (92,93). These findings support the idea that building physiological reserve prior to surgery through aerobic conditioning, strength training or combined modalities can optimise the body's ability to withstand the stress of surgery and facilitate recovery.

Postoperatively, the prescription must be amended to protect against deconditioning and support recovery, with early emphasis on frequency rather than duration. Brief, repeated bouts of walking or low intensity activity, often as short as 5–10 minutes in the early days, may improve markers of recovery such as insulin sensitivity, aerobic function and wound healing (94,95). While longer or higher volume sessions can be considered later in convalescence, early rehabilitation frequently benefits from multiple short sessions per day rather than fewer, prolonged efforts. The literature emphasises dose responsiveness, meaning that the "when, how often and how long" of exercise must be aligned with the body's current physiological state and individual patient vulnerability. Overall, exercise dosing around surgery reflects a continuum: In the lead-up to surgery, efforts focus on maximising capacity and physiological reserve; in the immediate postoperative phase, the goal is to preserve decline and promote recovery; and across both phases, responsiveness to individual capacity, surgical risk and recovery trajectory is essential. Effective prescription, therefore, hinges on aligning the timing and volume of exercise with the unique treatment-specific demands and the patient's evolving health status.

PATIENT VIGNETTE 7.1 "Dan"—fatigue and personal threshold

Dan, a 50-year-old lung cancer survivor, described fatigue as his biggest hurdle, likening it to "walking through concrete." On good days, he'd do a short walk, on bad days, simple stretches. He found pacing essential and believes exercise should be seen as flexible and responsive, not a rigid prescription. "There wasn't anything out there that felt like it was made for me. I had to adapt what I knew and trust my body."

7.4.2 Baseline fitness and comorbidities

The second critical modifier in exercise prescription for patients with cancer is the individual's starting point: That is, their baseline cardiorespiratory fitness, muscle strength, functional mobility and the burden of existing comorbidities (e.g., CVD, diabetes, arthritis). These factors strongly influence what constitutes a safe and effective "dose" of exercise at any treatment and survivorship phase. Fit, younger patients with few comorbidities may tolerate, and indeed benefit from, longer sessions and higher frequencies (e.g., four to six sessions per week, 30–60 minutes), even during active treatment. In contrast, older adults, deconditioned patients or those with multiple and/or significant comorbidities often require lower initial doses (e.g., 10–20 minutes per day, three to four times per week), with careful progression and monitoring. Evidence shows that survivors with higher baseline cardiopulmonary fitness and functional status are more likely to adhere to target training loads and achieve greater gains (96). Moreover, even modest, consistent exercise interventions appear capable of shifting metabolic profiles, supporting immune competence and reducing systemic inflammation, despite falling below more traditional guideline thresholds (97). To guide safe and effective prescription, baseline functional assessments, such as the 6-minute walk test, sit-to-stand and grip strength tests, in addition to patient-reported outcomes, should inform initial dosing and enable dynamic adjustment of exercise volume, intensity and frequency according to evolving capacity and comorbidity burden.

7.4.3 Age, sex, cancer type

Age, sex and cancer type represent three fundamental modifiers of exercise response and tolerance, particularly when considering appropriate frequency and duration of activity. These factors must be integrated into prescription to ensure both safety and efficacy.

7.4.3.1 Age

Older adults frequently experience age-related declines in cardiorespiratory fitness, muscular strength, joint mobility and balance. These changes are often compounded by cancer-related fatigue, sarcopenia and treatment-related side effects. For example, a recent systematic review of exercise training in elderly cancer patients confirmed that tailored interventions are safe and yield meaningful gains in functional independence even in the presence of comorbidities (98,99). Given this context, older or deconditioned patients are likely to better tolerate and adhere to shorter, more frequent sessions (e.g., 10–20 minutes daily) rather than longer workouts, especially during active treatment. Importantly, exercise is feasible across the cancer continuum in older adults with the right screening and supervision (99,100).

7.4.3.2 Sex

Biological sex may influence exercise response via hormonal profiles, intrinsic muscle fibre composition, body composition differences and immune modulation. Although direct data in oncology are limited, studies suggest that female survivors may derive greater benefit from equivalent amounts of physical activity than males. For instance, a nationally representative cohort found that women achieved similar mortality risk reductions with lower volumes of activity compared to men (101,102). In cancer biology, sex-specific patterns of muscle wasting (cachexia) have been noted, with males typically exhibiting higher prevalence and more severe muscle loss (103). While current exercise guidelines do not differentiate prescription by sex, it is prudent to individualise dosing based on sex-linked comorbidity profile (e.g., post-menopausal women and osteoporosis risk; men and cardiovascular risk) as well as recovery capacity and personal preferences.

7.4.3.3 Cancer type

The nature of the tumour, its anatomical location and its treatment also shape exercise dosing. For instance, patients with lung or head and neck cancer often present with substantially reduced aerobic capacity, impaired swallowing or compromised airways and may require shorter bouts with longer recovery intervals. In contrast, breast and prostate cancer survivors typically tolerate moderate-frequency aerobic and resistance training well, but may need adaptations for treatment-specific issues, such as post-surgical lymphoedema in breast cancer or androgen-deprivation-induced muscle loss in prostate cancer. For colorectal or abdominal cancers, practitioners must pay attention to intra-abdominal pressure, stoma care or anastomatic healing when selecting modalities and doses. Interestingly, an exercise study comparing heterogeneous cancer types found no major differences in the magnitude of training-induced adaptations between tumour sites when dosing was individually prescribed (104). Ultimately, cancer-specific physiology and treatment effects must be factored into dosing, while recognising that individual variability often exceeds tumour type as a predictor of exercise tolerance.

7.4.4 Psychosocial readiness and preferences

In addition to physiological capacity, an individual's psychosocial readiness and personal preferences play a crucial role in shaping the frequency and duration of exercise that are both realistic and sustainable. After a cancer diagnosis, many patients face emotional and cognitive challenges, including anxiety, depression, fear of recurrence or reduced motivation, which may influence their willingness or ability to engage in regular physical activity. A systematic review of programming and counselling preferences in adult cancer survivors found that walking was the most preferred modality and that flexibility (timing, home-based delivery) was key for adherence (105). For some, particularly those with no prior exercise history, the prospect of structured sessions several times a week may feel overwhelming. In such cases, shorter, more flexible sessions (e.g., 10–20 minutes per day) can help build confidence and reduce perceived barriers, making frequency more feasible than extended durations.

Conversely, patients with a strong pre-existing exercise habit or athletic identity may engage more effectively with higher frequency and longer sessions, using exercise as a means of self-efficacy and emotional regulation. Tailoring prescriptions to reflect what patients enjoy, feel competent doing and can realistically fit into their lifestyles is key to supporting adherence, especially when motivation is low. Social and environmental factors further influence what is possible. Access to safe exercise spaces, transport options, time availability and peer support networks all matter. Recent evidence suggests that social support, peer-led programmes and community-based exercise enhance adherence and frequency over time, particularly among women and older adults (106,107). Others may prefer self-paced, home-based interventions to maintain autonomy and privacy. Crucially, co-designing exercise prescriptions, where patients are active participants in shaping their routines, strengthens commitment and ensures that frequency and duration are aligned with both personal goals and existing constraints. Motivational interviewing, behavioural coaching and goal-setting techniques have been shown to facilitate the shift from intention to sustained action in cancer survivors (106,108). Table 7.2. summarises the impact of frequency and duration on adherence to physical activity and psychosocial outcomes in cancer survivors.

7.5 Balancing intensity, frequency and duration

An effective exercise prescription for people with cancer is rarely about maximising one variable in isolation. Instead, it is about finding the right balance between intensity, frequency and duration—a balance that shifts depending on treatment status, health status and individual goals. While high-intensity exercise may stimulate powerful acute biological responses (see Chapter 6, Section 6.3), this form of training is not always feasible or desirable, particularly during treatment. As shown in a series of in vitro experiments using exercise-conditioned serum, short bouts of high-intensity exercise can exert anti-tumour effects (11,15,112). However, these benefits may be achieved without needing long sessions or high cumulative weekly volumes. Conversely, low- to moderate-intensity exercise, when performed more frequently and for longer durations, supports cardiovascular health, muscle preservation, fatigue management and QoL. In these cases, the cumulative dose built from consistent daily, or near-daily, activity becomes the primary mechanism of benefit. Importantly, intensity, frequency and duration are

TABLE 7.2 How frequency and duration impact adherence and psychosocial outcomes in cancer survivors

Study	*Details*	*Population and dose*	*Key findings*	*Implication for frequency/duration*
Bell et al., 2021 (109)	Target 2 sessions per week but median 1.2 per week over ~20 weeks	Breast cancer survivors, median 1.2 sessions per week	VO_2peak improved by ~7% and strength by ~7–9% despite low frequency	Suggests even very low frequency (~1 per week) can yield meaningful benefits; reinforces feasibility of short/less frequency sessions
Brooke et al., 2022 (110)	Intervention with resistance + endurance training, reporting adherence by FITT	Mixed—breast, colorectal, prostate (n = 577) during treatment	Adherence to "time" and "frequency" principles varied widely; older age and fatigue predicted lower adherence	Highlights that frequency and session duration are key "adherence" variables, and shorter, more frequent sessions may support better adherence
Pedroso et al., 2024 (111)	Home-based aerobic + resistance during treatment	Lung/head and neck cancer, median age ~61yrs, treatment concurrent	Overall adherence ~47%; greater symptom burden (malaise) strongly predicted lower adherence	Indicates that treatment-related symptoms modulate ability to adhere, so shorter and more manageable sessions (in terms of duration) may be critical in such contexts

interdependent variables: When intensity is high, both duration and frequency may need to be reduced to allow for adequate recovery. By contrast, when intensity is low to moderate, exercise may be safely performed more often and for longer periods. For deconditioned or treatment-fatigued individuals, short, low-intensity sessions performed frequently (even in 5- to 10-minute blocks) may be the most sustainable and beneficial strategy.

This principle mirrors the dose-response curve observed in both clinical and behavioural exercise studies: Too little activity confers little benefit, but too much, especially if poorly timed, can cause harm, including excessive fatigue, injury or immune suppression (113–115). Therefore, individualised programming must consider the trade-offs between frequency, intensity and time. For example, a patient undergoing chemotherapy may benefit more from daily light walking (10–15 minutes) than from trying to meet weekly exercise targets in two to three larger sessions. A fit survivor in the post-treatment phase might safely engage in moderate-intensity sessions (30–45 minutes) four to five times per week, gradually increasing both volume and intensity as tolerated. Someone with bone metastases may need to reduce intensity and duration while maintaining frequency to preserve function without increasing fracture risk. In all cases, the priority is not simply reaching a numerical threshold but preserving autonomy, reducing symptom burden and maintaining both physiological and psychological resilience (Table 7.3).

TABLE 7.3 Quick reference guide to suggested frequency and duration of exercise across the cancer continuum

Cancer Phase	*Suggested Frequency*	*Suggested Duration*	*Key considerations*
Pre-treatment	3–5 sessions per week	20–60 minutes	Build physiological reserve; higher intensities often tolerated
During treatment	Most days of the week (light-to-moderate)	10–30 minutes	Prioritise consistency; adapt to fatigue; [watch out for] immune suppression
Post-treatment	3–5 sessions per week	30–60 minutes	Restore fitness and function; gradually progress volume
Advanced/metastatic	Daily light movement or 3–4 sessions per week	10–30 minutes	Emphasise mobility; symptom relief; QoL

7.6 Summary and key takeaways

This chapter has explored the important but often underappreciated components of exercise prescription: Frequency (how often) and time (how long). While intensity and modality have received greater focus in the literature, frequency and duration directly influence the biological, functional and psychosocial outcomes of exercise for individuals living with and beyond cancer. From a biological perspective, both acute and chronic exercise sessions drive systemic and tumour-specific responses, including modulation of inflammation, immune cell mobilisation, cytokine secretion and tumour suppression activation. Serum transfer studies show that even short bouts of high-intensity exercise can transiently reprogramme the systemic environment in ways that inhibit tumour cell proliferation. However, regular repetition of these bouts is necessary to sustain adaptations and cumulative benefits, highlighting the importance of both session duration and exercise frequency as key dosing variables.

Clinical and preclinical data suggest that ≥3 sessions per week, even if short in duration (10–30 minutes), may be sufficient to improve fatigue, functional outcomes and treatment tolerance, particularly when aligned with an individual's treatment phase, fitness level and psychosocial readiness. Short, frequent sessions are also better tolerated during chemotherapy or radiotherapy and may support immune recovery and treatment adherence. Conversely, during prehabilitation and post-treatment phases, longer sessions and higher frequencies may be feasible and beneficial. Throughout the cancer continuum, tailored exercise interventions offer distinct benefits at each phase, from improving treatment readiness and reducing side effects, through to promoting functional recovery and potentially lowering recurrence risk, exercise plays an important role. Timing also matters, both in terms of when exercise is initiated and how its dose evolves with the patient's changing physiological capacity. Clearly, there is a need for individualised, phase-specific exercise dosing, balancing frequency and time with intensity and modality, which takes into account a patient's individual needs to maximise safety, adherence and therapeutic benefit. The next chapter will pull all the evidence from this and the previous two chapters together, summarising the current guidelines and recommendations.

Chapter 7 Test your understanding question bank

1. What are the two main physiological distinctions between acute and chronic exercise effects in cancer care?
2. Why is frequency an important variable in exercise prescription for cancer patients?

3. What does current evidence suggest is the minimum effective frequency of exercise for cancer survivors?
4. How does session duration influence biological and behavioural outcomes in cancer patients?
5. In which phases of the cancer continuum might high-frequency or longer-duration exercise be most appropriate?
6. How can exercise prescriptions be adapted during active treatment to support adherence and safety?
7. What are some patient-specific factors that influence how frequency and duration should be prescribed?
8. Why might shorter, more frequent exercise sessions be more beneficial than fewer longer sessions?

References

1. Sever E, Yılmaz S, Koz M. Acute and chronic immunological responses to different exercise modalities: A narrative review. Healthcare [Internet]. 2025 Sep 1 [cited 2025 Nov 22];13(17):2244. Available from: https://pmc.ncbi.nlm.nih.gov/articles/PMC12428347/
2. Egan B, Sharples AP. Molecular responses to acute exercise and their relevance for adaptations in skeletal muscle to exercise training. Physiol Rev [Internet]. 2023 [cited 2025 Nov 22];103(3):2057–170. Available from: https://journals.physiology.org/doi/10.1152/physrev.00054.2021
3. Bettariga F, Taaffe DR, Galvão DA, Newton RU. Effects of short- and long-term exercise training on cancer cells in vitro: Insights into the mechanistic associations. J Sport Health Sci [Internet]. 2024 Dec 1 [cited 2025 Nov 22];14:100994. Available from: https://pmc.ncbi.nlm.nih.gov/articles/PMC11863286/
4. Michou V, Zervoudis S, Eskitzis P, Tsamos G, Vasdeki D, Vouxinou A, et al. Exercise interventions in breast cancer: Molecular mechanisms, physical benefits, and practical recommendations. Medicina [Internet]. 2025 Jun 27 [cited 2025 Nov 22];61(7):1167. Available from: https://www.mdpi.com/1648-9144/61/7/1167/htm
5. Sheill G, Guinan E, Brady L, Hevey D, Hussey J. Exercise interventions for patients with advanced cancer: A systematic review of recruitment, attrition, and exercise adherence rates. Palliat Support Care [Internet]. 2019 Dec 1 [cited 2025 Nov 22];17(6):686–96. Available from: https://www.cambridge.org/core/journals/palliative-and-supportive-care/article/abs/exercise-interventions-for-patients-with-advanced-cancer-a-systematic-review-of-recruitment-attrition-and-exercise-adherence-rates/CCE298BA3977D0E676D8E2AAFF07049A
6. Feng Y, Feng X, Wan R, Luo Z, Qu L, Wang Q. Impact of exercise on cancer: Mechanistic perspectives and new insights. Front Immunol [Internet]. 2024 [cited 2025 Nov 22];15. Available from: https://pubmed.ncbi.nlm.nih.gov/39346906/
7. Hojman P, Gehl J, Christensen JF, Pedersen BK. Molecular mechanisms linking exercise to cancer prevention and treatment. Cell Metab [Internet]. 2018 Jan 9 [cited 2019 May 31];27(1):10–21. Available from: https://linkinghub.elsevier.com/retrieve/pii/S1550413117305673
8. Wang Q, Zhou W. Roles and molecular mechanisms of physical exercise in cancer prevention and treatment. J Sport Health Sci [Internet]. 2020 Mar

1 [cited 2025 Nov 22];10(2):201. Available from: https://pmc.ncbi.nlm.nih.gov/articles/PMC7987556/

9. Simpson RJ, Kunz H, Agha N, Graff R. Exercise and the regulation of immune functions. Prog Mol Biol Transl Sci [Internet]. 2015 [cited 2025 Nov 22];135:355–80. Available from: https://pubmed.ncbi.nlm.nih.gov/26477922/
10. Bettariga F, Taaffe DR, Crespo-Garcia C, Clay TD, De Santi M, Baldelli G, et al. A single bout of resistance or high-intensity interval training increases anti-cancer myokines and suppresses cancer cell growth in vitro in survivors of breast cancer. Breast Cancer Res Treat [Internet]. 2025 Aug 1 [cited 2025 Nov 22];213(1):171–80. Available from: https://pubmed.ncbi.nlm.nih.gov/40608178/
11. Dethlefsen C, Hansen LS, Lillelund C, Andersen C, Gehl J, Christensen JF, et al. Exercise-induced catecholamines activate the hippo tumor suppressor pathway to reduce risks of breast cancer development. Cancer Res [Internet]. 2017 Sep 15 [cited 2019 Dec 6];77(18):4894–904. Available from: http://cancerres.aacrjournals.org/lookup/doi/10.1158/0008-5472.CAN-16-3125
12. Pedersen L, Idorn M, Olofsson GH, Lauenborg B, Nookaew I, Hansen RH, et al. Voluntary running suppresses tumor growth through epinephrine- and IL-6-dependent NK cell mobilization and redistribution. Cell Metab. 2016 Mar 8;23(3):554–62.
13. Furrer R, Hawley JA, Handschin C. The molecular athlete: Exercise physiology from mechanisms to medals. Physiol Rev [Internet]. 2023 Jul 1 [cited 2025 Nov 22];103(3):1693. Available from: https://pmc.ncbi.nlm.nih.gov/articles/PMC10110736/
14. Huang Q, Wu M, Wu X, Zhang Y, Xia Y. Muscle-to-tumor crosstalk: The effect of exercise-induced myokine on cancer progression. Biochim Biophys Acta Rev Cancer [Internet]. 2022 Sep 1 [cited 2025 Nov 22];1877(5). Available from: https://pubmed.ncbi.nlm.nih.gov/35850277/
15. Baldelli G, De Santi M, Gervasi M, Annibalini G, Sisti D, Højman P, et al. The effects of human sera conditioned by high-intensity exercise sessions and training on the tumorigenic potential of cancer cells. Clin Transl Oncol [Internet]. 2021 Jan 1 [cited 2025 Nov 16];23(1):22–34. Available from: https://pubmed.ncbi.nlm.nih.gov/32447643/
16. Rundqvist H, Augsten M, Strömberg A, Rullman E, Mijwel S, Kharaziha P, et al. Effect of acute exercise on prostate cancer cell growth. PLoS One [Internet]. 2013 Jul 5 [cited 2025 Nov 22];8(7):e67579. Available from: https://journals.plos.org/plosone/article?id=10.1371/journal.pone.0067579
17. Orange ST, Jordan AR, Odell A, Kavanagh O, Hicks KM, Eaglen T, et al. Acute aerobic exercise-conditioned serum reduces colon cancer cell proliferation in vitro through interleukin-6-induced regulation of DNA damage. Int J Cancer [Internet]. 2022 Jul 15 [cited 2025 Nov 22];151(2):265–74. Available from: https://pubmed.ncbi.nlm.nih.gov/35213038/
18. Kurgan N, Tsakiridis E, Kouvelioti R, Moore J, Klentrou P, Tsiani E. Inhibition of human lung cancer cell proliferation and survival by post-exercise serum is associated with the inhibition of Akt, mTOR, p70 S6K, and Erk1/2. Cancers [Internet]. 2017 May 8 [cited 2025 Nov 22];9(5):46. Available from: https://www.mdpi.com/2072-6694/9/5/46/htm
19. Jones LW, Eves ND, Scott JM. Bench-to-bedside approaches for personalized exercise therapy in cancer. Am Soc Clin Oncol Educ Book [Internet]. 2017 May [cited 2025 Nov 22];37(37):684–94. Available from: https://pubmed.ncbi.nlm.nih.gov/28561646/
20. American College of Sports Medicine. ACSM's guidelines for exercise testing and prescription / [Internet]. Wolters Kluwer. 2022 [cited 2025 Nov 14].

Available from: https://books.google.com/books/about/ACSM_s_Guidelines_for_Exercise_Testing_a.html?hl=sl&id=hTKvzgEACAAJ
21. Eschke RCKR, Lampit A, Schenk A, Javelle F, Steindorf K, Diel P, et al. Impact of physical exercise on growth and progression of cancer in rodents—A systematic review and meta-analysis. Front Oncol [Internet]. 2019 Feb [cited 2025 Nov 22];9:35. Available from: https://pmc.ncbi.nlm.nih.gov/articles/PMC6370688/
22. Faustino-Rocha AI, Silva A, Gabriel J, Gil da Costa RM, Moutinho M, Oliveira PA, et al. Long-term exercise training as a modulator of mammary cancer vascularization. Biomed Pharmacother [Internet]. 2016 Jul 1 [cited 2025 Nov 22];81:273–80. Available from: https://pubmed.ncbi.nlm.nih.gov/27261604/
23. Tsai MS, Kuo ML, Chang CC, Wu YT. The effects of exercise training on levels of vascular endothelial growth factor in tumor-bearing mice. Cancer Biomark [Internet]. 2013 [cited 2025 Nov 22];13(5):307–13. Available from: https://pubmed.ncbi.nlm.nih.gov/24440969/
24. Whittal-Strange KS, Chadau S, Parkhouse WS. Exercise during puberty and NMU induced mammary tumorigenesis in rats. Breast Cancer Res Treat [Internet]. 1998 [cited 2025 Nov 22];47(1):1–8. Available from: https://pubmed.ncbi.nlm.nih.gov/9493970/
25. Zhu Z, Jiang W, Sells JL, Neil ES, McGinley JN, Thompson HJ. Effect of nonmotorized wheel running on mammary carcinogenesis: Circulating biomarkers, cellular processes, and molecular mechanisms in rats. Cancer Epidemiol Biomarkers Prev. 2008 Aug;17(8):1920–9.
26. Brown JC, Winters-Stone K, Lee A, Schmitz KH. Cancer, physical activity, and exercise. In: Comprehensive Physiology [Internet]. Hoboken, NJ, USA: John Wiley & Sons, Inc. 2012 [cited 2019 May 31]. pp. 2775–809. Available from: http://www.ncbi.nlm.nih.gov/pubmed/23720265
27. Chen X, Li J, Chen C, Zhang Y, Zhang S, Zhang Y, et al. Effects of exercise interventions on cancer-related fatigue and quality of life among cancer patients: A meta-analysis. BMC Nursing [Internet]. 2023 Jun 13 [cited 2025 Nov 22];22(1):200. Available from: https://bmcnurs.biomedcentral.com/articles/10.1186/s12912-023-01363-0
28. Campbell KL, Winters-Stone KM, Wiskemann J, May AM, Schwartz AL, Courneya KS, et al. Exercise guidelines for cancer survivors: Consensus statement from international multidisciplinary roundtable. Med Sci Sports Exerc [Internet]. 2019 Nov 1 [cited 2025 Nov 14];51(11):2375–90. Available from: https://pubmed.ncbi.nlm.nih.gov/31626055/
29. Tyldesley-Marshall N, Greenfield SM, Parretti HM, Gokal K, Greaves C, Jolly K, et al. SnacktivityTM to promote physical activity: A qualitative study. Int J Behav Med [Internet]. 2022 Oct 1 [cited 2025 Nov 22];29(5):553–64. Available from: https://link.springer.com/article/10.1007/s12529-021-10040-y
30. Koivula T, Lempiäinen S, Rinne P, Rannikko JH, Hollmén M, Sundberg CJ, et al. The effect of acute exercise on circulating immune cells in newly diagnosed breast cancer patients. Sci Rep [Internet]. 2023 Apr 21 [cited 2025 Nov 22];13(1):6561. Available from: https://www.nature.com/articles/s41598-023-33432-4
31. Lima C, Alves LE, Iagher F, Machado AF, Bonatto SJ, Kuczera D, et al. Anaerobic exercise reduces tumor growth, cancer cachexia and increases macrophage and lymphocyte response in Walker 256 tumor-bearing rats. Eur J Appl Physiol [Internet]. 2008 [cited 2025 Nov 22];104(6):957–64. Available from: https://pubmed.ncbi.nlm.nih.gov/18688637/

32. Zhang QB, Meng XT, Jia QA, Bu Y, Ren ZG, Zhang BH, et al. Herbal compound songyou yin and moderate swimming suppress growth and metastasis of liver cancer by enhancing immune function. Integr Cancer Ther [Internet]. 2016 Sep 1 [cited 2025 Nov 22];15(3):368–75. Available from: https://pubmed.ncbi.nlm.nih.gov/26699805/
33. Hwang CL, Yu CJ, Shih JY, Yang PC, Wu YT. Effects of exercise training on exercise capacity in patients with non-small cell lung cancer receiving targeted therapy. Support Care Cancer [Internet]. 2012 Dec [cited 2025 Nov 22];20(12): 3169–77. Available from: https://pubmed.ncbi.nlm.nih.gov/22526147/
34. Gokal K, Wallis D, Ahmed S, Boiangiu I, Kancherla K, Munir F. Effects of a self-managed home-based walking intervention on psychosocial health outcomes for breast cancer patients receiving chemotherapy: A randomised controlled trial. Support Care Cancer [Internet]. 2016 Mar 1 [cited 2025 Nov 22];24(3): 1139–66. Available from: https://pubmed.ncbi.nlm.nih.gov/26275768/
35. Shi X, Hu L, Nieman DC, Li F, Chen P, Shi H, et al. Exercise workload: A key determinant of immune health—A narrative review. Front Immunol. 2025 Jul 24;16:1617261.
36. Syed M, Parmar C, Pouwels S. The effects of exercise therapy on immune cells and function in patients with overweight or obesity: A systematic review. Brain Behavior and Immunity Integrative. 2024 Dec 1;8:100093.
37. Siewierska K, Malicka I, Kobierzycki C, Paslawska U, Cegielski M, Grzegrzolka J, et al. The impact of exercise training on breast cancer. In Vivo [Internet]. 2018 [cited 2025 Nov 22];32(2):249–54. Available from: https://pubmed.ncbi.nlm.nih.gov/29475906/
38. van Doorslaer de Ten Ryen S, Deldicque L. The regulation of the metastatic cascade by physical activity: A narrative review. Cancers (Basel) [Internet]. 2020 Jan 8 [cited 2025 Jan 10];12(1):153. Available from: http://www.ncbi.nlm.nih.gov/pubmed/31936342
39. Mishra SI, Scherer RW, Geigle PM, Berlanstein DR, Topaloglu O, Gotay CC, et al. Exercise interventions on health-related quality of life for cancer survivors. Cochrane Database Syst Rev [Internet]. 2012 Aug 15 [cited 2025 Nov 22];2012(8):CD007566. Available from: https://pmc.ncbi.nlm.nih.gov/articles/PMC7387117/
40. Hong F, Ye W, Kuo CH, Zhang Y, Qian Y, Korivi M. Exercise intervention improves clinical outcomes, but the "time of session" is crucial for better quality of life in breast cancer survivors: A systematic review and meta-analysis. Cancers (Basel) [Internet]. 2019 May 1 [cited 2025 Nov 22];11(5):706. Available from: https://pmc.ncbi.nlm.nih.gov/articles/PMC6562879/
41. Avancini A, Borsati A, Toniolo L, Ciurnelli C, Belluomini L, Budolfsen T, et al. Physical activity guidelines in oncology: A systematic review of the current recommendations. Crit Rev Oncol Hematol. 2025 Jun 1;210:104718.
42. Spada GE, Masiero M, Pizzoli SFM, Pravettoni G. Heart rate variability biofeedback in cancer patients: A scoping review. Behav Sci [Internet]. 2022 Oct 1 [cited 2025 Nov 22];12(10):389. Available from: https://pmc.ncbi.nlm.nih.gov/articles/PMC9598295/
43. Mustian KM, Alfano CM, Heckler C, Kleckner AS, Kleckner IR, Leach CR, et al. Comparison of pharmaceutical, psychological, and exercise treatments for cancer-related fatigue a meta-analysis. JAMA Oncol [Internet]. 2017 Jul 1 [cited 2025 Nov 22];3(7):961. Available from: https://pmc.ncbi.nlm.nih.gov/articles/PMC5557289/
44. Cormie P, Galvão DA, Spry N, Joseph D, Chee R, Taaffe DR, et al. Can supervised exercise prevent treatment toxicity in patients with prostate cancer

initiating androgen-deprivation therapy: A randomised controlled trial. BJU Int [Internet]. 2015 Feb 1 [cited 2025 Nov 22];115(2):256–66. Available from: https://pubmed.ncbi.nlm.nih.gov/24467669/
45. Pelzer F, Leisge K, Schlüter K, Schneider J, Wiskemann J, Rosenberger F. Effects of exercise mode and intensity on patient-reported outcomes in cancer survivors: A four-arm intervention trial. Supportive Care in Cancer [Internet]. 2023 May 1 [cited 2025 Nov 22];31(5):315. Available from: https://pmc.ncbi.nlm.nih.gov/articles/PMC10154283/
46. Van Waart H, Stuiver MM, Van Harten WH, Geleijn E, Kieffer JM, Buffart LM, et al. Effect of low-intensity physical activity and moderate- to high-intensity physical exercise during adjuvant chemotherapy on physical fitness, fatigue, and chemotherapy completion rates: Results of the PACES randomized clinical trial. J Clin Oncol [Internet]. 2015 Jun 10 [cited 2025 Nov 22];33(17):1918–27. Available from: https://ascopubs.org/doi/10.1200/JCO.2014.59.1081
47. Booth CM, Vardy JL, O'Callaghan CJ, Gill S, Friedenreich C, Wong RK, et al. A randomized phase III trial of the impact of a structured exercise program on Disease-Free Survival (DFS) in stage 3 or high-risk stage 2 colon cancer: Canadian Cancer Trials Group (CCTG) CO.21 (CHALLENGE). J Clin Oncol [Internet]. 2025 Jun 10 [cited 2025 Nov 22];43(17_suppl). Available from: https://ascopubs.org/doi/10.1200/JCO.2025.43.17_suppl.LBA3510
48. Newton RU, Lopez P, Hart NH, Galvao DA, Taaffe DR, Clay TD, et al. Intense exercise for survival among men with metastatic prostate cancer: 12 months feasibility results from the INTERVAL-GAP4 trial. JCO Glob Oncol [Internet]. 2023 Aug [cited 2025 Nov 22];9(Supplement_1):81–81. Available from: https://ascopubs.org/doi/10.1200/GO.2023.9.Supplement_1.81
49. Holmen Olofsson G, Mikkelsen MK, Ragle AM, Christiansen AB, Olsen AP, Heide-Ottosen L, et al. High intensity aerobic exercise training and immune cell mobilization in patients with lung cancer (HI AIM)-a randomized controlled trial. BMC Cancer [Internet]. 2022 Dec 1 [cited 2025 Nov 25];22(1). Available from: https://pubmed.ncbi.nlm.nih.gov/35247994/
50. Courneya KS, Friedenreich CM. Framework PEACE: An organizational model for examining physical exercise across the cancer experience. Ann Behav Med [Internet]. 2001 [cited 2025 Nov 23];23(4):263–72. Available from: https://pubmed.ncbi.nlm.nih.gov/11761343/
51. Jones LW, Alfano CM. Exercise-oncology research: Past, present, and future. Acta Oncol (Madr) [Internet]. 2013 Feb 17 [cited 2019 Dec 10];52(2):195–215. Available from: http://www.ncbi.nlm.nih.gov/pubmed/23244677
52. An KY, Min J, Lee DH, Kang DW, Courneya KS, Jeon JY. Exercise across the phases of cancer survivorship: A narrative review. Yonsei Med J [Internet]. 2024 Jun 1 [cited 2025 Nov 23];65(6):315–23. Available from: https://doi.org/10.3349/ymj.2023.0638
53. Jones LW, Peddle CJ, Eves ND, Haykowsky MJ, Courneya KS, Mackey JR, et al. Effects of presurgical exercise training on cardiorespiratory fitness among patients undergoing thoracic surgery for malignant lung lesions. Cancer [Internet]. 2007 Aug 1 [cited 2025 Nov 25];110(3):590–8. Available from: https://pubmed.ncbi.nlm.nih.gov/17582629/
54. Bobbio A, Chetta A, Ampollini L, Primomo GL, Internullo E, Carbognani P, et al. Preoperative pulmonary rehabilitation in patients undergoing lung resection for non-small cell lung cancer. Eur J Cardiothorac Surg [Internet]. 2008 Jan [cited 2025 Nov 25];33(1):95–8. Available from: https://pubmed.ncbi.nlm.nih.gov/18006327/

55. Cesario A, Ferri L, Galetta D, Cardaci V, Biscione G, Pasqua F, et al. Pre-operative pulmonary rehabilitation and surgery for lung cancer. Lung Cancer [Internet]. 2007 Jul [cited 2025 Nov 14];57(1):118–9. Available from: https://pubmed.ncbi.nlm.nih.gov/17475363/
56. Steffens D, Beckenkamp PR, Young J, Solomon M, da Silva TM, Hancock MJ. Is preoperative physical activity level of patients undergoing cancer surgery associated with postoperative outcomes? A systematic review and meta-analysis. Eur J Surg Oncol [Internet]. 2019 Apr 1 [cited 2025 Nov 25];45(4): 510–8. Available from: https://pubmed.ncbi.nlm.nih.gov/30910052/
57. Roman M, Monaghan A, Serraino GF, Miller D, Pathak S, Lai F, et al. Meta-analysis of the influence of lifestyle changes for preoperative weight loss on surgical outcomes. Br J Surg [Internet]. 2019 Feb 1 [cited 2025 Nov 25];106(3):181–9. Available from: https://pubmed.ncbi.nlm.nih.gov/30328098/
58. Dhanis J, Keidan N, Blake D, Rundle S, Strijker D, van Ham M, et al. Prehabilitation to improve outcomes of patients with gynaecological cancer: A new window of opportunity? Cancers (Basel) [Internet]. 2022 Jul 1 [cited 2025 Nov 25];14(14). Available from: https://pubmed.ncbi.nlm.nih.gov/35884512/
59. Molenaar CJL, Minnella EM, Coca-Martinez M, Ten Cate DWG, Regis M, Awasthi R, et al. Effect of multimodal prehabilitation on reducing postoperative complications and enhancing functional capacity following colorectal cancer surgery: The PREHAB randomized clinical trial. JAMA Surg [Internet]. 2023 Jun 14 [cited 2025 Nov 14];158(6):572. Available from: https://pmc.ncbi.nlm.nih.gov/articles/PMC10061316/
60. Ikeda T, Noma K, Maeda N, Tanabe S, Sakamoto Y, Katayama Y, et al. Effectiveness of early exercise on reducing skeletal muscle loss during preoperative neoadjuvant chemotherapy for esophageal cancer. Surg Today [Internet]. 2022 Aug 1 [cited 2025 Nov 25];52(8):1143–52. Available from: https://pubmed.ncbi.nlm.nih.gov/34988678/
61. Avancini A, Cavallo A, Trestini I, Tregnago D, Belluomini L, Crisafulli E, et al. Exercise prehabilitation in lung cancer: Getting stronger to recover faster. Eur J Surg Oncol [Internet]. 2021 Aug 1 [cited 2025 Nov 25];47(8):1847–55. Available from: https://pubmed.ncbi.nlm.nih.gov/33757650/
62. Carayol M, Bernard P, Boiché J, Riou F, Mercier B, Cousson-gélie F, et al. Psychological effect of exercise in women with breast cancer receiving adjuvant therapy: What is the optimal dose needed? Ann Oncol [Internet]. 2013 Feb [cited 2025 Nov 25];24(2):291–300. Available from: https://pubmed.ncbi.nlm.nih.gov/23041586/
63. Van Vulpen JK, Peeters PHM, Velthuis MJ, Van Der Wall E, May AM. Effects of physical exercise during adjuvant breast cancer treatment on physical and psychosocial dimensions of cancer-related fatigue: A meta-analysis. Maturitas [Internet]. 2016 Mar 1 [cited 2025 Nov 25];85:104–11. Available from: https://pubmed.ncbi.nlm.nih.gov/26857888/
64. Furmaniak AC, Menig M, Markes MH. Exercise for women receiving adjuvant therapy for breast cancer. Cochrane Database Syst Rev [Internet]. 2016 Sep 21 [cited 2025 Nov 25];9(9). Available from: https://pubmed.ncbi.nlm.nih.gov/27650122/
65. Lipsett A, Barrett S, Haruna F, Mustian K, O'Donovan A. The impact of exercise during adjuvant radiotherapy for breast cancer on fatigue and quality of life: A systematic review and meta-analysis. Breast [Internet]. 2017 Apr 1 [cited 2025 Nov 25];32:144–55. Available from: https://pubmed.ncbi.nlm.nih.gov/28189100/

66. Lund CM, Dolin TG, Mikkelsen MK, Juhl CB, Vinther A, Nielsen DL. Effect of exercise on physical function and psychological well-being in older patients with colorectal cancer receiving chemotherapy-A systematic review. Clin Colorectal Cancer [Internet]. 2020 Dec 1 [cited 2025 Nov 25];19(4): e243–57. Available from: https://pubmed.ncbi.nlm.nih.gov/32828706/
67. Dun L, Xian-Yi W, Xiao-Ying J. Effects of moderate-to-vigorous physical activity on cancer-related fatigue in patients with colorectal cancer: A systematic review and meta-analysis. Arch Med Res [Internet]. 2020 Feb 1 [cited 2025 Nov 25];51(2):173–9. Available from: https://pubmed.ncbi.nlm.nih.gov/32111495/
68. Lopez P, Galvão DA, Taaffe DR, Newton RU, Souza G, Trajano GS, et al. Resistance training in breast cancer patients undergoing primary treatment: A systematic review and meta-regression of exercise dosage. Breast Cancer [Internet]. 2021 Jan 1 [cited 2025 Nov 25];28(1):16–24. Available from: https://pubmed.ncbi.nlm.nih.gov/32815096/
69. Bland KA, Zadravec K, Landry T, Weller S, Meyers L, Campbell KL. Impact of exercise on chemotherapy completion rate: A systematic review of the evidence and recommendations for future exercise oncology research. Crit Rev Oncol Hematol [Internet]. 2019 Apr 1 [cited 2025 Nov 25];136:79–85. Available from: https://pubmed.ncbi.nlm.nih.gov/30878132/
70. Courneya KS, Segal RJ, McKenzie DC, Dong H, Gelmon K, Friedenreich CM, et al. Effects of exercise during adjuvant chemotherapy on breast cancer outcomes. Med Sci Sports Exerc [Internet]. 2014 [cited 2025 Nov 22];46(9):1744–51. Available from: https://journals.lww.com/acsm-msse/fulltext/2014/09000/effects_of_exercise_during_adjuvant_chemotherapy.9.aspx
71. Morielli AR, Usmani N, Boulé NG, Severin D, Tankel K, Joseph K, et al. Feasibility, safety, and preliminary efficacy of exercise during and after neoadjuvant rectal cancer treatment: A phase II randomized controlled trial. Clin Colorectal Cancer [Internet]. 2021 Sep 1 [cited 2025 Nov 25];20(3):216–26. Available from: https://pubmed.ncbi.nlm.nih.gov/34158253/
72. An KY, Arthuso FZ, Kang DW, Morielli AR, Ntoukas SM, Friedenreich CM, et al. Exercise and health-related fitness predictors of chemotherapy completion in breast cancer patients: Pooled analysis of two multicenter trials. Breast Cancer Res Treat [Internet]. 2021 Jul 1 [cited 2025 Nov 25];188(2):399–407. Available from: https://pubmed.ncbi.nlm.nih.gov/33779887/
73. Stout NL, Baima J, Swisher AK, Winters-Stone KM, Welsh J. A systematic review of exercise systematic reviews in the cancer literature. (2005–2017). PM R [Internet]. 2017 Sep 1 [cited 2025 Nov 22];9(9 Suppl 2):S347. Available from: https://pmc.ncbi.nlm.nih.gov/articles/PMC5679711/
74. Mustian KM, Sprod LK, Palesh OG, Peppone LJ, Janelsins MC, Mohile SG, et al. Exercise for the management of side effects and quality of life among cancer survivors. Curr Sports Med Rep [Internet]. 2009 Nov [cited 2025 Nov 25];8(6):325. Available from: https://pmc.ncbi.nlm.nih.gov/articles/PMC2875185/
75. Misiąg W, Piszczyk A, Szymańska-Chabowska A, Chabowski M. Physical activity and cancer care—A review. Cancers (Basel) [Internet]. 2022 Sep 1 [cited 2025 Nov 22];14(17):4154. Available from: https://pmc.ncbi.nlm.nih.gov/articles/PMC9454950/
76. Spence RR, Heesch KC, Brown WJ. Exercise and cancer rehabilitation: A systematic review. Cancer Treat Rev [Internet]. 2010 Apr [cited 2025 Nov 25];36(2):185–94. Available from: https://pubmed.ncbi.nlm.nih.gov/19962830/

77. Gao R, Yu T, Liu L, Bi J, Zhao H, Tao Y, et al. Exercise intervention for post-treatment colorectal cancer survivors: A systematic review and meta-analysis. J Cancer Surviv [Internet]. 2020 Dec 1 [cited 2025 Nov 25];14(6):878–93. Available from: https://pubmed.ncbi.nlm.nih.gov/32533468/
78. An KY, Min J, Lee DH, Kang DW, Courneya KS, Jeon JY. Exercise across the phases of cancer survivorship: A narrative review. Yonsei Med J [Internet]. 2024 Jun 1 [cited 2025 Nov 25];65(6):315–23. Available from: https://doi.org/10.3349/ymj.2023.0638
79. Ballard-Barbash R, Friedenreich CM, Courneya KS, Siddiqi SM, McTiernan A, Alfano CM. Physical activity, biomarkers, and disease outcomes in cancer survivors: A systematic review. J Natl Cancer Inst [Internet]. 2012 Jun [cited 2025 Nov 25];104(11):815–40. Available from: https://pubmed.ncbi.nlm.nih.gov/22570317/
80. Rock CL, Thomson CA, Sullivan KR, Howe CL, Kushi LH, Caan BJ, et al. American cancer society nutrition and physical activity guideline for cancer survivors. CA Cancer J Clin [Internet]. 2022 May [cited 2025 Nov 25];72(3):230–62. Available from: https://pubmed.ncbi.nlm.nih.gov/35294043/
81. Frikkel J, Götte M, Beckmann M, Kasper S, Hense J, Teufel M, et al. Fatigue, barriers to physical activity and predictors for motivation to exercise in advanced cancer patients. BMC Palliat Care [Internet]. 2020 Mar 31 [cited 2025 Nov 25];19(1):43. Available from: https://link.springer.com/article/10.1186/s12904-020-00542-z
82. Hussey C, Gupta A. Exercise interventions to combat cancer-related fatigue in cancer patients undergoing treatment: A review. Cancer Invest [Internet]. 2022 Oct 21 [cited 2025 Nov 25];40(9):822–38. Available from: https://www.tandfonline.com/doi/abs/10.1080/07357907.2022.2105349
83. Metcalfe JW, Orange ST, Madden LA, Marshall P, Vince R V. Effects of resistance training on quality of life, fatigue, physical function, and muscular strength during chemotherapy treatment: A systematic review and meta-analysis. Supportive Care in Cancer [Internet]. 2024 Sep 1 [cited 2025 Nov 25];32(9):593. Available from: https://pmc.ncbi.nlm.nih.gov/articles/PMC11330399/
84. Bay ML, Unterrainer N, Stagaard R, Pedersen KS, Schauer T, Staffeldt MM, et al. Voluntary wheel running can lead to modulation of immune checkpoint molecule expression. Acta Oncol [Internet]. 2020 Dec 1 [cited 2025 Nov 25];59(12):1447–54. Available from: https://pubmed.ncbi.nlm.nih.gov/32935602/
85. Kurz E, Hirsch CA, Dalton T, Shadaloey SA, Khodadadi-Jamayran A, Miller G, et al. Exercise-induced engagement of the IL-15/IL-15Rα axis promotes anti-tumor immunity in pancreatic cancer. Cancer Cell. 2022 Jul 11;40(7):720–37.e5.
86. Liu XF, Zhu XD, Feng LH, Li XL, Xu B, Li KS, et al. Physical activity improves outcomes of combined lenvatinib plus anti-PD-1 therapy in unresectable hepatocellular carcinoma: A retrospective study and mouse model. Exp Hematol Oncol [Internet]. 2022 Dec 1 [cited 2025 Nov 25];11(1). Available from: https://pubmed.ncbi.nlm.nih.gov/35379324/
87. Gomes-Santos IL, Amoozgar Z, Kumar AS, Ho WW, Roh K, Talele NP, et al. Exercise training improves tumor control by increasing CD8+ T-cell infiltration via CXCR3 signaling and sensitizes breast cancer to immune checkpoint blockade. Cancer Immunol Res [Internet]. 2021 Jul 1 [cited 2025 Nov 16];9(7):765. Available from: https://pmc.ncbi.nlm.nih.gov/articles/PMC8295193/
88. Wennerberg E, Lhuillier C, Rybstein MD, Dannenberg K, Rudqvist NP, Koelwyn GJ, et al. Exercise reduces immune suppression and breast cancer progression in a preclinical model. Oncotarget [Internet]. 2020 [cited 2025 Nov 16];11(4):452–61. Available from: www.oncotarget.com

89. Buss LA, Williams T, Hock B, Ang AD, Robinson BA, Currie MJ, et al. Effects of exercise and anti-PD-1 on the tumour microenvironment. Immunol Lett [Internet]. 2021 Nov 1 [cited 2025 Nov 25];239:60–71. Available from: https://pubmed.ncbi.nlm.nih.gov/34480981/
90. Study Details | NCT03171064 | Exercise as a supportive measure for patients undergoing checkpoint-inhibitor treatment | ClinicalTrials.gov [Internet]. [cited 2025 Nov 25]. Available from: https://clinicaltrials.gov/study/NCT03171064
91. Gouez M, Pérol O, Pérol M, Caux C, Ménétrier-Caux C, Villard M, et al. Effect of acute aerobic exercise before immunotherapy and chemotherapy infusion in patients with metastatic non-small-cell lung cancer: Protocol for the ERICA feasibility trial. BMJ Open [Internet]. 2022 Apr 7 [cited 2025 Nov 25];12(4). Available from: https://pubmed.ncbi.nlm.nih.gov/35393316/
92. Steffens D, Hancock M, Jiang W, Solomon M, Koh C, Hirst N, et al. An updated systematic review and meta-analysis of unimodal prehabilitation with exercise intervention to enhance postoperative outcomes in cancer surgery. Anesth Analg [Internet]. 2025 Apr 1 [cited 2025 Nov 25];140(4):811–20. Available from: https://pubmed.ncbi.nlm.nih.gov/39383108/
93. Gennuso D, Baldelli A, Gigli L, Ruotolo I, Galeoto G, Gaburri D, et al. Efficacy of prehabilitation in cancer patients: An Rcts systematic review with meta-analysis. BMC Cancer [Internet]. 2024 Dec 1 [cited 2025 Nov 25];24(1):1302. Available from: https://link.springer.com/article/10.1186/s12885-024-13023-w
94. Minnella EM, Awasthi R, Loiselle SE, Agnihotram RV., Ferri LE, Carli F. Effect of exercise and nutrition prehabilitation on functional capacity in esophagogastric cancer surgery: A randomized clinical trial. JAMA Surg [Internet]. 2018 Dec 1 [cited 2025 Nov 25];153(12):1081–9. Available from: https://jamanetwork.com/journals/jamasurgery/fullarticle/2698681
95. Waterland JL, McCourt O, Edbrooke L, Granger CL, Ismail H, Riedel B, et al. Efficacy of prehabilitation including exercise on postoperative outcomes following abdominal cancer surgery: A systematic review and meta-analysis. Front Surg [Internet]. 2021 Mar 19 [cited 2025 Nov 25];8:628848. Available from: https://pmc.ncbi.nlm.nih.gov/articles/PMC8017317/
96. Saleh AY, Shareef A, Bishoyi AK, Jyothi SR, Panigrahi R, Pargaien A, et al. Personalized exercise programs in oncology. Oncol Rev [Internet]. 2025 [cited 2025 Nov 25];19:1645505. Available from: https://pmc.ncbi.nlm.nih.gov/articles/PMC12463836/
97. Musanti, PhD, APN-BC R, Chao, PhD, GNP-BC YY, Collins, BS, RDN K. Fitness and quality of life outcomes of cancer survivor participants in a community exercise program. J Adv Pract Oncol [Internet]. 2019 Feb 1 [cited 2025 Nov 25];10(1):24. Available from: https://pmc.ncbi.nlm.nih.gov/articles/PMC6605700/
98. Giallauria F, Testa C, Cuomo G, Di Lorenzo A, Venturini E, Lauretani F, et al. Exercise training in elderly cancer patients: A systematic review. Cancers (Basel) [Internet]. 2023 Mar 1 [cited 2025 Nov 25];15(6):1671. Available from: https://pmc.ncbi.nlm.nih.gov/articles/PMC10046194/
99. Macías-Valle A, Rodríguez-López C, González-Senac NM, Mayordomo-Cava J, Vidán MT, Cruz-Arnés ML, et al. Exercise effects on functional capacity and quality of life in older patients with colorectal cancer: Study protocol for the ECOOL randomized controlled trial. BMC Geriatr [Internet]. 2023 Dec 1 [cited 2025 Nov 25];23(1):314. Available from: https://link.springer.com/article/10.1186/s12877-023-04026-6
100. Drouin JP. Exercise in older individuals with cancer: Topics in geriatric rehabilitation. Top Geriatr Rehabil. 2004;20(2):81–97.

101. Ji H, Gulati M, Huang TY, Kwan AC, Ouyang D, Ebinger JE, et al. Sex differences in association of physical activity with all-cause and cardiovascular mortality. J Am Coll Cardiol [Internet]. 2024 Feb 27 [cited 2025 Nov 25];83(8):783–93. Available from: https://www.jacc.org/doi/10.1016/j.jacc.2023.12.019
102. He A, Wang Y, Du C, Wang Y, Wu J, Kuang D, et al. Sex differences in the association of physical activity patterns with all-cause and cardiovascular mortality: A prospective cohort study from NHANES 2007–2018. Sci Rep 2025 15:1 [Internet]. 2025 Jul 1 [cited 2025 Nov 25];15(1):22197. Available from: https://www.nature.com/articles/s41598-025-06056-z
103. Zhong X, Zimmers TA. Sex differences in cancer cachexia. Curr Osteoporos Rep [Internet]. 2020 Dec 1 [cited 2025 Nov 25];18(6):646–54. Available from: https://link.springer.com/article/10.1007/s11914-020-00628-w
104. Repka CP, Peterson BM, Brown JM, Lalonde TL, Schneider CM, Hayward R. Cancer type does not affect exercise-mediated improvements in cardiorespiratory function and fatigue. Integr Cancer Ther [Internet]. 2014 Nov 19 [cited 2025 Nov 25];13(6):473–81. Available from: https://journals.sagepub.com/doi/full/10.1177/1534735414547108
105. Wong JN, McAuley E, Trinh L. Physical activity programming and counseling preferences among cancer survivors: A systematic review. Int J Behav Nutr Phys Act [Internet]. 2018 Jun 7 [cited 2025 Nov 25];15(1):48. Available from: https://link.springer.com/article/10.1186/s12966-018-0680-6
106. Kampshoff CS, Jansen F, van Mechelen W, May AM, Brug J, Chinapaw MJM, et al. Determinants of exercise adherence and maintenance among cancer survivors: A systematic review. Int J Behav Nutr Phys Act [Internet]. 2014 Jul 2 [cited 2025 Nov 25];11(1):80. Available from: https://pmc.ncbi.nlm.nih.gov/articles/PMC4096543/
107. Ranes M, Wiestad TH, Thormodsen I, Arving C. Determinants of exercise adherence and maintenance for cancer survivors: Implementation of a community-based group exercise program: A qualitative feasibility study. PEC Innovation. 2022 Dec 1;1:100088.
108. Felser S, Behrens M, Lampe H, Henze L, Grosse-Thie C, Murua Escobar H, et al. Motivation and preferences of cancer patients to perform physical training. Eur J Cancer Care (Engl) [Internet]. 2020 Jul 1 [cited 2025 Nov 25];29(4):e13246. Available from: https://onlinelibrary.wiley.com/doi/full/10.1111/ecc.13246
109. Bell KE, Pfeiffer AG, Schmidt S, Bos L, Russell C, Barnes T, et al. Low-frequency exercise training improves cardiovascular fitness and strength during treatment for breast cancer: A single-arm intervention study. Sci Rep [Internet]. 2021 Nov 23 [cited 2025 Nov 25];11(1):22758. Available from: https://www.nature.com/articles/s41598-021-01962-4
110. Brooke HL, Mazzoni AS, Buffart LM, Berntsen S, Nordin K, Demmelmaier I. Patterns and determinants of adherence to resistance and endurance training during cancer treatment in the Phys-Can RCT. BMC Sports Sci Med Rehabil [Internet]. 2022 Dec 1 [cited 2025 Nov 25];14(1):155. Available from: https://link.springer.com/article/10.1186/s13102-022-00548-5
111. Pedroso M, Grigoletto I, Oliveira L, Martins S, Costa L, Pozo K, et al. Adherence to exercise in people with lung or head and neck cancer: Self-reported symptoms and motivation during cancer treatment need to be considered. J Clin Med [Internet]. 2024 Oct 21 [cited 2025 Nov 25];13(20):6267. Available from: https://www.mdpi.com/2077-0383/13/20/6267/htm

112. Orange ST, Jordan AR, Saxton JM. The serological responses to acute exercise in humans reduce cancer cell growth in vitro: A systematic review and meta-analysis. Physiol Rep [Internet]. 2020 Nov 1 [cited 2025 Nov 25];8(22):e14635. Available from: https://onlinelibrary.wiley.com/doi/full/10.14814/phy2.14635
113. Diao X, Ling Y, Zeng Y, Wu Y, Guo C, Jin Y, et al. Physical activity and cancer risk: A dose-response analysis for the Global Burden of Disease Study 2019. Cancer Commun (Lond) [Internet]. 2023 Nov 1 [cited 2025 Nov 25];43(11): 1229–43. Available from: https://pubmed.ncbi.nlm.nih.gov/37743572/
114. Ekelund U, Sanchez-Lastra MA, Dalene KE, Tarp J. Dose–response associations, physical activity intensity and mortality risk: A narrative review. J Sport Health Sci [Internet]. 2023 Jan 1 [cited 2025 Nov 25];13(1):24. Available from: https://pmc.ncbi.nlm.nih.gov/articles/PMC10818107/
115. Geidl W, Schlesinger S, Mino E, Miranda L, Pfeifer K. Dose-response relationship between physical activity and mortality in adults with noncommunicable diseases: A systematic review and meta-analysis of prospective observational studies. Int J Behav Nutr Phys Act [Internet]. 2020 Aug 26 [cited 2025 Nov 25];17(1):109. Available from: https://link.springer.com/article/10.1186/s12966-020-01007-5

PART III

Current guidelines

8

EXERCISE GUIDELINES AND RECOMMENDATIONS

8.1 Introduction

Exercise oncology has evolved from a promising adjunct to a recognised element of modern cancer care. Regular physical activity has been shown to improve physical function, reduce treatment-related side effects, enhance psychological wellbeing, and increasingly, to influence survival outcomes. While integration into routine oncology care remains inconsistent, the role of exercise as a supportive intervention is gaining traction across the continuum. Yet, despite decades of research, the translation of this evidence into consistent clinical practice remains uneven. Patients still report uncertainty about what kinds of exercise are safe, how much is enough and when it should be undertaken (1,2). Similarly, clinicians often express concern about when and how to make appropriate referrals (3–5). The need for clear, evidence-informed guidance has therefore never been greater.

This chapter summarises current global and cancer-specific physical activity guidelines, outlining the minimum levels of activity required for health and the rationale for their application in oncology. It then considers how these guidelines can be adapted across the cancer continuum, from prehabilitation through to survivorship and palliative care. Subsequent sections address the importance of individualisation, behavioural support and system-level implementation, while also highlighting the research priorities needed to refine and personalise exercise prescription in the years ahead. In essence, this chapter moves from principle to practice: From broad public health recommendations to the realities of helping individuals living with and beyond cancer move safely, confidently and meaningfully throughout their cancer pathway.

DOI: 10.4324/9781003511519-11

8.2 Global physical activity guidelines

Physical activity is a cornerstone of public health, with strong evidence linking regular movement to reduced morbidity and improved longevity. While recommendations vary slightly across organisations, there is a broad consensus on the minimum levels of activity required to support overall health and these form the foundation for exercise guidelines in oncology.

8.2.1 General guidelines for health

The WHO recommends that all adults, including those living with chronic conditions such as cancer, engage in at least 150–300 minutes of moderate-intensity aerobic activity, or 75–150 minutes of vigorous-intensity activity per week, in addition to muscle-strengthening activities involving major muscle groups on two or more days per week. These recommendations are based on a compelling body of evidence showing that regular physical activity reduces the risk of CVD, type 2 diabetes, depression and at least 13 types of cancer (6).

8.2.2 Cancer-specific guidelines

Cancer-specific exercise recommendations have evolved significantly over the past two decades, informed by an expanding evidence base and clinical consensus. Key bodies such as the ACSM, the American Society of Clinical Oncology (ASCO) and Macmillan Cancer Support provide aligned guidance (7–9). ACSM's 2019 roundtable concluded that exercise is safe during and after cancer treatment and should be considered a standard part of care (10). ASCO supports the integration of physical activity into survivorship care plans, recognising its role in reducing fatigue, improving physical function and enhancing QoL (8). Macmillan Cancer Support recommends that people living with cancer "move more" throughout treatment and recovery, echoing the WHO guidance in terms of frequency, intensity and duration (9,11). Despite some variation in language and emphasis, these guidelines consistently advocate for 150 minutes of moderate-intensity aerobic activity per week (or 75 minutes of vigorous intensity) and two strength-based sessions targeting major muscle groups (Figure 8.1). This convergence in recommendations reflects the robust evidence showing benefits across cancer types and stages.

8.2.3 Practical emphasis: Every move counts

While global guidelines provide a clear benchmark for weekly physical activity, they should be viewed as flexible targets rather than rigid prescriptions,

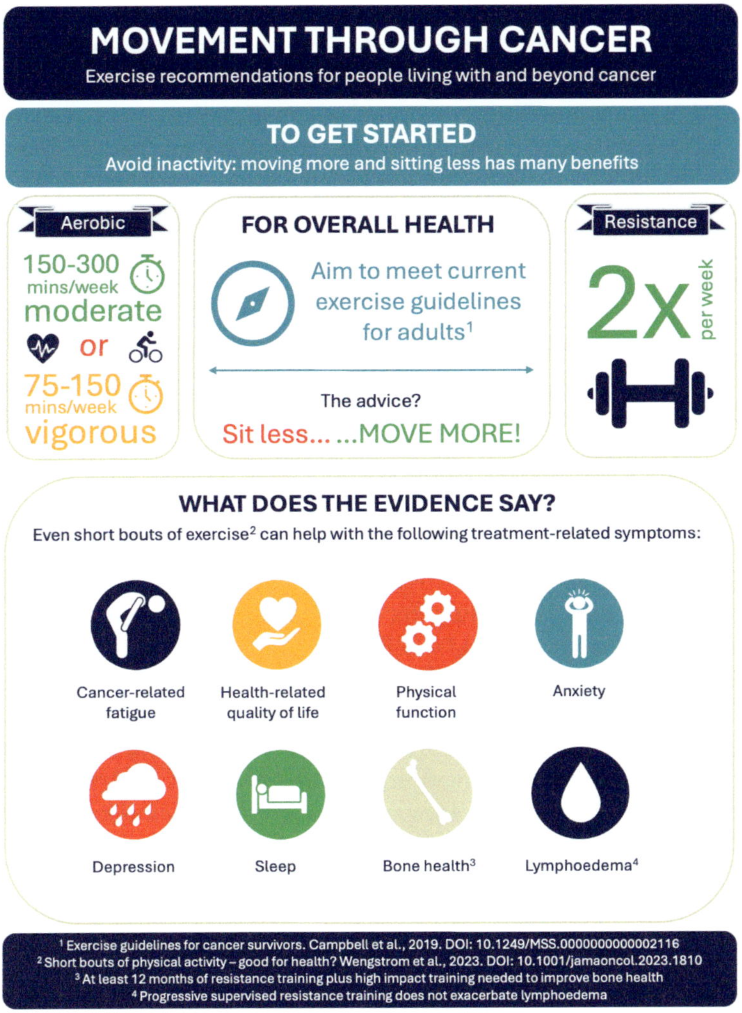

FIGURE 8.1 Physical activity and exercise recommendations and benefits for people living with and beyond cancer. This infographic, adapted from the ACSM roundtable on exercise and cancer (12), summarises current exercise guidelines and the evidence base for physical activity in cancer care. People affected by cancer are encouraged to aim for 150–300 minutes of moderate-intensity aerobic activity, or 75–150 minutes of vigorous activity per week, alongside muscle strengthening resistance training twice weekly, in line with general adult health recommendations. Avoiding inactivity is emphasised as a crucial first step. Even short bouts of movement have been shown to improve a range of treatment-related symptoms, including fatigue, anxiety, depression, sleep quality, bone health, lymphoedema and overall physical function and quality of life. This evidence-based approach highlights the role of exercise as a supportive therapy across the cancer continuum.

especially in the context of cancer. For many individuals living with or beyond cancer, achieving the recommended 150 minutes of moderate-intensity activity per week may not be immediately feasible. Fatigue, pain, treatment-related side effects and fluctuating physical capacity often make sustained or structured exercise challenging. However, compelling evidence supports the idea that any amount of movement is beneficial and that accumulated activity, even in short or lighter bouts, can confer measurable health benefits.

Studies show that breaking physical activity into smaller increments (e.g., 3 × 10 minutes) yields comparable outcomes to continuous sessions of the same total duration, particularly in terms of cardiovascular fitness, fatigue reduction and psychological wellbeing (13–16). This is especially relevant for individuals coping with cancer-related fatigue, one of the most pervasive and debilitating symptoms during and after treatment. Several studies acknowledge that even light-intensity or incidental activity, such as gentle walking, stretching or household tasks, can help mitigate fatigue and improve functional capacity over time (17–19). A "something is better than nothing" approach also aligns with the evolving clinical emphasis on personalised and adaptive movement (20,21). Tailoring activity to daily energy levels, individual levels of side effects and personal goals supports engagement and long-term adherence. This perspectivity underpins Macmillan Cancer Support's message to "move more," encouraging individuals to start where they are and build gradually, even if that means beginning with just a few minutes a day (22). Overall, the goal is not to meet an idealised weekly quota, but to embed movement into daily life in a way that is achievable, safe and meaningful. Over time, these small steps can lead to significant gains in physical and emotional wellbeing.

8.3 Exercise prescriptions across the cancer continuum

Exercise is not a one-off intervention but a dynamic, adaptive component of cancer care. Across the continuum, from diagnosis through treatment, into recovery and beyond, exercise serves different yet overlapping purposes: To prepare, to protect, to restore and to sustain (Table 8.1). Recognising where a patient sits on this continuum is key to tailoring an appropriate and safe exercise prescription.

8.3.1 Prehabilitation: Preparing for treatment

Prehabilitation refers to structured exercise (often combined with nutritional and psychological support) undertaken between diagnosis and the start of treatment (23). Its primary aim is to enhance physical and psychological resilience before exposure to the stresses of surgery, chemotherapy or radiotherapy. Patients and their clinicians may have many different goals for

TABLE 8.1 Exercise goals and adaptations across the cancer continuum

Cancer Phase	*Primary Goals*	*Typical Prescription*	*Adaptations/Notes*
Prehabilitation	Build fitness and resilience before treatment	3–5 days per week moderate aerobic and 2 resistance sessions	Short, targeted programmes; focus on major muscle groups
During treatment	Maintain function, reduce fatigue	Daily light-moderate aerobic; resistance 1–2 × per week	Flexible intensity; adapt to treatment side effects
Post-treatment and/or survivorship	Restore strength, endurance and wellbeing	Gradual progression to 150 min per week and 2 strength sessions	Emphasise enjoyment and sustainability
Advanced stage or palliative care	Preserve mobility and independence	Gentle movement, stretching, light resistance	Prioritise comfort, autonomy and social engagement

prehabilitation: To improve aerobic capacity, muscle strength or functional reserve; to reduce post-operative complications; to shorten hospital stays; and/or to promote psychological readiness. Studies show that prehabilitation can significantly improve cardiorespiratory fitness, muscle strength and post-operative recovery in colorectal, lung, breast and prostate cancer patients (24–29). In terms of prescription, this does not differ from general recommendations: Moderate-intensity aerobic training (e.g., brisk walking, cycling) three to five times per week, combined with resistance training for major muscle groups twice weekly. Time is often limited between the point of diagnosis and the start of treatment; however short, targeted interventions (even 2–3 weeks) can yield benefits and should not be ruled out.

8.3.2 During treatment: Maintaining function and mitigating side effects

During chemotherapy, radiotherapy or immunotherapy, the main objective shifts from optimisation to maintenance and symptom control. Exercise helps counteract the well-documented effects of deconditioning, fatigue and muscle loss. RCTs demonstrate improvements in physical function, fatigue and emotional wellbeing in patients who exercise during active treatment (30–32). The goals during this phase of the continuum include maintaining cardiorespiratory fitness, preserving lean muscle mass, reducing patient fatigue and enhancing mood. During active treatment, exercise prescriptions may include 20–30 minutes of moderate-intensity activity on most days, with light to moderate resistance exercises (1–2 sets of 10–15 reps) twice a week, depending on individual capacity and clinical status. Gentle stretching, yoga or Tai chi may promote mobility and relaxation. Overall, exercise prescriptions may need to be adapted based on fatigue, pain or treatment side effects, where shorter bouts (5–10 minutes) accumulated through the day could be adopted instead.

8.3.3 Post-treatment: Recovery and survivorship

Following treatment, exercise becomes central to rehabilitation and long-term survivorship care. The focus here is on rebuilding strength, endurance, confidence and identity. During this phase, the main goals are to restore pre-diagnosis fitness and body composition, manage late treatment side effects (e.g., neuropathy, lymphoedema) and support psychological wellbeing. Evidence demonstrates that post-treatment exercise can reduce cancer-related fatigue, improve cardiorespiratory fitness and may reduce recurrence in breast, colorectal and prostate cancers (33–37). From a prescription standpoint, the focus is on gradual progression towards WHO/ACSM guidelines: 150 minutes of moderate or 75 minutes of vigorous aerobic activity per week plus two strength sessions. Longer-term, a variety of exercise types (aerobic, strength and flexibility) are encouraged, incorporating patient preference to ensure sustainability and enhance adherence.

8.3.4 Advanced cancer and palliative contexts: Enhancing quality of life

In advanced or metastatic cancer, the goal is not fitness optimisation but functional preservation, comfort and dignity. Exercise can still play an important role in enhancing QoL, mobility and psychological wellbeing. In this phase, the primary goals are to maintain patient independence, reduce their symptom burden and support their emotional health and wellbeing. Gentle, low-impact activities (walking, stretching, seated resistance bands) should be tailored to their individual tolerance, with an emphasis on flexibility, balance and breathing exercises. Frequency and duration are highly individualised at this stage. Even minimal physical activity can improve fatigue, mood and a sense of control in palliative care populations (38–41).

8.4 Tailoring exercise to the individual

While global exercise guidelines provide an essential foundation, the reality of exercise oncology practice is that no two patients are alike. Cancer, and its treatment, significantly alter physiology, function and motivation, rendering the “one-size-fits-all” approach inadequate. Individualisation is therefore central to safe, effective and sustainable exercise prescription in oncology.

8.4.1 The limits of a "one-size-fits-all" model

As Jones and colleagues (2017) highlight, most exercise interventions in cancer survivors have historically adopted a generic model—typically moderate-intensity aerobic and resistance exercise following WHO recommendations (42). While these regimens are safe, tolerable and beneficial across broad populations, they overlook the nuances that define each patient's cancer experience. This approach would be akin, as the authors memorably framed it, to prescribing the same dose and schedule of chemotherapy to every patient regardless of tumour type, stage or genetic profile. Just as oncological treatments are becoming increasingly precision-based, exercise prescriptions would also benefit from a move towards precision exercise medicine, taking into account the biological, clinical and psychosocial diversity of each individual.

8.4.2 Factors shaping an individualised prescription

A tailored approach considers the interplay of medical, physiological and behavioural factors. Effective exercise oncology prescriptions require more than simply applying generic dosage guidelines (e.g., 150 minutes per week). They must reflect tumour- and treatment-specific side effects, an individual's baseline physiological capacity, the presence of comorbidities, symptom burden, preferences and psychosocial context (21,43).

8.4.2.1 Cancer type and stage

Patients' ability to tolerate exercise and the benefits they receive from engaging in activity differ across diagnoses. Tumour type, anatomical site and stage influence risk (e.g., bone metastases, lymph node dissection, lymphoedema) and determine specific exercise considerations. For example, women with breast cancer may require careful consideration of lymphoedema risk and upper-body loading, whereas those with prostate cancer may experience androgen-deprivation-related sarcopenia and bone density loss, thus placing the emphasis on heavier loading and muscle-preserving resistance exercise (43). Furthermore, individuals with advanced or metastatic disease may require more conservative loading due to skeletal involvement, fracture risk or widespread muscle wasting (44).

8.4.2.2 Treatment modality and phase

The mode and timing of treatment (surgery, chemotherapy, radiotherapy, hormone therapy, immunotherapy and targeted agents) substantially shape exercise capacity, recovery dynamics and risk profile. Chemotherapy may cause fatigue, anaemia, and neuropathy (45,46). Radiotherapy may contribute to cardiotoxicity or pulmonary changes (47,48). Hormone therapy may alter body composition and bone health (49,50). As such, exercise prescription should be dynamic, adapting "in-cycle" (between rounds), "off-cycle" (during recovery) and transitioning into survivorship. The phase of treatment (prehabilitation, during treatment, early survivorship, long-term survivorship or palliative care) requires different loading, monitoring and progression strategies (51) (see Section 8.3).

8.4.2.3 Comorbidities and baseline fitness

Many cancer patients enter treatment with pre-existing CVD, diabetes, obesity, musculoskeletal limitations or low cardiorespiratory fitness, all of which affect safety, tolerance and response to exercise (52,53). Baseline screening (for cardiac risk, bone health, neuropathy and musculoskeletal integrity) and functional assessments (e.g., 6-minute walk test, sit-to-stand, grip strength) are essential to individualise load and mode (21,54). In practice, having lower fitness or multiple comorbidities may necessitate a more gradual build-up, more frequent rest, lower-intensity exercise or alternative modes (e.g., seated cycling, water-based exercise interventions) until adaptation occurs.

8.4.2.4 Symptoms and treatment sequelae

Ongoing issues such as pain, fatigue, peripheral neuropathy, cognitive impairment ("chemobrain") or fear of movement (kinesiophobia) represent barriers to sustained exercise participation (1,55–57). A symptom-led or autoregulatory approach to exercise allows the individual to adjust volume or intensity based on daily energy levels, side-effects and comfort, which promotes adherence and reduces risk of exacerbation (51). For example, on days of high fatigue, the plan may switch to a light aerobic or mobility session rather than full-intensity training. This flexibility supports long-term sustainability of the exercise intervention.

8.4.2.5 Patient preference and psychosocial context

Engagement and adherence depend heavily on psychosocial factors: Enjoyment, autonomy, social support, meaning and alignment with personal goals. Tailoring the mode of exercise (e.g., home-based versus group, walking versus resistance machine) to the individual's interests, lifestyle and environment boosts the likelihood of persistence and maintenance of activity (58). Moreover, behavioural strategies, such as self-monitoring, goal-setting, motivational interviewing and linking with peer exercise groups, are integral to embedding exercise into oncological care pathways (see Section 8.5).

BOX-OUT 8.1 CASE STUDY: PERSONALISED PREHABILITATION IN LUNG CANCER

Patient profile

A 70-year-old-male with stage IIIA non-small cell lung cancer (NSCLC) is preparing for curative surgery. He has mild COPD, borderline pulmonary function, sarcopenia, low cardiorespiratory fitness (VO_2max <15 mL/kg/min) and recent unintentional weight loss. Fatigue and appetite loss are present, and he has no prior exercise history.

Goal

To optimise surgical eligibility, reduce perioperative risk, and improve recovery through a personalised 8-week prehabilitation programme.

Exercise intervention

A parallel periodised approach was implemented over two 4-week blocks:
Block 1 (weeks 1–4):

- Aerobic: 2 × per week moderate-intensity continuous training (MICT) at ~70% HRmax (e.g., walking, cycling)
- Resistance: 1 session per week for hypertrophy (40–60% 1RM, 12–15 reps, 2–3 sets) and 1 session per week for strength (60–80% 1RM, 6–8 reps, 3 sets)

Block 2 (weeks 5–8):

- Aerobic: MICT continues with increased intensity (75% HRmax) and duration (≥40 min); 1 × per week HIIT introduced (5 × 60s high:120s low, 3 sets)
- Resistance: Hypertrophy: 50–70% 1RM, 10–12 reps, 3–4 sets; strength: 70–90% 1RM, 6–8 reps, 4 sets

Additional considerations

Tailored nutrition support was provided to address malnutrition and support body composition goals.

Outcomes and relevance

This comprehensive programme aimed to enhance both cardiorespiratory fitness and muscle function, reduce surgical risk and promote recovery. It illustrates how structured, individualised exercise, paired with nutritional support, can be safely and effectively integrated into the pre-treatment phase of cancer care, even in patients with comorbidities and functional decline.

Source: Periodizing exercise medicine prescription for patients with cancer: A narrative opinion (51).

8.4.3 Approaches to personalisation

Practical tailoring involves modifying the type, intensity, frequency and duration of exercise to match the individual's condition and goals. Three key strategies include:

1. Symptom-led programming:
   Allowing daily symptom monitoring (e.g., fatigue, pain, nausea scales) to guide whether to reduce, maintain or skip sessions. The "2-day rule," whereby an individual can rest or modify activity if symptoms worsen over two consecutive days, can be a helpful guiding principle.
2. Intensity modulation:
   Using self-perceived exertion (e.g., Borg Rating of Perceived Exertion, or RPE, scale) or talk-test methods rather than fixed heart rate zones allows real-time adjustment. During active treatment, light-to-moderate activity (RPE 11–13) is generally safe and effective.
3. Pacing and energy budgeting:
   Especially relevant for individuals with chronic fatigue or advanced disease, pacing encourages short bouts of activity interspersed with rest. A structured approach of "plan, prioritise, pace" helps patients balance energy expenditure across daily activities.

For example, a patient recovering from chemotherapy might begin with 10-minute walks twice daily, combined with seated resistance-band exercise. Over time, duration and load are gradually increased as fatigue lessens and confidence grows. An individualised prescription begins with a comprehensive understanding of the patient's physiological status, disease pathophysiology and treatment-related limitations. Objective measures, such as CPET, provide insight into cardiovascular, pulmonary and neuromuscular function, and help determine safe and effective exercise intensity through metabolic or ventilatory thresholds (42). Such assessments allow clinicians to move beyond generic targets (e.g., $\%VO_2max$ or HRmax), towards prescriptions that reflect the individual's unique training zones.

Principles such as specificity, progressive overload, periodisation and rest are key to optimising adaptation and ensuring both efficacy and safety, particularly in populations with multimorbidity or treatment-related impairments.

8.4.4 From generic to precision exercise oncology

The evolving ambition within exercise oncology is to transition from broad, "one-size-fits-all" prescriptions towards precision exercise oncology, where the dose, timing, modality and progression of physical activity are prescribed with a level of granularity approaching that of pharmacologic therapy. This means moving beyond generic guidance (e.g., 150 minutes per week of moderate aerobic activity) to prescriptions that reflect individual tumour biology, treatment history, biomarker profiles and real-time physiological response. Several emerging lines of research underpin this: Reviews highlight that exercise interventions in cancer populations are beginning to report biomarker changes (e.g., the insulin-IGF axis, inflammatory cytokines) and that the nature of the exercise prescription (intensity, frequency, modality) influences these responses. This suggests the possibility of dose-response tuning and incremental optimisation of exercise prescription (59,60). A framework has been proposed in which exercise may modulate tumour perfusion, hypoxia, immune response and the TME, and where tailoring exercise according to tumour type, treatment phase and systemic context might enhance synergy with conventional therapies (61,62).

However, the practical translation of precision exercise prescriptions is still in its early stages. In clinical practice, this should include recording baseline biomarkers or physiological indices (where available) and using them to inform the setting of exercise targets. Moreover, there needs to be a tailoring of exercise modalities for individual patients: For example, higher-intensity aerobic training or resistance training may be indicated based on individual response patterns or tumour/treatment characteristics. Monitoring individual responses and exercise tolerances is also critical. Through accurate measurement and recording of symptoms, side effects, functional tests, perhaps even biomarker changes or tracking wearable device data, individual load, volume and recovery time can be adapted as needed. Finally, incorporating patient preference is equally important, taking into consideration their individual circumstances as well as physical and emotional constraints, such that their individualised plan balances an optimal exercise prescription with feasibility, adherence and safety. Here, the "art" of personalisation complements the "science."

8.4.4.1 Key takeaway

Exercise guidelines offer a framework, but the route to recovery is personal. The goal is not to meet fixed targets, but to support each individual in making meaningful progress toward improved health, function and QoL.

8.5 Adherence considerations

Even the most well-designed exercise prescription is only effective if it is adhered to over time. In the context of cancer, where physical, emotional and logistical challenges are often heightened, understanding and addressing the factors that influence adherence is essential to achieving meaningful outcomes.

8.5.1 Perceived barriers to regular exercise

Many individuals living with or beyond cancer face a complex array of barriers that limit their ability to engage in regular physical activity. These barriers are often multifactorial, spanning physiological symptoms, psychological states and environmental constraints. Despite the growing evidence base supporting the benefits of physical activity and exercise during both active treatment and cancer survivorship (2), most survivors do not meet the current minimum exercise guidelines of 150 minutes per week of moderate-intensity exercise (63). Approximately two-thirds of cancer patients reduce their activity levels during active treatment, largely due to side effects such as fatigue, pain and treatment-related burden (1). This presents a major challenge to ensure cancer survivors are taking the necessary steps to improve their physical and mental health and wellbeing (2,63,64), underscoring the importance of identifying and mitigating barriers to promote meaningful engagement with physical activity. Addressing mental health is also central to supporting exercise adherence. Depression has been directly linked to reduced engagement in physical activity programmes (65). Interventions that support mood, such as group-based activity or integration with psychosocial care, may indirectly but significantly improve exercise uptake and retention.

8.5.1.1 Fatigue

Cancer-related fatigue is the most prevalent and persistent physical barrier to exercise for cancer survivors, with up to 70% of patients reporting difficulties, particularly during active treatment (1,55,66). Even 3 years after active treatment ceases, 30% of cancer survivors continue to experience fatigue that hinders their participation in exercise (67). In a similar vein, most individuals cite both disease- and treatment-related side effects as highly significant barriers to exercising, including nausea (68), pain (55), weight gain (69) and joint stiffness (1). Unlike normal tiredness, cancer-related fatigue is not alleviated by rest and can be extremely demotivating, reducing an individual's capacity for physical activity. While regular exercise can reduce fatigue over time, the initial effort required to begin or maintain activity can feel insurmountable for many.

8.5.1.2 Pain

Post-surgical pain, chemotherapy-induced neuropathy, or pre-existing musculoskeletal issues can act as a significant deterrent to movement. For some, pain is episodic and manageable, but for others it is chronic, unpredictable and closely associated with fear of exacerbating pain or injury, especially if they have not received professional guidance. The term "kinesiophobia," which means excessive fear of motion, can arise during cancer therapy in relation to various symptoms, including pain, fatigue and lymphoedema (56,70–72). Without reassurance and tailored support, pain can become a self-reinforcing barrier, where avoidance leads to further deconditioning and functional decline. Furthermore, some individuals may avoid exercise because of the assumption that it will be uncomfortable or painful, or that it could worsen their condition, or increase their risk of injury, leading to more avoidance and overall lower levels of activity (1,55,69).

8.5.1.3 Time constraints

Time is another frequently cited barrier, particularly for individuals managing multiple demands, such as treatment schedules, medical appointments, work and household responsibilities, and caregiving roles (73). The time cost of exercise may be perceived as high, especially when energy and attention are already stretched. For these patients, long or inflexible exercise sessions may feel unrealistic, particularly if they require travel or equipment. In such cases, short, flexible bouts of activity can be an effective alternative. Accumulating activity in 5- to 10-minute increments throughout the day may be more feasible and still offer physiological benefits (74). Embedding movement into daily routines, such as walking during phone calls or stretching while watching TV, can help overcome this barrier.

8.5.1.4 Lack of support

Many patients report insufficient guidance or encouragement from their healthcare team regarding the benefits and safety of exercise during and after treatment, as an essential part of their recovery (58,75). Smaradottir et al. (2017) demonstrated that more than half of the participants in their study were unaware of the benefits of exercise, highlighting the disconnect observed between current exercise guidelines and patient/survivor adherence (68). A common theme in the literature is the perceived lack of PA recommendations for cancer survivors coming from their healthcare providers directly (1,2,68). Fernandez et al. (2015) reported that 51.9% of cancer survivors were unaware of specialist PA programmes (1). These observations point to a systemic issue, where limited clinical training, time constraints and resource availability contribute to under-referral and missed opportunities for engagement (68,76).

8.5.1.5 Misinformation or uncertainty

If exercise is not positioned as a legitimate part of the care plan, it may be perceived as optional or even risky. In some settings, patients are told to rest rather than move, reinforcing inactivity. Moreover, fear of doing the wrong thing and confusion around what is safe, especially after surgery or in the presence of medical devices (e.g., ports) or with metastatic disease, can lead patients to avoid exercise altogether (77). In the absence of clear, evidence-based guidance, uncertainty often fosters inactivity (78). This is especially true for individuals with more complex clinical presentations, who may benefit most from professional support to build confidence and ensure safety.

Another significant barrier to PA participation is a lack of self-discipline and/or motivation due to exercise not being a priority for cancer survivors (66). This may also be exacerbated by a lack of awareness around whether it is safe to exercise (1). Where patients and survivors do participate in PA and/or exercise, there is often limited knowledge of the correct PA guidelines (2). Collectively, these psychological barriers can cause survivors to become fearful of exercise, which supports the need to consider all aspects of an individual's cancer experience when designing exercise interventions (79). These barriers are not insurmountable, but they require acknowledgement and proactive strategies. With appropriate education, empathy and co-designed interventions, patients can be empowered to engage in physical activity in ways that are safe, meaningful and sustainable. The following sections will explore behavioural strategies and the role of the clinical team in supporting adherence.

PATIENT VIGNETTE 8.1 "Jas"—lost in the system

Jas, 48, underwent treatment for colorectal cancer. He wanted to stay active but didn't know if it was safe. "No one told me whether I could or should exercise," he noted. Fatigue and muscle pain kept him mostly sedentary, and when he tried doing more, he worried it would make things worse. The only information he received was "basic and vague." Now in remission, Jas reflects that if there had been a dedicated specialist or clearer guidance, he would have felt more confident.

8.5.2 Behavioural and psychological strategies

To improve adherence, exercise recommendations must move beyond the purely clinical and into the realm of behavioural support and psychological empowerment. For many individuals living with or beyond cancer, the key to sustained engagement lies not in more information, but in greater personal relevance, support and autonomy. Surveys consistently show that patients want more personalised exercise advice (80). In one study, over two-thirds of cancer survivors expressed a preference for tailored exercise programmes aligned to their specific needs, treatment stage and baseline fitness (81). This underscores the importance of ensuring personal relevance in programme design, a key factor in enhancing long-term adherence. Several evidence-based strategies have been shown to support regular physical activity in oncology populations, including goal setting, social support, motivational interviewing and guidance from health professionals.

8.5.2.1 Goal setting

Collaborative, achievable goal setting is a key driver of exercise adherence. Studies in exercise oncology populations show that interventions which include specific, measurable goals, regular review of progress and self-monitoring are associated with higher adherence rates (82,83). Goals that are relevant and meaningful to the individual (e.g., walking the dog daily, completing a 10-minute morning routine, or attending a weekly class) can provide structure, motivation and a sense of accomplishment. Tracking progress towards these goals also reinforces behaviour change, builds self-efficacy and helps maintain engagement over time. Qualitative work with cancer survivors further emphasises that being able to set and monitor small, short-term goals helps to initiate movement and develop sustainable routines (84). Indeed, results from a randomised controlled trial investigating the effect of self-regulatory behaviour change techniques, including goal setting, review of behavioural goals and self-monitoring, support the hypothesis that goal setting can help improve long-term physical activity maintenance in cancer survivors (85).

8.5.2.2 Social support

Social support is a consistently reported facilitator of exercise participation among individuals living with and beyond cancer. Encouragement and assistance from family, peers, healthcare professionals and exercise specialists not only enhance motivation but can also significantly reduce dropout rates. Social support helps patients overcome emotional, logistical and psychological barriers by fostering accountability, reducing isolation and reinforcing the belief that exercise is both safe and worthwhile (86,87). Group-based exercise programmes, buddy systems and community classes offer structure, connection and mutual encouragement, which are particularly valuable for those navigating the physical and emotional aftermath of treatment. Participants in group interventions often cite peer support as a key motivator, describing a sense of belonging and shared understanding that boosts confidence and adherence (87,88).

In one qualitative study of a group walking programme for cancer survivors, social connectedness and the informal support provided by fellow participants were central to sustaining participation over time (88). In another mixed-methods study, a volunteer-led walking group for women living with and beyond breast cancer ("Best Foot Forward") demonstrated that the combination of walking, talking and natural outdoor environments created a therapeutic setting of "shoulder-to-shoulder support," enabling meaningful peer connection and promoting wellbeing in ways that more formal or sedentary settings may not (89). In a study examining physical activity interventions for cancer survivors and their caregivers, higher perceived social support was linked to increased physical activity participation and self-efficacy (86). By contrast, a systematic review of determinants of exercise adherence and maintenance revealed moderate evidence of a positive association between exercise history and exercise adherence, and although there was insufficient evidence, the few studies included in this review all point to a social and supportive environment being positively associated with adherence and maintenance (90).

Importantly, social support is not limited to in-person settings. Remote coaching, online platforms and virtual communities can also provide meaningful connection and accountability, especially for those facing geographical or health-related barriers to attendance. A study analysing the efficacy of a home-based DVD-delivered exercise intervention found that cancer survivors experienced clinically meaningful improvements in functional health and balance over a 24-month period, suggesting that such programmes may offer accessible, scalable options for promoting physical activity during survivorship (91). Taken together, these findings support the idea that integrating social support into physical activity and exercise programmes, whether through trained professionals, exercise buddies, family-inclusive interventions or remote platforms, can strengthen commitment, reduce psychological barriers and promote sustained engagement with exercise longer-term.

8.5.2.3 Motivational interviewing and other behaviour change techniques

This patient-centred communication approach helps individuals explore and resolve ambivalence about physical activity. Rather than prescribing behaviour, motivational interviewing uses reflective listening and open-ended questions to draw out a person's own reasons for change, reinforcing their sense of control. It is especially useful in populations who feel uncertain or discouraged. Many individuals lack confidence, not because they doubt the benefits of exercise, but because they are uncertain about what is safe (78). Several studies report that a substantial proportion of cancer survivors avoid or reduce physical activity due to limited knowledge or guidance on safe participation (5,92–94). Behavioural interventions should therefore not only motivate but also educate and reassure.

Other behavioural techniques, such as self-monitoring (e.g., using pedometers or activity diaries), positive reinforcement and problem-solving planning, can also increase adherence, particularly when integrated into supervised programmes or survivorship care plans. Crucially, these strategies must be tailored to the individual's stage of change, cultural context and values. For some, a structured programme may feel empowering; for others, autonomy and flexibility are more motivating. When behaviour change techniques are embedded within cancer care, rather than treated as optional extras, adherence improves, and with it, the potential for meaningful clinical benefit.

8.5.3 Role of clinicians and exercise professionals

Embedding cancer-specialist exercise professionals directly into oncology settings to provide real-time support, answer safety questions and adjust exercise plans as needed can foster accountability, reduce uncertainty and increase confidence, which are all important drivers of behavioural change. When exercise is framed not as a lifestyle recommendation but as an integral part of the treatment pathway, patients are more likely to take it seriously and therefore more likely to follow through (95). Clinicians (including oncologists, nurses and general practitioners) play a pivotal role in this process. Their endorsement carries weight: A simple statement such as "Exercise is safe and beneficial for you during treatment" can significantly increase patient willingness to participate. Yet, many clinicians feel under-prepared to make tailored exercise recommendations due to time constraints, competing priorities or lack of specific training (3–5). To bridge this gap, exercise professionals, such as clinical exercise physiologists, physiotherapists, or cancer rehabilitation specialists, can provide individualised assessment, programme design and supervision. These professionals are best placed to adjust frequency, intensity and duration to match patient needs, monitor progress and troubleshoot barriers in real time. Models that integrate exercise professionals into oncology services, whether through prehabilitation clinics, survivorship programmes or community-based referrals, have shown promise (96). Importantly, these models normalise exercise as a routine part of cancer care, not an optional wellness add-on. A visual summary of this approach is presented in Figure 8.2, outlining a pathway to support tailored, timely and person-centred physical activity advice.

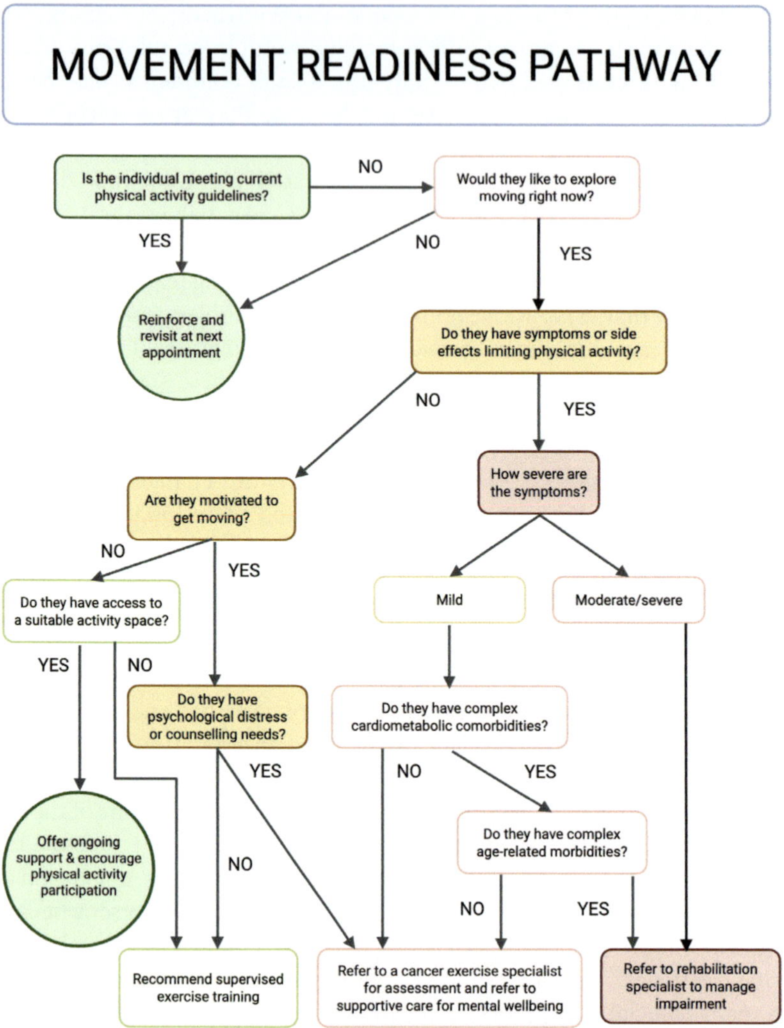

FIGURE 8.2 Movement readiness pathway for people living with and beyond cancer. This visual decision-making tool, adapted from Stout et al. (2020) (20), outlines a structured approach to identifying and supporting readiness for physical activity in individuals living with and beyond cancer. The pathway encourages clinicians to assess current activity levels, motivation and potential barriers such as treatment side effects, comorbidities, psychological distress, or limited access to exercise facilities. The flowchart supports tailored referrals and recommendations. The aim is to guide person-centred conversations around movement to ensure that each individual receives safe, timely and appropriate support to be physically active. Created in Biorender.com.

A systems-level approach to embedding exercise includes:

1. Incorporating physical activity assessment into standard oncology assessments
2. Training clinicians in brief exercise counselling techniques
3. Establishing referral pathways to certified professionals or programmes
4. Co-locating exercise services with oncology clinics or treatment centres
5. Advocating for policy support and reimbursement for exercise interventions

When exercise is championed by the care team, tailored to the individual and delivered by trained professionals, adherence improves and the full therapeutic potential of exercise in cancer care can begin to be realised.

8.6 Research gaps and priorities

Despite the growing maturity of exercise oncology as a discipline, the evidence base underpinning exercise prescription in cancer care remains comparatively young. Most of what we know stems from small to medium-sized RCTs conducted in highly selected populations—predominantly younger, fitter and often female survivors of early-stage breast cancer. These studies have been instrumental in establishing safety and feasibility, yet they leave critical questions unanswered about the optimal type, dose and timing of exercise across the full spectrum of malignancies, treatment regimens and survivorship stages.

A clear research priority is the development of large-scale, multicentre RCTs that can robustly evaluate personalised exercise dosing. As previously discussed, exercise oncology has reached the point where "one-size-fits-all" approaches are no longer sufficient. Determining the most effective and sustainable combinations of frequency, intensity, time and type (the FITT principle) for different cancers, and even different treatment phases within the same diagnosis, will be key to translating exercise into a precision therapeutic. Such trials should adopt stratified designs that account for tumour biology, treatment modality, comorbidities and genetic or metabolic variability, mirroring the sophistication of modern oncology research.

Related to this is the urgent need to delineate dose-response relationships between exercise exposure and outcomes such as recurrence, survival and QoL. While epidemiological data demonstrate a strong inverse association between physical activity and cancer mortality, the precise threshold for benefit remains elusive. Does "more" exercise always confer "better" outcomes, or is there a ceiling effect beyond which benefits plateau or even reverse? Or might the J-shaped curve, as described in exercise immunology (97) also apply in exercise oncology—where moderate-intensity exercise yields the greatest benefit, while both insufficient and excessive volumes could attenuate or even negate positive effects? These questions carry not only mechanistic importance but also practical relevance for survivors striving to balance recovery with realistic, sustainable activity levels.

The field must also confront its sampling bias. Research has overwhelmingly focused on a narrow subset of the cancer population, leaving those with rare tumours, metastatic disease, advanced age, or multiple comorbidities vastly underrepresented. Sampling bias also extends along lines of race, ethnicity and geography. People from global majority groups remain underrepresented in all areas of oncology research, including exercise oncology, despite well-documented disparities in cancer incidence, outcomes and access to supportive care (98–102). Similarly, individuals living in rural or remote communities often face structural barriers, such as limited access to exercise facilities, specialist services, or transport, which restrict their participation in clinical trials (103–105). Addressing these inequalities through inclusive research design, recruitment, community-based programmes and culturally sensitive interventions is essential for truly representative and equitable evidence. These groups stand to benefit greatly from physical activity interventions but are often excluded due to safety concerns or logistical barriers. Future studies must adopt inclusive designs and pragmatic trial methodologies that reflect the diversity of real-world oncology care.

PATIENT VIGNETTE 8.2 "Peter"—lack of access and rural barriers

Living in a rural area, Peter, a 65-year-old non-Hodgkin lymphoma survivor, had little access to cancer-specific exercise classes. Travel fatigue and time constraints were major barriers. "The nearest class was an hour's drive. After chemo, even 10 minutes felt like a marathon." He found online resources helpful but still missed the value of face-to-face support. He recommends investment in digital support platforms tailored to remote patients.

Equally critical is the need for longitudinal data that track adherence and outcomes over years rather than weeks or months. Exercise is not a single intervention but a behavioural process that unfolds over time, influenced by changing motivation, life circumstances and disease status. Understanding how survivors sustain or abandon activity, and how patterns of engagement relate to long-term physiological and psychological outcomes, requires integrated follow-up and data-sharing frameworks that extend well beyond traditional trial endpoints.

Emerging technologies hold promise for addressing several of these gaps. The rapid evolution of wearable devices, digital health platforms and artificial intelligence offers unprecedented opportunities to collect continuous, real-world data on physical activity, physiological responses and recovery patterns. With appropriate validation and ethical oversight, these tools could enable highly personalised, adaptive exercise prescriptions that respond dynamically to an individual's condition, much as modern oncology tailors treatment to molecular signatures.

The next phase of research, then, must move beyond establishing that exercise *works* to understanding *how*, *for whom* and *under what conditions* it works best. Only through this precision-oriented, inclusive and technologically informed agenda can exercise fulfil its full therapeutic potential as a critical component of modern cancer care.

BOX-OUT 8.2 THE FUTURE OF DIGITAL PRECISION EXERCISE ONCOLOGY

In the coming decades, advances in wearable sensors and AI-driven analytics could transform how exercise is prescribed and monitored in cancer care. Continuous data on heart rate, sleep, movement and fatigue could allow real-time adjustment of exercise dose, while machine learning models integrating clinical, genomic and behavioural data could be used to predict individual responses. Such systems could make personalised exercise medicine a part of routine cancer care.

8.7 From guidelines to action: Implementation in practice

Turning guidelines into everyday practice remains one of the greatest challenges in exercise oncology. Although the evidence for the safety and efficacy of exercise is now overwhelming, the infrastructure to deliver it routinely within oncology care pathways is still emerging. The translation from knowledge to action requires not only clinical endorsement but also organisational commitment, inter-professional collaboration and cultural change.

8.7.1 Translating evidence into clinical settings

In most healthcare systems, exercise is still perceived as an *adjunct* rather than an *integral component* of cancer treatment. This perception persists despite the robust evidence base demonstrating that regular physical activity can mitigate treatment side effects, improve physical function and enhance survival (3,106,107). Bridging this evidence-practice gap demands a step change: From viewing exercise as optional lifestyle advice to prescribing it as *standard supportive care*. Implementation begins with embedding physical activity screening and referral into oncology workflows. Simple prompts, such as a "physical activity vital sign" incorporated into routine assessments, can normalise conversations about exercise from the point of diagnosis (3,108). Electronic medical record systems can then facilitate automatic referrals to exercise professionals in the same way that dieticians or psychologists are routinely involved. Integrating exercise into survivorship care plans and multidisciplinary team discussions reinforces its legitimacy as part of comprehensive cancer care. Successful translation also relies on accessible delivery models. Hospital-based prehabilitation and rehabilitation programmes remain the gold standard for complex cases, but scalable community- and home-based options are essential for long-term sustainability. Hybrid models combining initial supervised sessions with remote monitoring or online support can maintain safety while enhancing reach, especially for rural or time-constrained patients.

8.7.2 The role of multidisciplinary teams in exercise referral

Exercise oncology is inherently multidisciplinary. No single clinician or professional group can deliver the full spectrum of expertise required to assess, prescribe and support physical activity safely across the cancer continuum. Oncologists and cancer nurses are often the first point of contact. Their role is to initiate the conversation, reinforce safety and endorse exercise as part of standard care. A brief, confident recommendation ("It's safe and beneficial to be active during treatment,") can have a profound impact on patient perception and motivation (3). Physiotherapists and clinical exercise physiologists translate this endorsement into actionable prescriptions. They perform pre-exercise screening, tailor programmes to the patient's medical and functional status and monitor progress. Their involvement ensures that exercise remains evidence-based, individualised and responsive to treatment side effects. Psychologists, dieticians and occupational therapists contribute by addressing motivational, nutritional and practical barriers, helping to embed exercise within broader lifestyle and recovery plans. Community exercise professionals, once appropriately trained, play a vital role in sustaining activity beyond the clinical setting, facilitating social engagement and lifelong participation (3,20,109–111). Collaborative communication between these disciplines is key. Shared referral pathways, integrated documentation and mutual respect for expertise create continuity for the patient and cohesion across services.

8.7.3 Case examples: Translating theory into reality

Real-world programmes illustrate how these principles can be enacted. In the UK, Macmillan's Move More initiative and NHS Prehabilitation for Cancer pilots have demonstrated the feasibility of integrating exercise screening and referral into routine oncology care. Early evidence shows improvements in fitness, treatment tolerance and psychological wellbeing when patients are referred to exercise services soon after diagnosis (9,112–114).

At the more grassroots level, community-led organisations such as Battle Cancer have pioneered innovative models of exercise rehabilitation that combine structured training with peer support and empowerment. Their programmes, delivered in collaboration with exercise professionals, emphasise inclusivity and identity rebuilding, helping participants reconnect with strength and self-efficacy after cancer treatment. These examples highlight that implementation need not be confined to clinical environments; meaningful engagement can happen wherever people move together with purpose and support. For further examples of these and other organisations driving innovation in exercise oncology in both clinical and community settings, see Chapter 10.

BOX-OUT 8.3 BATTLE CANCER: FROM COMPETITION TO COMMUNITY

The Battle Cancer Program is a charitable initiative offering 12-week, fully funded exercise rehabilitation programmes for people recovering from cancer. Launched in 2021, the program supports individuals in rebuilding physical confidence, mobility and self-belief through structured, progressive training designed by experts in oncology and exercise. With over 500 participants to date, its impact reaches beyond physical health, creating connection, identity and hope after treatment (see Figure 8.3). To learn more about the Battle Cancer Program, see Chapter 10 or visit www.battlecancerprogram.com.

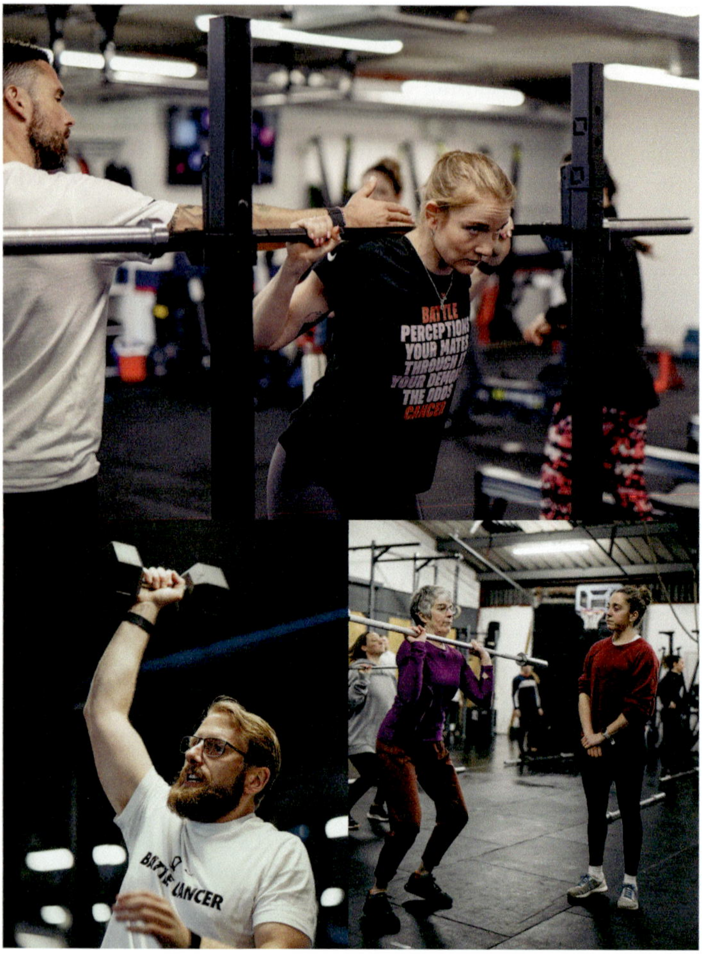

FIGURE 8.3 Participants engaging in the Battle Cancer Program. Participants involved in the structured, progressive exercise sessions on the Battle Cancer Program designed to support recovery after cancer treatment. The programme emphasises physical empowerment, community connection and rebuilding confidence through movement. Photos reproduced with kind permission from the Battle Cancer Program.

8.7.4 From pathways to practice: A systems view

Implementation should be viewed as a pathway rather than a point of care. The process begins at diagnosis, when patients are informed about the role of physical activity and continues through referral, assessment, programme design and ongoing support. Sustaining these pathways requires alignment across policy, funding and education. Health systems must invest in training for exercise professionals, establish reimbursement models for exercise prescription and embed outcome monitoring to demonstrate value. Implementation science frameworks, such as RE-AIM (Reach, Effectiveness, Adoption, Implementation, Maintenance), can guide evaluation and scale-up (115). Ultimately, bringing guidelines to life is about creating environments where movement becomes the norm rather than the exception. When clinicians, researchers, policymakers and communities work together, exercise ceases to be an afterthought and becomes central to modern cancer care.

8.8 Conclusion

Exercise has become one of the most powerful and versatile tools in cancer care. The collective evidence now demonstrates that regular physical activity and exercise can improve treatment tolerance, reduce fatigue, preserve physical function and enhance QoL—benefits that extend well beyond the clinic into survivorship and daily living. Whether performed in a hospital gym, a community centre or at home, movement remains an inherently accessible form of medicine. What this chapter has underscored is that guidelines are only the beginning. The true challenge lies in translating recommendations into personalised, sustainable action, helping each person find a level and type of activity that is both achievable and meaningful. The future of exercise oncology will depend on precision: Matching the right exercise "dose" to the right individual, at the right time. It will also depend on inclusivity: Ensuring that opportunities for movement are available to everyone, regardless of diagnosis, background or circumstance. As the field matures, a shift in mindset is needed: From asking "Should I exercise?" to asking "How can I exercise safely and meaningfully today?" For clinicians, that means integrating physical activity as a routine part of care; for researchers, it means continuing to refine and personalise recommendations; and for survivors, it means recognising that every movement, no matter how small, is an act of resilience and recovery. Ultimately, the message is simple: Keep moving. Not just to live longer, but to live better; to reclaim agency, restore strength and reimagine what life after cancer can look like.

Chapter 8 Test your understanding question bank

1. What are the general WHO physical activity recommendations for adults, including those with chronic conditions such as cancer?

2. Name three key benefits of regular exercise for individuals undergoing cancer treatment.
3. What is the primary goal of prehabilitation in cancer care?
4. What does a symptom-led approach to exercise involve?
5. List two common barriers to exercise adherence among cancer patients.
6. What principle supports the idea that exercise should be adapted to a patient's current energy and side-effect levels?
7. What type of training is recommended for post-treatment cancer survivors aiming to restore fitness?
8. What role do community exercise professionals play in cancer care?
9. Define "precision exercise oncology."
10. What is the "2-day rule" in symptom-led programming?
11. What behavioural strategies can enhance exercise adherence in cancer survivors?
12. Why is patient preference important in exercise prescription?
13. List two functions of cardiopulmonary exercise testing (CPET) in exercise oncology.
14. In the context of exercise oncology, what is meant by "training periodisation"?

References

1. Fernandez S, Franklin J, Amlani N, DeMilleVille C, Lawson D, Smith J. Physical activity and cancer: A cross-sectional study on the barriers and facilitators to exercise during cancer treatment. Can Oncol Nurs J [Internet]. 2015 [cited 2023 Dec 13];25(1):37–48. Available from: http://www.ncbi.nlm.nih.gov/pubmed/26642493
2. Eng L, Pringle D, Su J, Shen X, Mahler M, Niu C, et al. Patterns, perceptions, and perceived barriers to physical activity in adult cancer survivors. Supportive Care in Cancer [Internet]. 2018 Nov 29 [cited 2023 Dec 13];26(11):3755–63. Available from: http://link.springer.com/10.1007/s00520-018-4239-5
3. Schmitz KH, Campbell AM, Stuiver MM, Pinto BM, Schwartz AL, Morris GS, et al. Exercise is medicine in oncology: Engaging clinicians to help patients move through cancer. CA Cancer J Clin [Internet]. 2019 Nov 16 [cited 2020 Jan 10];69(6):468–84. Available from: https://onlinelibrary.wiley.com/doi/abs/10.3322/caac.21579
4. Caperchione CM, English M, Sharp P, Agar MR, Phillips JL, Liauw W, et al. Exploring the practicality and acceptability a brief exercise communication and clinician referral pathway in cancer care: A feasibility study. BMC Health Serv Res [Internet]. 2023 Dec 1 [cited 2025 Nov 25];23(1):1023. Available from: https://link.springer.com/article/10.1186/s12913-023-10003-x
5. Ramsey I, Chan A, Charalambous A, Cheung YT, Darling HS, Eng L, et al. Exercise counselling and referral in cancer care: An international scoping survey of health care practitioners' knowledge, practices, barriers, and facilitators. Supportive Care in Cancer [Internet]. 2022 Nov 1 [cited

2025 Nov 25];30(11):9379–91. Available from: https://link.springer.com/article/10.1007/s00520-022-07342-6
6. WHO guidelines on physical activity and sedentary behaviour [Internet]. [cited 2025 Nov 14]. Available from: https://www.who.int/publications/i/item/9789240015128
7. American College of Sports Medicine. ACSM's guidelines for exercise testing and prescription / [Internet]. Wolters Kluwer. 2022 [cited 2025 Nov 14]. Available from: https://books.google.com/books/about/ACSM_s_Guidelines_for_Exercise_Testing_a.html?hl=sl&id=hTKvzgEACAAJ
8. Ligibel JA, Bohlke K, May AM, Clinton SK, Demark-Wahnefried W, Gilchrist SC, et al. Exercise, diet, and weight management during cancer treatment: ASCO guideline. J Clin Oncol [Internet]. 2022 May 1 [cited 2025 Nov 25];348. Available from: https://ascopubs.org/doi/10.1200/JCO.22.00687
9. Physical activity and cancer | Macmillan Cancer Support [Internet]. [cited 2025 Nov 25]. Available from: https://www.macmillan.org.uk/cancer-information-and-support/treatment/preparing-for-treatment/physical-activity-and-cancer
10. Patel AV., Friedenreich CM, Moore SC, Hayes SC, Silver JK, Campbell KL, et al. American college of sports medicine roundtable report on physical activity, sedentary behavior, and cancer prevention and control. Med Sci Sports Exerc [Internet]. 2019 Nov 1 [cited 2025 Nov 25];51(11):2391–402. Available from: https://pubmed.ncbi.nlm.nih.gov/31626056/
11. Webb J, Fife-Schaw C, Ogden J, Foster J. The effect of the move more pack on the physical activity of cancer survivors: Protocol for a randomized waiting list control trial with process evaluation. JMIR Res Protoc [Internet]. 2017 Nov 1 [cited 2025 Nov 25];6(11):e220. Available from: https://pmc.ncbi.nlm.nih.gov/articles/PMC5701086/
12. Home—Exercise is medicine [Internet]. [cited 2025 Dec 1]. Available from: https://www.exerciseismedicine.org/
13. Stamatakis E, Ahmadi MN, Gill JMR, Thøgersen-Ntoumani C, Gibala MJ, Doherty A, et al. Association of wearable device-measured vigorous intermittent lifestyle physical activity with mortality. Nat Med [Internet]. 2022 Dec 8 [cited 2025 Nov 25];28(12):2521–9. Available from: https://www.nature.com/articles/s41591-022-02100-x
14. Wengström Y, Fornander T, Lindström LS. Short bouts of physical activity—Good for health? JAMA Oncol. 2023 Sep 21;9(9):1199–201.
15. Yin M, Li Y, Aziz AR, Buffey A, Bishop DJ, Bao D, et al. Short bouts of accumulated exercise: Review and consensus statement on definition, efficacy, feasibility, practical applications, and future directions. J Sport Health Sci. 2025 Sep 18;101088.
16. Jenkins DG, Devin JL, Weston KL, Jenkins JG, Skinner TL. Benefits beyond cardiometabolic health: The potential of frequent high intensity "exercise snacks" to improve outcomes for those living with and beyond cancer. J Physiol [Internet]. 2023 Nov 1 [cited 2025 Nov 25];601(21):4691–7. Available from: https://pubmed.ncbi.nlm.nih.gov/37732418/
17. van Roekel EH, Duchâteau J, Bours MJL, van Delden L, Breedveld-Peters JJL, Koole JL, et al. Longitudinal associations of light-intensity physical activity with quality of life, functioning and fatigue after colorectal cancer. Qual Life Res [Internet]. 2020 Nov 1 [cited 2025 Nov 25];29(11):2987–98. Available from: https://pubmed.ncbi.nlm.nih.gov/32617891/

18. Ferrer S, Roekel van, Serdà Ferrer BC, van Roekel E, Lynch BM. The role of physical activity in managing fatigue in cancer survivors. Curr Nutr Rep. 2018;7(3):59.
19. Tanaka R, Matsunaga-Myoji Y, Kubo S, Nagao N, Fujita K. Effects of light-intensity physical activity on health-related outcomes in cancer survivors: A systematic review. Jpn J Nurs Sci [Internet]. 2025 Apr 1 [cited 2025 Nov 25];22(2):e12653. Available from: https://onlinelibrary.wiley.com/doi/full/10.1111/jjns.12653
20. Stout NL, Brown JC, Schwartz AL, Marshall TF, Campbell AM, Nekhlyudov L, et al. An exercise oncology clinical pathway: Screening and referral for personalized interventions. Cancer [Internet]. 2020 Jun 15 [cited 2025 Nov 25];126(12):2750–8. Available from: https://onlinelibrary.wiley.com/doi/full/10.1002/cncr.32860
21. Campbell KL, Winters-Stone KM, Wiskemann J, May AM, Schwartz AL, Courneya KS, et al. Exercise guidelines for cancer survivors. Med Sci Sports Exerc [Internet]. 2019 Nov [cited 2019 Dec 6];51(11):2375–90. Available from: http://www.ncbi.nlm.nih.gov/pubmed/31626055
22. Move more.
23. Silver JK, Baima J. Cancer prehabilitation: An opportunity to decrease treatment-related morbidity, increase cancer treatment options, and improve physical and psychological health outcomes. Am J Phys Med Rehabil [Internet]. 2013 Aug [cited 2025 Nov 25];92(8):715–27. Available from: https://journals.lww.com/ajpmr/fulltext/2013/08000/cancer_prehabilitation__an_opportunity_to_decrease.9.aspx
24. Avancini A, Cavallo A, Trestini I, Tregnago D, Belluomini L, Crisafulli E, et al. Exercise prehabilitation in lung cancer: Getting stronger to recover faster. Eur J Surg Oncol [Internet]. 2021 Aug 1 [cited 2025 Nov 25];47(8):1847–55. Available from: https://pubmed.ncbi.nlm.nih.gov/33757650/
25. Gennuso D, Baldelli A, Gigli L, Ruotolo I, Galeoto G, Gaburri D, et al. Efficacy of prehabilitation in cancer patients: An Rcts systematic review with meta-analysis. BMC Cancer [Internet]. 2024 Dec 1 [cited 2025 Nov 25];24(1):1302. Available from: https://link.springer.com/article/10.1186/s12885-024-13023-w
26. Michael CM, Lehrer EJ, Schmitz KH, Zaorsky NG. Prehabilitation exercise therapy for cancer: A systematic review and meta-analysis. Cancer Med [Internet]. 2021 Jul 1 [cited 2025 Nov 25];10(13):4195–205. Available from: https://onlinelibrary.wiley.com/doi/full/10.1002/cam4.4021
27. Singh F, Newton RU, Taaffe DR, Lopez P, Thavaseelan J, Brown M, et al. Prehabilitative versus rehabilitative exercise in prostate cancer patients undergoing prostatectomy. J Cancer Res Clin Oncol [Internet]. 2023 Dec 1 [cited 2025 Nov 25];149(18):16563–73. Available from: https://link.springer.com/article/10.1007/s00432-023-05409-3
28. Hennessy DT, Miller KJ, Khan N, Edo SM, Bell L, Areerob P, et al. Effects of perioperative exercise therapy on cardiorespiratory fitness and postoperative complications in patients with colorectal cancer: A systematic review and meta-analysis. Supportive Care in Cancer [Internet]. 2025 Jul 1 [cited 2025 Nov 25];33(7):551. Available from: https://pmc.ncbi.nlm.nih.gov/articles/PMC12144058/
29. Guerra-Londono CE, Cata JP, Nowak K, Gottumukkala V. Prehabilitation in adults undergoing cancer surgery: A comprehensive review on rationale, methodology, and measures of effectiveness. Curr Oncol [Internet]. 2024 Apr 9 [cited 2025 Nov 25];31(4):2185–200. Available from: https://www.mdpi.com/1718-7729/31/4/162/htm

30. Brown JC, Huedo-Medina TB, Pescatello LS, Pescatello SM, Ferrer RA, Johnson BT. Efficacy of exercise interventions in modulating cancer-related fatigue among adult cancer survivors: A meta-analysis. Cancer Epidemiol Biomarkers Prev [Internet]. 2011 Jan [cited 2025 Nov 25];20(1):123–33. Available from: https://www.ncbi.nlm.nih.gov/books/NBK81248/
31. Meneses-Echávez JF, González-Jiménez E, Ramírez-Vélez R. Effects of supervised multimodal exercise interventions on cancer-related fatigue: Systematic review and meta-analysis of randomized controlled trials. Biomed Res Int [Internet]. 2015 [cited 2025 Nov 25];2015:328636. Available from: https://pmc.ncbi.nlm.nih.gov/articles/PMC4488083/
32. Hagstrom AD, Marshall PWM, Lonsdale C, Cheema BS, Fiatarone Singh MA, Green S. Resistance training improves fatigue and quality of life in previously sedentary breast cancer survivors: A randomised controlled trial. Eur J Cancer Care (Engl) [Internet]. 2016 Sep 1 [cited 2025 Nov 25];25(5):784–94. Available from: https://pubmed.ncbi.nlm.nih.gov/26593858/
33. Friedenreich CM, Stone CR, Cheung WY, Hayes SC. Physical activity and mortality in cancer survivors: A systematic review and meta-analysis. JNCI Cancer Spectr [Internet]. 2020 Feb 1 [cited 2025 Nov 25];4(1). Available from: https://dx.doi.org/10.1093/jncics/pkz080
34. Morishita S, Hamaue Y, Fukushima T, Tanaka T, Fu JB, Nakano J. Effect of exercise on mortality and recurrence in patients with cancer: A systematic review and meta-analysis. Integr Cancer Ther [Internet]. 2020 [cited 2025 Nov 25];19. Available from: https://journals.sagepub.com/doi/10.1177/1534735420917462
35. Brown JC, Gilmore LA. Physical activity reduces the risk of recurrence and mortality in cancer patients. Exerc Sport Sci Rev [Internet]. 2020 Apr 1 [cited 2025 Nov 25];48(2):67–73. Available from: https://pubmed.ncbi.nlm.nih.gov/31913187/
36. Filis P, Markozannes G, Chan DS, Mauri D, Foukakis T, Matikas A, et al. Grading the evidence for physical activity and any outcome in cancer survivors: An Umbrella review of 740 meta-analytic associations. Crit Rev Oncol Hematol. 2025 Mar 1;207:104602.
37. Beyer M, Bischoff C, Lässing J, Gockel I, Falz R. Effects of postoperative physical exercise rehabilitation on cardiorespiratory fitness, functional capacity and quality of life in patients with colorectal, breast, and prostate cancer—A systematic review and meta-analysis. J Cancer Res Clin Oncol [Internet]. 2024 Jan 1 [cited 2025 Nov 25];151(1):13. Available from: https://pmc.ncbi.nlm.nih.gov/articles/PMC11668849/
38. Eyigor S, Akdeniz S. Is exercise ignored in palliative cancer patients? World J Clin Oncol [Internet]. 2014 Aug 10 [cited 2025 Nov 25];5(3):554. Available from: https://pmc.ncbi.nlm.nih.gov/articles/PMC4127625/
39. Schwonke I, Freitag N, Aschendorf P, Wucharz K, Thieme J, Appelmann I, et al. Feasibility of a physical exercise intervention for patients on a palliative care unit: A critical analysis. BMC Palliat Care [Internet]. 2024 Dec 1 [cited 2025 Nov 25];23(1):58. Available from: https://link.springer.com/article/10.1186/s12904-024-01388-5
40. Oldervoll LM, Loge JH, Paltiel H, Asp MB, Vidvei U, Wiken AN, et al. The effect of a physical exercise program in palliative care: A phase II study. J Pain Symptom Manage. 2006 May 1;31(5):421–30.
41. Physical activity and cancer | Macmillan Cancer Support [Internet]. [cited 2025 Nov 25]. Available from: https://www.macmillan.org.uk/cancer-information-and-support/treatment/preparing-for-treatment/physical-activity-and-cancer

42. Jones LW, Eves ND, Scott JM. Bench-to-bedside approaches for personalized exercise therapy in cancer. Am Soc Clin Oncol Educ Book [Internet]. 2017 May [cited 2025 Nov 22];37(37):684–94. Available from: https://pubmed.ncbi.nlm.nih.gov/28561646/
43. Wagoner CW, Capozzi LC, Culos-Reed SN. Tailoring the evidence for exercise oncology within breast cancer care. Curr Oncol [Internet]. 2022 Jul 1 [cited 2025 Nov 25];29(7):4827. Available from: https://pmc.ncbi.nlm.nih.gov/articles/PMC9322354/
44. Campbell KL, Cormie P, Weller S, Alibhai SMH, Bolam KA, Campbell A, et al. Exercise recommendation for people with bone metastases: Expert consensus for health care providers and exercise professionals. JCO Oncol Pract [Internet]. 2022 May [cited 2025 Nov 25];18(5):e697. Available from: https://pmc.ncbi.nlm.nih.gov/articles/PMC9810134/
45. Groopman JE, Itri LM. Chemotherapy-induced anemia in adults: Incidence and treatment. J Natl Cancer Inst [Internet]. 1999 Oct 6 [cited 2025 Nov 25];91(19):1616–34. Available from: https://pubmed.ncbi.nlm.nih.gov/10511589/
46. Zajaczkowską R, Kocot-Kępska M, Leppert W, Wrzosek A, Mika J, Wordliczek J. Mechanisms of chemotherapy-induced peripheral neuropathy. Int J Mol Sci [Internet]. 2019 Mar 2 [cited 2025 Nov 25];20(6):1451. Available from: https://pmc.ncbi.nlm.nih.gov/articles/PMC6471666/
47. Siaravas KC, Katsouras CS, Sioka C. Radiation treatment mechanisms of cardiotoxicity: A systematic review. Int J Mol Sci [Internet]. 2023 Apr 1 [cited 2025 Nov 25];24(7):6272. Available from: https://pmc.ncbi.nlm.nih.gov/articles/PMC10094086/
48. Niezink AGH, de Jong RA, Muijs CT, Langendijk JA, Widder J. Pulmonary function changes after radiotherapy for lung or esophageal cancer: A systematic review focusing on dose-volume parameters. Oncologist [Internet]. 2017 Oct 1 [cited 2025 Nov 25];22(10):1257. Available from: https://pmc.ncbi.nlm.nih.gov/articles/PMC5634763/
49. Malagrinò M, Zavatta G. Review of bone health in women with estrogen receptor–positive breast cancer receiving endocrine therapy. Women's Health [Internet]. 2023 Jan 1 [cited 2025 Nov 25];19:17455057221149492. Available from: https://pmc.ncbi.nlm.nih.gov/articles/PMC9846301/
50. Owen PJ, Daly RM, Livingston PM, Fraser SF. Lifestyle guidelines for managing adverse effects on bone health and body composition in men treated with androgen deprivation therapy for prostate cancer: an update. Prostate Cancer Prostatic Dis [Internet]. 2017 Jan 24 [cited 2025 Nov 25];20(2):137–45. Available from: https://www.nature.com/articles/pcan201669
51. Bettariga F, Newton RU, Bishop C, Maestroni L, Borsati A, Avancini A, et al. Periodizing exercise medicine prescription for patients with cancer: A narrative opinion. Sports Med [Internet]. 2025 Dec 1 [cited 2025 Nov 25];55(12):2987–99. Available from: https://link.springer.com/article/10.1007/s40279-025-02311-5
52. Subramaniam S, Kong YC, Zaharah H, Uiterwaal CSPM, Richard A, Taib NA, et al. Baseline cardiovascular comorbidities, and the influence on cancer treatment decision-making in women with breast cancer. Ecancermedicalscience. 2021;15.
53. Viamonte SG, Joaquim AV, Alves AJ, Vilela E, Capela A, Ferreira C, et al. Cardio-oncology rehabilitation for cancer survivors with high cardiovascular risk: A randomized clinical trial. JAMA Cardiol [Internet]. 2023 Dec 1 [cited

2025 Nov 25];8(12):1119–28. Available from: https://jamanetwork.com/journals/jamacardiology/fullarticle/2810101
54. White KR, Lu J, Ibrahim Z, Furth PA. Enabling exercise prescription for survivors of cancer. Sci Rep [Internet]. 2021 May 5 [cited 2025 Nov 25];11(1):9557. Available from: https://www.nature.com/articles/s41598-021-89021-w
55. Cole SF, Skaczkowski G, Wilson C. The role of illness perceptions and exercise beliefs in exercise engagement during treatment for cancer. Support Care Cancer [Internet]. 2021 Sep [cited 2023 Dec 13];29(9):5065–73. Available from: http://www.ncbi.nlm.nih.gov/pubmed/33594512
56. Velthuis MJ, Peeters PH, Gijsen BC, Van Den Berg JP, Koppejan-Rensenbrink RA, Vlaeyen JW, et al. Role of fear of movement in cancer survivors participating in a rehabilitation program: A longitudinal cohort study. Arch Phys Med Rehabil [Internet]. 2012 Feb [cited 2025 Nov 25];93(2):332–8. Available from: https://pubmed.ncbi.nlm.nih.gov/22289246/
57. Can AG, Can SS, Ekşioğlu E, Çakcı FA. Is kinesiophobia associated with lymphedema, upper extremity function, and psychological morbidity in breast cancer survivors? Turk J Phys Med Rehabil [Internet]. 2018 [cited 2025 Nov 25];65(2):139. Available from: https://pmc.ncbi.nlm.nih.gov/articles/PMC6706825/
58. Humphreys L, Humphreys, Liam J, Greenfield DM. An integrated model of exercise support for people affected by cancer: Consensus through scoping. [cited 2025 Nov 25]. Available from: http://shura.shu.ac.uk/information.html
59. Sabiston CM, Brunet J. Reviewing the benefits of physical activity during cancer survivorship. Am J Lifestyle Med [Internet]. 2012 Mar [cited 2025 Nov 26];6(2):167–77. Available from: https://journals.sagepub.com/doi/10.1177/1559827611407023
60. Blanchard CM, Courneya KS, Stein K, American Cancer Society's SCS-II. Cancer survivors' adherence to lifestyle behavior recommendations and associations with health-related quality of life: Results from the American Cancer Society's SCS-II. J Clin Oncol [Internet]. 2008 May 1 [cited 2023 Dec 13];26(13):2198–204. Available from: https://ascopubs.org/doi/10.1200/JCO.2007.14.6217
61. Gho SA, Munro BJ, Jones SC, Steele JR. Perceived exercise barriers explain exercise participation in Australian women treated for breast cancer better than perceived exercise benefits. Phys Ther [Internet]. 2014 Dec [cited 2023 Dec 13];94(12):1765–74. Available from: http://www.ncbi.nlm.nih.gov/pubmed/25060956
62. Velthuis MJ, May AM, Koppejan-Rensenbrink RA, Gijsen BCM, van Breda E, de Wit GA, et al. Physical Activity during Cancer Treatment (PACT) study: Design of a randomised clinical trial. BMC Cancer [Internet]. 2010 Jun 9 [cited 2023 Dec 13];10:272. Available from: http://www.ncbi.nlm.nih.gov/pubmed/20534147
63. Smaradottir A, Smith AL, Borgert AJ, Oettel KR. Are we on the same page? Patient and provider perceptions about exercise in cancer care: A focus group study. J Natl Compr Canc Netw [Internet]. 2017 May [cited 2023 Dec 13];15(5):588–94. Available from: http://www.ncbi.nlm.nih.gov/pubmed/28476738
64. Husebø AML, Dyrstad SM, Mjaaland I, Søreide JA, Bru E. Effects of scheduled exercise on cancer-related fatigue in women with early breast cancer. Sci

World J [Internet]. 2014 [cited 2023 Dec 13];2014:271828. Available from: http://www.ncbi.nlm.nih.gov/pubmed/24563628
65. SH K. Kinesiophobia: A new view of chronic pain behavior. Pain Manage [Internet]. 1990 [cited 2025 Nov 26];3:35–43. Available from: https://cir.nii.ac.jp/crid/1572824501081889280
66. Van der Gucht E, Dams L, Meeus M, Devoogdt N, Beintema A, Penen F, et al. Kinesiophobia contributes to pain-related disability in breast cancer survivors: A cross-sectional study. Support Care Cancer [Internet]. 2020 Sep 1 [cited 2025 Nov 26];28(9):4501–8. Available from: https://pubmed.ncbi.nlm.nih.gov/31953624/
67. Can AG, Can SS, Ekşioğlu E, Çakcı FA. Is kinesiophobia associated with lymphedema, upper extremity function, and psychological morbidity in breast cancer survivors? Turk J Phys Med Rehabil [Internet]. 2018 [cited 2025 Nov 26];65(2):139. Available from: https://pmc.ncbi.nlm.nih.gov/articles/PMC6706825/
68. Clifford BK, Mizrahi D, Sandler CX, Barry BK, Simar D, Wakefield CE, et al. Barriers and facilitators of exercise experienced by cancer survivors: A mixed methods systematic review. Support Care Cancer [Internet]. 2018 Mar 1 [cited 2025 Nov 26];26(3):685–700. Available from: https://pubmed.ncbi.nlm.nih.gov/29185105/
69. Bettariga F, Taaffe DR, Crespo-Garcia C, Clay TD, De Santi M, Baldelli G, et al. A single bout of resistance or high-intensity interval training increases anti-cancer myokines and suppresses cancer cell growth in vitro in survivors of breast cancer. Breast Cancer Res Treat [Internet]. 2025 Aug 1 [cited 2025 Nov 22];213(1):171–80. Available from: https://pubmed.ncbi.nlm.nih.gov/40608178/
70. Humphreys L, Crank H, Frith G, Speake H, Reece LJ. Bright spots, physical activity investments that work: Active everyday, Sheffield's physical activity service for all people living with and beyond cancer. Br J Sports Med [Internet]. 2019 Jul [cited 2023 Dec 13];53(13):837–8. Available from: http://www.ncbi.nlm.nih.gov/pubmed/29212766
71. Blaney JM, Lowe-Strong A, Rankin-Watt J, Campbell A, Gracey JH. Cancer survivors' exercise barriers, facilitators and preferences in the context of fatigue, quality of life and physical activity participation: A questionnaire-survey. Psychooncology [Internet]. 2013 Jan [cited 2023 Dec 13];22(1):186–94. Available from: http://www.ncbi.nlm.nih.gov/pubmed/23296635
72. Murray J, Perry R, Pontifex E, Selva-Nayagam S, Bezak E, Bennett H. The impact of breast cancer on fears of exercise and exercise identity. Patient Educ Couns. 2022 Jul 1;105(7):2443–9.
73. Chan A, Ports K, Neo P, Ramalingam MB, Lim AT, Tan B, et al. Barriers and facilitators to exercise among adult cancer survivors in Singapore. Supportive Care in Cancer [Internet]. 2022 Jun 1 [cited 2025 Nov 26];30(6):4867. Available from: https://pmc.ncbi.nlm.nih.gov/articles/PMC9046302/
74. Sabiston CM, Brunet J. Reviewing the benefits of physical activity during cancer survivorship. Am J Lifestyle Med [Internet]. 2012 Mar 26 [cited 2023 Dec 13];6(2):167–77. Available from: http://journals.sagepub.com/doi/10.1177/1559827611407023
75. Jones LW, Courneya KS. Exercise discussions during cancer treatment consultations. Cancer Pract [Internet]. 2002 [cited 2023 Dec 13];10(2):66–74. Available from: http://www.ncbi.nlm.nih.gov/pubmed/11903271

76. Peeters C, Stewart A, Segal R, Wouterloot E, Scott CG, Aubry T. Evaluation of a cancer exercise program: Patient and physician beliefs. Psychooncology [Internet]. 2009 Aug [cited 2023 Dec 13];18(8):898–902. Available from: http://www.ncbi.nlm.nih.gov/pubmed/19117271
77. Ormel HL, van der Schoot GGF, Sluiter WJ, Jalving M, Gietema JA, Walenkamp AME. Predictors of adherence to exercise interventions during and after cancer treatment: A systematic review. Psychooncology [Internet]. 2018 Mar 1 [cited 2025 Nov 26];27(3):713–24. Available from: https://onlinelibrary.wiley.com/doi/full/10.1002/pon.4612
78. Finne E, Glausch M, Exner AK, Sauzet O, Stölzel F, Seidel N. Behavior change techniques for increasing physical activity in cancer survivors: A systematic review and meta-analysis of randomized controlled trials. Cancer Manag Res [Internet]. 2018 Oct 30 [cited 2025 Nov 26];10:5125–43. Available from: https://www.dovepress.com/behavior-change-techniques-for-increasing-physical-activity-in-cancer--peer-reviewed-fulltext-article-CMAR
79. Tsai E, Robertson MC, Lyons EJ, Swartz MC, Basen-Engquist K. Physical activity and exercise self-regulation in cancer survivors: A qualitative study. Psychooncology [Internet]. 2017 Feb 1 [cited 2025 Nov 26];27(2):563. Available from: https://pmc.ncbi.nlm.nih.gov/articles/PMC5929476/
80. Mazzoni AS, Brooke HL, Berntsen S, Nordin K, Demmelmaier I. Effect of self-regulatory behaviour change techniques and predictors of physical activity maintenance in cancer survivors: A 12-month follow-up of the Phys-Can RCT. BMC Cancer [Internet]. 2021 Dec 1 [cited 2025 Nov 26];21(1):1272. Available from: https://link.springer.com/article/10.1186/s12885-021-08996-x
81. Fedricker D, Barber A®. Effects of social support on physical activity, self-efficacy, and quality of life in sdult vancer durvivors and their caregivers. Oncology Nursing Forum. 2013;40(5).
82. McDonough MH, Beselt LJ, Kronlund LJ, Albinati NK, Daun JT, Trudeau MS, et al. Social support and physical activity for cancer survivors: A qualitative review and meta-study. J Cancer Surviv [Internet]. 2021 Oct 1 [cited 2025 Nov 26];15(5):713–28. Available from: https://pubmed.ncbi.nlm.nih.gov/33128705/
83. Price J, Brunet J. Exploring cancer survivors' experiences in a group-based walking program before and during the COVID-19 pandemic: A qualitative study. Supportive Care in Cancer [Internet]. 2021 Feb 1 [cited 2025 Nov 26];30(2):1355. Available from: https://pmc.ncbi.nlm.nih.gov/articles/PMC8426160/
84. Ireland AV, Finnegan-John J, Hubbard G, Scanlon K, Kyle RG. Walking groups for women with breast cancer: Mobilising therapeutic assemblages of walk, talk and place. Soc Sci Med. 2019 Jun 1;231:38–46.
85. Kampshoff CS, Jansen F, van Mechelen W, May AM, Brug J, Chinapaw MJM, et al. Determinants of exercise adherence and maintenance among cancer survivors: A systematic review. Int J Behav Nutr Phys Act [Internet]. 2014 Jul 2 [cited 2025 Nov 25];11(1):80. Available from: https://pmc.ncbi.nlm.nih.gov/articles/PMC4096543/
86. Salerno EA, Gothe NP, Fanning J, Peterson LL, Colditz GA, McAuley E. Effects of a DVD-delivered randomized controlled physical activity intervention on functional health in cancer survivors. BMC Cancer [Internet]. 2021 Dec 1 [cited 2025 Nov 26];21(1):870. Available from: https://link.springer.com/article/10.1186/s12885-021-08608-8
87. Sita-Lumsden A, Howlett S, Garritt C, Cole S, Howells L, Rehman F. Identifying and managing the barriers to exercise during and following breast cancer

treatment. Clin Oncol [Internet]. 2019 Jul 1 [cited 2025 Nov 26];31(7):e114. Available from: https://www.clinicaloncologyonline.net/action/showFullText?pii=S0936655519301347

88. Elshahat S, Treanor C, Donnelly M. Factors influencing physical activity participation among people living with or beyond cancer: A systematic scoping review. Int J Behav Nutr Phys Act [Internet]. 2021 Apr 6 [cited 2025 Nov 26];18(1):50. Available from: https://link.springer.com/article/10.1186/s12966-021-01116-9
89. Orange ST, Gilbert SE, Brown MC, Saxton JM. Recall, perceptions and determinants of receiving physical activity advice amongst cancer survivors: A mixed-methods survey. Supportive Care in Cancer [Internet]. 2021 Nov 1 [cited 2025 Nov 26];29(11):6369–78. Available from: https://link.springer.com/article/10.1007/s00520-021-06221-w
90. Stout NL, Brown JC, Schwartz AL, Marshall TF, Campbell AM, Nekhlyudov L, et al. An exercise oncology clinical pathway: Screening and referral for personalized interventions. Cancer [Internet]. 2020 Jun 15 [cited 2025 Nov 26];126(12):2750. Available from: https://pmc.ncbi.nlm.nih.gov/articles/PMC7258139/
91. A scoping review examining the integration of exercise services in clinical oncology settings | BMC Health Services Research [Internet]. [cited 2025 Nov 26]. Available from: https://link.springer.com/article/10.1186/s12913-022-07598-y
92. Nieman DC. Risk of upper respiratory tract infection in athletes: An epidemiologic and immunologic perspective. J Athl Train [Internet]. 1997 Oct [cited 2025 Nov 22];32(4):344. Available from: https://pmc.ncbi.nlm.nih.gov/articles/PMC1320353/
93. Esnaola NF, Ford ME. Racial differences and disparities in cancer care and outcomes: Where's the rub? Surg Oncol Clin N Am [Internet]. 2012 Jul [cited 2025 Nov 26];21(3):417. Available from: https://pmc.ncbi.nlm.nih.gov/articles/PMC4180671/
94. Hirko KA, Rocque G, Reasor E, Taye A, Daly A, Cutress RI, et al. The impact of race and ethnicity in breast cancer—Disparities and implications for precision oncology. BMC Med [Internet]. 2022 Dec 1 [cited 2025 Nov 26];20(1):72. Available from: https://link.springer.com/article/10.1186/s12916-022-02260-0
95. Scott ECS, Hoskin PJ. Health inequalities in cancer care: A literature review of pathways to diagnosis in the United Kingdom. EClinicalMedicine [Internet]. 2024 Oct 1 [cited 2025 Nov 26];76:102864. Available from: https://www.thelancet.com/action/showFullText?pii=S2589537024004437
96. Abuali I, Patel S, Kiel L, Meza K, Florez N. Disparities in cancer care—A call to action. Cancer Cell [Internet]. 2023 Jan 9 [cited 2025 Nov 26];41(1):1–4. Available from: https://www.cell.com/action/showFullText?pii=S1535610822005505
97. Winn R, Winkfield K, Mitchell E. Addressing disparities in cancer care and incorporating precision medicine for minority populations. J Natl Med Assoc. 2023 May 1;115(2):S2–7.
98. Hirko KA, Dorn JM, Dearing JW, Alfano CM, Wigton A, Schmitz KH. Implementation of physical activity programs for rural cancer survivors: Challenges and opportunities. Int J Environ Res Public Health [Internet]. 2021 Dec 7 [cited 2025 Nov 26];18(24):12909. Available from: https://www.mdpi.com/1660-4601/18/24/12909/htm

99. Culos-Reed N, Wagoner CW, Dreger J, McNeely ML, Keats M, Santa Mina D, et al. Implementing an exercise oncology model to reach rural and remote individuals living with and beyond cancer: A hybrid effectiveness-implementation protocol for project EXCEL (EXercise for Cancer to Enhance Living Well). BMJ Open [Internet]. 2022 Dec 1 [cited 2025 Nov 26];12(12):e063953. Available from: https://bmjopen.bmj.com/content/12/12/e063953
100. Gell NM, Dittus K, Caefer J, Martin A, Bae M, Patel K V. Remotely delivered exercise to older rural cancer survivors: A randomized controlled pilot trial. J Cancer Surviv [Internet]. 2024 Apr 1 [cited 2025 Nov 26];18(2):596–605. Available from: https://link.springer.com/article/10.1007/s11764-022-01292-y
101. Kennedy MA, Bayes S, Newton RU, Zissiadis Y, Spry NA, Taaffe DR, et al. Implementation barriers to integrating exercise as medicine in oncology: An ecological scoping review. J Cancer Surviv [Internet]. 2021 Aug 1 [cited 2025 Nov 26];16(4):865. Available from: https://pmc.ncbi.nlm.nih.gov/articles/PMC9300485/
102. Campbell KL, Winters-Stone KM, Wiskemann J, May AM, Schwartz AL, Courneya KS, et al. Exercise guidelines for cancer survivors: Consensus statement from international multidisciplinary roundtable. Med Sci Sports Exerc [Internet]. 2019 Nov 1 [cited 2025 Nov 26];51(11):2375. Available from: https://pmc.ncbi.nlm.nih.gov/articles/PMC8576825/
103. Moving Medicine—The ultimate resource for healthcare professionals [Internet]. [cited 2025 Nov 26]. Available from: https://movingmedicine.ac.uk/
104. Mizrahi D, Murnane A, Quinn S, Crowe J, Rosenbaum S, Adams D, et al. Exercise recommendations and referral patterns of oncology professionals. Asia Pac J Clin Oncol [Internet]. 2022 Jun 1 [cited 2025 Nov 26];18(3):295–302. Available from: https://pubmed.ncbi.nlm.nih.gov/34187099/
105. Santa Mina D, Alibhai SMH, Matthew AG, Guglietti CL, Steele J, Trachtenberg J, et al. Exercise in clinical cancer care: A call to action and program development description. Curr Oncol [Internet]. 2012 [cited 2025 Nov 26];19(3):e136. Available from: https://pmc.ncbi.nlm.nih.gov/articles/PMC3364774/
106. Roberts AL, Potts HWW, Stevens C, Lally P, Smith L, Fisher A. Cancer specialist nurses' perspectives of physical activity promotion and the potential role of physical activity apps in cancer care. [cited 2025 Nov 26]. Available from: https://doi.org/10.1007/s11764-019-00801-w
107. Humphreys L, Frith G, Humphreys H, Crank H, Dixey J, Greenfield DM, et al. Evaluation of a city-wide physical activity pathway for people affected by cancer: The active everyday service. Supportive Care in Cancer [Internet]. 2023 Feb 1 [cited 2025 Nov 26];31(2):101. Available from: https://pmc.ncbi.nlm.nih.gov/articles/PMC9829638/
108. Bloom E. Prehabilitation evidence and insight review. 2017.
109. Macmillan Cancer Support. Principles and guidance for prehabilitation within the management and support of people with cancer In partnership with acknowledgements. 2020. https://www.macmillan.org.uk/healthcare-professionals/news-and-resources/guides/principles-and-guidance-for-prehabilitation
110. RE-AIM—Home—Reach effectiveness adoption implementation maintenance [Internet]. [cited 2025 Nov 26]. Available from: https://re-aim.org/
111. Roberts AL, Potts HWW, Stevens C, Lally P, Smith L, Fisher A. Cancer specialist nurses' perspectives of physical activity promotion and the

potential role of physical activity apps in cancer care [Internet]. doi:10.1007/s11764-019-00801-w

112. Humphreys L, Frith G, Humphreys H, Crank H, Dixey J, Greenfield DM, et al. Evaluation of a city-wide physical activity pathway for people affected by cancer: The active everyday service. Supportive Care in Cancer. [2023 Feb 1];31(2):101. doi:10.1007/S00520-022-07560-Y PubMed PMID: 36622460.
113. Bloom E. Prehabilitation evidence and insight review. 2017.
114. Cancer Support M. Principles and guidance for prehabilitation within the management and support of people with cancer In partnership with Acknowledgements.
115. RE-AIM – Home – Reach effectiveness adoption implementation maintenance [Internet]. [cited 2025 Nov 26]. Available from: https://re-aim.org/

9

A NEW PERSPECTIVE ON EXERCISE AND CANCER

9.1 Introduction

Throughout this book, the evolving and evidence-based role of physical activity and exercise across the cancer continuum has been explored. From prevention and treatment to survivorship and recurrence, the message has remained consistent and clear: Sit less, move more—every step counts. What began as a public health observation that physically active individuals experience better cancer outcomes, has now been substantiated by a growing body of evidence spanning epidemiology, clinical trials and molecular biology. In these pages, the field of exercise oncology has been examined from multiple angles, including large-scale population studies linking physical activity to reduced cancer incidence, and experimental findings detailing the molecular, cellular and microenvironmental mechanisms through which exercise exerts its effects.

9.2 Key takeaways from each chapter

This final chapter brings together the key learnings from each chapter to reaffirm this core message. It also invites the reader to consider how this knowledge can shape future research, clinical practice and public health strategies. The promise of exercise as a low-cost, accessible and biologically active tool against cancer is compelling. Realising its full impact now depends on translating this knowledge into systematic action across research, clinical practice and public health policy.

DOI: 10.4324/9781003511519-12

9.2.1 Chapter 1: Introduction to physical activity, exercise and cancer

The opening chapter laid the conceptual foundation of the field, defining physical activity and exercise, and highlighting their distinct yet overlapping roles in cancer prevention, treatment and survivorship. It traced the evolution of exercise oncology from an emerging discipline to a growing field of translational importance and set the stage for exploring both the breadth and depth of evidence supporting movement as medicine across the cancer continuum.

9.2.2 Chapter 2: The evidence behind exercise versus sedentary behaviour and cancer

Drawing on epidemiological studies and global health data, this chapter examined the contrasting effects of sedentary behaviour and physical activity on cancer incidence and mortality. It underscored how prolonged inactivity increases the risk of several common cancers, while regular physical activity is associated with reduced risk and improved survival. The chapter also introduced the socio-economic, demographic and behavioural factors that shape patterns of movement and sedentarism across populations.

9.2.3 Chapter 3: The cellular response to exercise in cancer

This chapter explored how exercise exerts its effects at the cellular level, particularly within the TME. Key themes included modulation of immune surveillance, remodelling of the vasculature and adipose tissue by counteracting the inflammatory microenvironment. Exercise-induced changes in the infiltration and function of NK cells, T cells and MDSCs demonstrated how movement reshapes the immunological profile associated with cancer.

9.2.4 Chapter 4: The molecular basis of exercise in cancer

At the molecular level, exercise induces a cascade of intracellular and extracellular signalling events. This chapter highlighted the role of myokines, such as IL-6 and irisin, EVs and key signalling regulators, such as AMPK, in mediating anti-tumour effects. It also examined how these signals influence angiogenesis, metabolism and inflammatory profiles, positioning exercise as a modulator of tumour-supportive and suppressive pathways alike.

9.2.5 Chapter 5: Types of exercise and their benefits

Focusing on the "how," this chapter unpacked the specific benefits of aerobic, resistance and endurance exercise, incidental physical activity and mind-body therapies. Using the FITT principle as the guiding framework, it detailed the physiological, psychological and oncological outcomes associated with each modality. Aerobic activity enhances cardiovascular and immune function, while resistance training supports muscle mass and bone health. The importance of integrating movement into daily life was emphasised as a means to reduce sedentary time and sustain long-term engagement.

9.2.6 Chapter 6: Differential effects of exercise intensities

Here, the discussion centred on intensity as a biological lever. Moderate-intensity emerged as particularly effective in promoting immune surveillance and reducing systemic inflammation, while high-intensity training showed potential to enhance anti-tumour immunity, albeit with caution regarding systemic stress and recovery needs. Preclinical and clinical data illustrated the nuanced effects of intensity on the TME, vascular adaptation and immune cell mobilisation.

9.2.7 Chapter 7: Frequency and length of exercise bouts

This chapter addressed how often and how long exercise should be performed to optimise benefit. Acute bouts were found to trigger transient but potent systemic effects, while chronic training facilitated sustained adaptations in metabolism, immune function and vascular health. Evidence from serum studies revealed that even single sessions can exert anti-tumour effects.

9.2.8 Chapter 8: Exercise guidelines and recommendations

The final body chapter translated the science into practice, outlining global and cancer-specific exercise guidelines, reinforcing the message that movement is safe, feasible and beneficial across all stages of cancer care. Attention was given to tailoring exercise prescriptions across the cancer continuum: From prehabilitation through to palliative care. The chapter concluded with a call for more personalised, inclusive and systems-informed approaches to implementation.

9.3 Future directions in exercise oncology research

While the field of exercise oncology has advanced significantly, important questions remain unanswered. To fully harness the therapeutic potential of exercise in cancer care, future research must address several critical gaps and embrace innovation in both methodology and application. Many traditional clinical trials in exercise oncology suffer from limitations in design, such as underpowered sample sizes, reliance on self-reported activity levels, and insufficient mechanistic endpoints. To advance the field, future trials should include biological surrogates of efficacy (e.g., tumour perfusion, immune profiling), explore prehabilitation (exercise before treatment) and peri-treatment timing to exploit windows of sensitivity. Moreover, they should consider using multimodal interventions (e.g., combining exercise with dietary or pharmacological agents) to enhance efficacy, and prioritise the real-world translation of exercise oncology research to evaluate cost-effectiveness, scalability and most importantly, equity of access.

9.3.1 Mechanistic pathways and dose-response relationships

Understanding how exercise exerts its anti-cancer effects at the molecular and cellular level remains a priority. Although key pathways involving immune activation, inflammation, metabolism and angiogenesis have been identified, the precise interactions within different tumour types, stages and treatment contexts are not yet fully characterised. A more granular understanding of how different exercise doses (defined by type, intensity, frequency and duration) affect tumour biology is essential for moving from general recommendations to precision exercise prescriptions.

Mechanistic studies have revealed that exercise can alter angiogenesis, immune surveillance, insulin signalling, inflammatory cytokine production and the composition of the TME. However, patients and clinicians alike are rightly asking: "What kind of exercise? How much? When? And for whom?" To answer these questions, translational research must go beyond establishing feasibility and efficacy. In particular, research should aim to clarify:

1. The minimum effective dose required to induce biological change.
2. The thresholds beyond which exercise may be counterproductive (e.g., through systemic stress or immunosuppression).
3. How these relationships vary by cancer type, treatment modality and individual patient characteristics.

9.3.2 Individualisation and personalised exercise medicine

Despite broad guidelines, one size does not fit all. Factors such as tumour burden, comorbidities, baseline fitness, psychological readiness and cultural context all influence how exercise is tolerated and how effective it can be. In the same way as oncology has embraced precision medicine, so too must precision exercise prescriptions be adopted. Key parameters for tailoring exercise include: (1) cancer type and treatment modality (e.g., chemotherapy, radiotherapy, immunotherapy); (2) patient baseline fitness level and prior activity history; (3) biological phenotype (e.g., inflammatory, metabolic or immunosuppressive profile); and (4) treatment stage and side-effect burden (e.g., fatigue, neutropenia, cachexia). Emerging evidence suggests that patients with obesity, insulin resistance or systemic inflammation may derive disproportionate benefit from exercise interventions (1). In such cases, targeting exercise to correct specific biological vulnerabilities (e.g., via myokines, metabolic competition or vascular normalisation) may enhance both cancer-specific and holistic outcomes. Developing biomarker-informed exercise prescriptions, similar to pharmacogenomics, represents a critical translational goal. For example, tracking changes in circulating IL-6, adiponectin, VEGF or NK cell activity could guide dose adjustment and monitor biological efficacy. Future studies should also investigate how individual factors (e.g., sex, age, genetics, immune phenotype) intersect with exercise variables to optimise outcomes. This could lead to adaptive exercise protocols that evolve with the patient's condition and treatment phase.

PATIENT VIGNETTE 9.1 "Maya"—body image and empowerment

Maya, 39, felt disconnected from her body during treatment for triple negative breast cancer. Starting dance-based workouts at home post-treatment helped her reconnect and rebuild confidence. Exercise was key in reclaiming her sense of identity and strength. "I started dancing in my kitchen, just 5 minutes at first. It was messy and brilliant. I felt alive again." She now mentors others navigating similar journeys.

9.3.3 Technology-enabled monitoring and delivery

Digital health tools offer new opportunities for scaling and refining exercise interventions. Wearable sensors, mobile apps and remote coaching platforms can enhance the precision, adherence and accessibility of exercise programmes, especially for those in rural or underserved settings. They can also provide continuous feedback on physiological responses, enabling dynamic adjustments to exercise prescriptions. Future research should explore how technology can support remote supervision and "tele-exercise," real-time monitoring of biomarkers (e.g., HRV, blood glucose, inflammatory markers), and gamification and behavioural nudges to improve engagement and adherence. Integration with electronic health records and cancer care pathways will also be crucial to embed exercise within routine care. Such innovative trials using wearables, remote coaching and machine learning-guided prescriptions to support personalised exercise delivery and real-time monitoring offer exciting avenues for future research in this area.

9.3.4 Inclusion of under-represented populations and cancer types

Much of the current literature focuses on breast, colorectal and prostate cancers, often in predominantly white, middle-aged populations. There is an urgent need to expand research to include less common or more aggressive cancers (e.g., pancreatic, brain and haematological malignancies), paediatric, adolescent and young adult cancer survivors, older adults and those with multiple chronic conditions, as well as ethnically and socioeconomically diverse populations. By broadening the scope of research and evaluating the equity of access to care, the field can ensure that future guidelines and interventions are equitable, relevant and inclusive.

9.3.5 Clinical implementation and systems-level integration

Despite widespread interest in exercise as a therapeutic adjunct, several practical and systemic barriers continue to hinder its implementation in routine cancer care. Firstly, lack of awareness, insufficient training or even scepticism among healthcare providers about the biological and clinical benefits of exercise can hinder uptake amongst patients and survivors. As a result, many are left fearful of causing harm and fall back on long-standing beliefs that "rest is best," rather than recognising the potential of physical activity and exercise to improve their outcomes. Moreover, with inconsistent referral pathways, exercise is not being routinely integrated into oncology care plans. In addition, the field of clinical exercise physiology is in its relative infancy and therefore patients have limited access to trained exercise oncology specialists, especially in rural or resource-limited settings. For exercise to become meaningfully integrated into oncology care, health systems must formally recognise exercise professionals as essential members of the multidisciplinary cancer care team. This includes investing in training programmes tailored to physiotherapists, fitness professionals and clinicians to build capacity in exercise oncology (2).

To further complicate matters, the wide heterogeneity in patient capacity, motivation, comorbidities and treatment-related side effects makes applying standardised protocols difficult. In addition, sustainable reimbursement pathways are needed to support the delivery of exercise assessment, prescription and monitoring. Digital platforms should also be prioritised to enable remote access, particularly for underserved or immunocompromised populations who may face barriers to attending in-person sessions. Despite guidelines from organisations like ACSM recommending exercise as standard of care (3–6), implementation is fragmented, often relying on local champions rather than being embedded through public health policy.

9.4 A call to action: Be part of the movement

As the scientific case for exercise in cancer care continues to strengthen, so too must the movement to translate this knowledge into everyday action. The responsibility for advancing exercise oncology does not lie with researchers alone: It belongs to a broad and diverse community of students, clinicians, scientists, policymakers and patients themselves. This is a shared opportunity to redefine the narrative and reframe how we think about cancer care.

9.4.1 Empowering the next generation

Whether you are an undergraduate student discovering this field for the first time, a postgraduate developing a thesis project, or a clinician wondering how to implement exercise prescriptions in your practice, your role matters. By asking questions, challenging assumptions and embracing interdisciplinary collaboration, the next generation of leaders can accelerate progress. Researchers are encouraged to design inclusive, pragmatic studies that answer real-world questions. Clinicians can advocate for exercise to be integrated into routine care, referring patients early and often to exercise professionals. Educators and course leaders can embed exercise oncology into core curricula, ensuring future healthcare professionals are equipped with the knowledge and confidence to promote movement as medicine.

9.4.2 Changing the narrative through education and communication

To date, public health messages about cancer prevention and survivorship have often focused on avoidance tactics: Avoidance of smoking, poor diet, or environmental exposures. However, a more proactive, empowering message of embracing movement could be the key to unlocking a new perspective on cancer care: That movement is not only safe but also beneficial; not only preventive but also therapeutic. Effective communication strategies are key to spreading this message. Whether through public campaigns, clinical conversations, social media channels, or school curricula, we must collectively redirect the story from fear to empowerment. Tailoring messages to different audiences, including patients, families, clinicians and policymakers, will ensure relevance and resonance. Importantly, these efforts must be grounded in empathy, cultural sensitivity and lived experience. Not every individual has equal access to green space, time, equipment or supportive care. Making exercise oncology truly inclusive means addressing these barriers and co-designing solutions that work in the real world. The movement toward active cancer care is already underway, but it needs more voices, more champions and more momentum. Whether you contribute through research, clinical practice, education, advocacy or personal example, you are part of the solution. By working together, across disciplines, sectors and systems, it is possible to ensure that the benefits of exercise are not reserved for a select few but are accessible to all.

9.5 Final thoughts

Exercise is not a magic bullet, but it is a powerful, pleiotropic and largely untapped ally in the fight against cancer. It offers measurable benefits across cancer prevention, treatment, recovery and survivorship: Benefits grounded in a growing body of evidence spanning epidemiology, cellular biology and clinical research. This volume has examined the field of exercise oncology from multiple angles: The population-level associations between movement and cancer risk; the cellular and molecular responses to different forms of exercise; and the practical considerations of prescribing activity throughout the cancer continuum. Collectively, these insights highlight the urgent need to bridge scientific discovery with clinical application.

Achieving this translation will require continued collaboration across research, healthcare and policy. Mechanistic findings must inform clinical trials; implementation science must guide the delivery of effective, scalable interventions; and education must equip professionals and the public with the tools and confidence to promote physical activity safely and inclusively. Fundamentally, the message is one of empowerment: Meaningful change does not depend on perfection or intensity, but on consistency and accessibility. Even small amounts of movement, adapted to individual capacity and context, can support physical and psychological resilience. Every step, whether in the lab, the clinic, or the community setting, contributes to a future where exercise is fully integrated into the standard of cancer care.

Chapter 9 Test your understanding question bank

1. How does the concept of "every step counts" align with both the molecular mechanisms and population-level benefits of exercise discussed throughout this book?

2. What challenges might a clinician face in implementing exercise as part of a standard cancer care pathway, and how could these be addressed at the system level?
3. Why is it important to move from general exercise guidelines to precision exercise prescriptions? What tools or biomarkers might support this shift?
4. What factors contribute to the underrepresentation of certain populations in exercise oncology research, and how can future studies become more inclusive?
5. Compare the role of physical activity in prehabilitation versus survivorship. How do goals, barriers and outcomes differ across these phases of care?
6. What role might wearable technology and remote platforms play in shaping the future of exercise oncology delivery and monitoring?
7. Reflect on your own role: How can you contribute to advancing the integration of exercise in cancer care?

References

1. Koelwyn GJ, Quail DF, Zhang X, White RM, Jones LW. Exercise-dependent regulation of the tumour microenvironment. Nat Rev Cancer [Internet]. 2017 Oct 25 [cited 2019 Dec 6];17(10):620–32. Available from: http://www.nature.com/articles/nrc.2017.78
2. Morris M, Crank H, Loosemore M, Stevinson C. Identification of research priorities in exercise oncology: A consensus study. J Cancer [Internet]. 2020 [cited 2024 Jul 25];11(9):2702–7. Available from: http://www.ncbi.nlm.nih.gov/pubmed/32201540
3. ACSM's guidelines for exercise testing and prescription—ACSM [Internet]. [cited 2025 Nov 18]. Available from: https://acsm.org/education-resources/books/guidelines-exercise-testing-prescription/
4. Aicr, WCRF. Diet, nutrition, physical activity and cancer: A global perspective a summary of the third expert report. [cited 2025 Nov 14]. Available from: http://gco.iarc.fr/today
5. WHO guidelines on physical activity and sedentary behaviour [Internet]. [cited 2025 Nov 14]. Available from: https://www.who.int/publications/i/item/9789240015128
6. Campbell KL, Winters-Stone KM, Wiskemann J, May AM, Schwartz AL, Courneya KS, et al. Exercise guidelines for cancer survivors: Consensus statement from international multidisciplinary roundtable. Med Sci Sports Exerc [Internet]. 2019 Nov 1 [cited 2025 Nov 14];51(11):2375–90. Available from: https://pubmed.ncbi.nlm.nih.gov/31626055/

10

ADDITIONAL RESOURCES

This directory is intended to support readers with further exploration, application and implementation of the concepts discussed throughout this book. It includes a wide range of reputable resources, from national charities and clinical services to professional bodies, guideline repositories and educational platforms. These entries are listed alphabetically within each category for ease of reference. Where applicable, social media handles are provided.

10.1 How to use this directory

This list includes both UK-based and international organisations. Many are open-access and freely available to students, clinicians, researchers and people living with and beyond cancer. This is not an exhaustive list, nor an endorsement, but a curated collection of high-quality, evidence-informed tools and services.

10.2 Charities and community support programmes

5K your way: Move against cancer

www.5kyourway.org
Community-based initiative encouraging people affected by cancer to walk, jog or run monthly 5k events at local parkruns, supported by healthcare professionals and ambassadors. See also Move Charity.
Instagram: @5kyourway

DOI: 10.4324/9781003511519-13

Battle Cancer program

www.battlecancerprogram.com

Founded in 2021, the Battle Cancer Program is a charitable organisation supporting individuals post-cancer through a 12-week, fully funded programme designed by experts in the field to aid cancer recovery. The Program works to engage people who have experienced cancer in a meaningful pathway of structured and progressive exercise rehabilitation that builds physical confidence and independence, and a belief in a better QoL and health for the future. The scheme has been built from research and studies around the benefit of physical exercise on the prevention and recovery from disease, in particular, cancer. In the short time the programme has been running, it has already helped over 500 people return to exercise post-cancer treatment and seen considerable changes in physical fitness, confidence, mobility and ability.

For more information, head to www.battlecancerprogram.com or follow the charity on social media, @thebcprogram.

Case study: Maintaining identity during melanoma treatment

Age: 50–59
Diagnosis: Melanoma
Treatment: Surgery and immunotherapy
Programme timing: During treatment

Uninspired by many traditional cancer support offerings, Matt wanted something physically challenging. Having always trained, Matt was used to coping through exercise. He discovered CrossFit through Battle Cancer, which provided exactly what was needed: intensity, challenge and functional fitness. The initial sessions felt intimidating and at first he doubted himself, but embracing discomfort became part of his coping strategy. Exercise during treatment became both a psychological anchor and a form of release. Workplace support allowed attendance, reinforcing the importance of structural support systems in enabling exercise participation.

"Give it a go, it might not suit all but at least you gave it a go . . .it can cater for all ages and abilities."

Case study: Regaining purpose and "me time" after breast cancer

Age: 60+
Diagnosis: Breast cancer
Treatment: Chemotherapy, surgery, radiotherapy, ongoing letrozole
Programme timing: After treatment

Susie described feeling as though cancer had aged her "ten years overnight". She felt physically weaker, emotionally drained and disconnected from her previous sense of vitality. Battle Cancer became more than exercise: it became structure, purpose and community. Participating in the programme improved her sleep and helped her rebuild strength, and the morning sessions provided a reason to get up. Emotionally, training alongside other women with similar experiences helped her reconnect socially after becoming fairly reclusive. As a carer for her husband with dementia, the programme also provided her with valuable "me time."

There were challenges, for example, being the oldest in the group, which made her feel like she struggled with feeling slower than the others, and later health issues prevented her from completing the course, which was disheartening. Yet her reflection is powerful: she recognises that waiting to feel better before restarting exercise may not be realistic since movement is part of the recovery process itself.

"Do it. Just do it. Don't put it off. . . You will feel a MILLION times better. You WILL be stronger, fitter, more energised, motivated. And if you are also a carer (as am I) it is a precious bit of 'me time' . . .you will find depths you didn't know you had. It's so rewarding in every way."

Case study: Rebuilding strength and confidence after breast cancer

Age: 30–39
Diagnosis: Breast cancer
Treatment: Surgery, chemotherapy, radiotherapy, hormone therapy
Programme timing: After treatment

After completing intensive treatment, this participant joined Battle Cancer with a simple goal: to regain fitness and strength. At first, joining a new group class felt daunting. The anxiety of stepping into an unfamiliar environment after cancer treatment was very real. However, the supportive coach and welcoming group quickly transformed that fear into connection. Being surrounded by other people with shared experiences created an immediate sense of belonging. Physically, the programme improved fitness and strength, but perhaps more importantly, it restored confidence and provided focus during a difficult transition period. The sessions offered structure, routine and a renewed sense of self.

"It's given me focus and a sense of self during a difficult time."

Case study: A safe route back to normality

Age: 40–49
Diagnosis: Breast cancer
Treatment: Chemotherapy, surgery, radiotherapy
Programme timing: After treatment

After treatment, this participant sought a safe, structured route back into exercise. The key factor was not simply returning to movement, but doing so in an environment sensitive to treatment-related changes in the body. The programme provided physical rebuilding within a psychologically safe space.

"Getting back to exercise was restoring another bit of normality post-treatment."

Case study: Rebuilding function and identity after throat cancer

Age: 50–59
Diagnosis: Throat cancer
Treatment: Surgery, radiotherapy, chemotherapy
Programme timing: After treatment

Following intensive treatment, Simon's primary goal was to regain sufficient strength and stamina to return to everyday life and enjoy the hobbies that mattered to him. Treatment had taken a significant physical toll on his body, with substantial weight loss and muscle wasting leading to reduced strength and stamina. Surgery had affected his shoulder mobility, and his cardiovascular fitness had declined during radiotherapy when fatigue became overwhelming. Although he attempted to walk throughout treatment to maintain a baseline level of fitness, he became too weak to continue by three weeks into his radiotherapy.

Recovery was gradual and deliberate. He resumed walking post-treatment, followed by physiotherapy to restore shoulder mobility. He then introduced light resistance exercises before joining Battle Cancer. The structured, scalable design of the programme allowed him to rebuild strength safely and progressively. Physically, he became stronger and more resilient. Socially, being part of a group navigating similar challenges was invaluable. The shared experience fostered bonds that have endured beyond the programme itself.

"Whatever your background in exercise, take the plunge. . .the bonds you form because you are on a shared journey are incredible and long-lasting."

Cancer research UK

www.cancerresearchuk.org
Includes dedicated guidance pages on physical activity during and after cancer treatment, with patient-friendly explanations and evidence summaries.

Macmillan cancer support

www.macmillan.org.uk
Offers booklets, physical activity toolkits, local services and exercise referral schemes through the "Move More" initiative.

Move charity

www.movecharity.org
Provides online exercise programmes for young people with cancer and cancer survivors through its 5K Your Way and other initiatives.

Pink ribbon program

www.pinkribbonprogram.com
Post-surgical rehabilitation programme for breast cancer recovery, focusing on posture, strength and confidence through specialist training.

Wessex cancer trust

www.wessexcancer.org.uk
Provides wellbeing and exercise support to people affected by cancer in the Wessex region, including links to trusted online exercise resources.

10.3 Clinical and rehabilitation services

Active against cancer (Harrogate and district)

www.activeagainstcancer.org.uk
Local NHS initiative providing supervised physical activity and wellbeing support for people living with or beyond cancer.

Move4You (North Central London Cancer Alliance)

https://gps.northcentrallondon.icb.nhs.uk/services/move4you-ncl-cancer-physical-activity-rehabilitation-service

Twelve-session-guided exercise programme for adults diagnosed with cancer in the past 5 years. Note, this website is for healthcare professionals and not intended for public use.

Prehab4Cancer (GM cancer)

www.gmcancer.org.uk
Pioneering prehabilitation programme offering tailored support for people preparing for cancer surgery in Greater Manchester.

Wales prehab/rehab service (Velindre cancer centre)

https://velindre.nhs.wales/
Supports cancer patients across Wales with access to tailored physical activity support before and after treatment.

10.4 Professional bodies and guidelines

American College of Sports Medicine (ACSM)

www.acsm.org
Publishes gold-standard cancer-specific exercise guidelines and offers Cancer Exercise Trainer certification.

British Association of Sport and Exercise Sciences (BASES)

www.bases.org.uk
Supports sport and exercise scientists, including cancer-focused practitioners and researchers.

Canadian Society for Exercise Physiology (CSEP)

www.csep.ca
Provides guidelines, certification and resources for exercise professionals working with clinical populations.

Exercise Is Medicine Global (EIM)

www.exerciseismedicine.org
Promotes physical activity as a standard in clinical care, including the Moving Through Cancer global initiative.

International Society of Exercise Oncology (ISEO)

www.exerciseoncology.org

A global network of researchers, clinicians and practitioners focused on advancing the science and practice of exercise oncology.

National Institute for Health and Care Excellence (NICE) guidelines (UK)

www.nice.org.uk
Provides evidence-based recommendations on physical activity in cancer care.

World Cancer Research Fund (WCRF)

www.wcrf.org
Evidence-based cancer prevention guidelines highlighting physical activity and weight management.

10.5 Education and learning resources

CanRehab

www.canrehab.co.uk
UK-based training provider for cancer and exercise qualifications (Level 4 accredited). Widely used in clinical and community settings.

Macmillan learning hub

https://www.macmillan.org.uk/healthcare-professionals/macmillan-professionals/learning-and-development
Free online learning platform with modules on physical activity and cancer.

Union for International Cancer Control (UICC) online learning

https://www.uicc.org/
Online resources and training for cancer professionals with growing emphasis on prevention and lifestyle interventions.

10.6 Online toolkits and practical platforms

Moving medicine (UK)

www.movingmedicine.ac.uk
Clinician-facing tool to support brief interventions about physical activity, including a dedicated cancer module.

RMP cancer alliance—physical activity resource hub

https://rmpartners.nhs.uk/
Resources for healthcare professionals and patients, including referral forms, videos and local activity options.

Active norfolk—getting active with cancer

www.activenorfolk.org
Local authority resource for people with cancer or long-term conditions seeking gentle, appropriate activity options.

This directory is intended to grow with the field. Readers are encouraged to explore these resources and share them within clinical, academic and community settings. For corrections or additions, please contact the author or publisher.

APPENDIX A

Test your understanding question bank with answers

Chapter 2 Test your understanding question bank with answers

1. Define sedentary behaviour and explain how it differs from physical inactivity.

   A. Sedentary behaviour refers to any waking behaviour done while sitting, reclining or lying down with an energy expenditure of ≤1.5 METs. Examples include TV watching, deskwork and driving.

   Physical inactivity describes not meeting physical activity guidelines (typically <150 minutes per week of moderate activity.

   A person can be active but highly sedentary (e.g., meets guidelines but sits for 10 hours per day) or inactive but not very sedentary (e.g., on their feet at work but does not exercise).

2. What MET categories classify light, moderate and vigorous physical activity? Provide one example of each.

   A. Light activity: 1.6–2.9 METs (e.g., slow walking, light household tasks)

   Moderate activity: 3–5.9 METs (e.g., brisk walking, steady cycling)
   Vigorous activity: ≥6 METs (e.g., running, aerobic dance)

3. Why is it important not to use the terms "physical activity" and "exercise" interchangeably when interpreting epidemiological evidence?

   A. Because they describe different behaviours with distinct metabolic and health effects. Sedentary behaviour concerns posture and energy expenditure, inactivity concerns failure to meet guidelines, and exercise refers to structured, purposeful physical activity. Conflating them can misinterpret risk and mechanisms.

4. Summarise two major global patterns in sedentary behaviour. Which populations are most sedentary?

   A. Koreans report the highest daily sedentary time (~8.3 hours per day). Americans follow closely (~7.7 hours per day). In Singapore, nearly half the population sits ≥7 hours per day. High income and urban populations tend to be more sedentary than rural or lower income groups.

5. Describe two socio-economic or demographic disparities in physical activity or sedentary behaviour identified in the UK.

   A. Individuals in the least deprived areas are more likely to be sufficiently active (70%) compared with those in the most deprived areas (55%). Older adults are less active: ~50% of adults >75 do <30 minutes of weekly moderate activity versus only 20% of adults aged 16–34. Women generally spend more time sedentary than men.

6. What evidence links sedentary time to increased cancer incidence or mortality?

   A. An umbrella review of 14 meta-analyses found sedentary behaviour increases risk for six cancers (colon, breast, endometrial, ovarian, prostate, rectal) and is linked to higher cancer mortality, even after adjusting for physical activity.

7. List three biological pathways through which sedentary behaviour increases cancer risk.

   A. Metabolic dysregulation (decrease in LPL and GLUT4, insulin resistance); hormonal imbalance (increased oestrogen and IGF-1, decreased SHBG); chronic inflammation and oxidative stress (increased cytokines, ROS and reduced DNA repair).

8. Explain the role of lipoprotein lipase (LPL) in metabolic health and describe what happens to LPL during prolonged sitting.

   A. LPL breaks down circulating triglycerides into free fatty acids for energy. During prolonged sitting, LPL activity decreases, leading to increased triglycerides, decreased HDL and impaired lipid metabolism, factors associated with metabolic syndrome and cancer risk.

9. How does reduced GLUT4 expression contribute to insulin resistance and why is this relevant for cancer development.

   A. GLUT4 transports glucose into muscle cells in response to insulin. Sedentary behaviour reduces GLUT4 expression, resulting in reduced glucose uptake and insulin resistance. This leads to higher circulating insulin and IGF-1, both of which promote cell proliferation and create cancer-promoting conditions.

10. Describe how adiposity and sedentary behaviour influence hormone levels in post-menopausal women.

    A. Adipose tissue becomes the main site of aromatase, converting androgens to oestrogen. Sedentary behaviour increases aromatase activity and raises circulating oestrogen, even independently of BMI. Lower SHBG further increases bioactive oestrogen, heightening risk for breast and endometrial cancers.

11. Explain how chronic, low-grade inflammation contributes to carcinogenesis. In your answer, refer to ROS and DNA repair.

    A. Chronic inflammation increases production of pro-inflammatory cytokines and ROS, which can cause DNA damage. Persistent ROS exposure, combined with reduced DNA repair, creates mutations. Chronic inflammatory signalling also promotes cell proliferation and inhibits apoptosis, enabling tumour growth.

12. Outline how sedentary behaviour could elevate risk for both endometrial and pancreatic cancer, despite differences in tissue type.

    A. Across tissues, sedentary behaviour drives: Hormonal dysregulation (increased oestrogen, increasing endometrial risk); metabolic dysfunction (insulin resistance, increased insulin/IGF-1, promotes proliferative signals); inflammation (increased cytokines, oxidative stress). These systemic changes create a shared pro-tumourigenic environment, regardless of organ.

13. Which three cancer types have the strongest evidence for risk reduction through physical activity, and what is the approximate percentage reduction?

    A. Colon: 20–30% reduction; Breast (post-menopausal): 15–25%; Endometrial: 20–30%

14. Why is the evidence for physical activity and lung cancer risk reduction considered limited?

    Because smoking is a strong confounder. Even with statistical adjustments, it is difficult to isolate the independent effect of physical activity on lung cancer risk.

15. Despite measurement challenges, what overall conclusions can be drawn about the dose-response relationship between physical activity and cancer risk?

    A. There is a general dose-response trend: Higher activity levels correlate with lower cancer risk. However, the exact activity "thresholds" remain unclear due to inconsistent measurement methods across studies.

16. Describe how becoming physically activate later in life can still reduce cancer risk. Provide one example from epidemiological studies.

    A. Even when activity increases after menopause, women can reduce their breast cancer risk, regardless of premenopausal activity. In general, adopting physical activity later in life still lowers risk by improving metabolic, hormonal and inflammatory profiles.

17. Define "cancer prehabilitation" and describe its purpose within the treatment pathway.

    A. Prehabilitation occurs between diagnosis and the start of treatment. It assesses baseline function and introduces interventions (exercise, nutrition, psychological support) to improve resilience, reduce complications and enhance treatment outcomes.

18. Explain two ways in which moderate-intensity exercise may reduce metastatic progression after a cancer diagnosis.

    A. Moderate exercise can:

    - Normalise tumour vasculature, reducing hypoxia and limiting opportunities for tumour cells to escape.
    - Enhance immune surveillance, particularly by mobilising NK cells, improving clearance of circulating tumour cells.

    These effects may collectively reduce metastatic spread.

Chapter 3 Test your understanding question bank with answers

1. What are the main cellular components of the TME, and how do they influence cancer progression?

A. The TME includes cancer-associated fibroblasts (CAFs), immune cells (e.g., T cells, macrophages, NK cells), endothelial cells, adipocytes and stem cells. These components can promote or suppress tumour growth through complex signalling and physical interactions (see Section 3.2. for individual details).

2. Describe the role of immune checkpoint proteins such as PD-1 and PD-L1 in tumour immune evasion.

   A. PD-1 on T cells binds PD-L1 on tumour cells, inhibiting T cell activity. This allows tumours to evade immune detection. Immune checkpoint inhibitors block this interaction to restore T cell function.

3. How does exercise influence the infiltration and function of natural killer (NK) cells and CD8+ T cells within the TME?

   A. Exercise increases mobilisation and infiltration of NK and CD8+ T cells into tumours, enhancing their cytotoxic function and contributing to tumour suppression.

4. What is the difference between M1-like and M2-like tumour-associated macrophages (TAMs), and how might exercise influence their polarisation?

   A. M1-like TAMs are pro-inflammatory and tumour-suppressive, while M2-like TAMs are anti-inflammatory and tumour-promoting. Exercise may shift macrophage polarisation towards the M1 phenotype.

5. Explain how regulatory T cells (Tregs) and myeloid-derived suppressor cells (MDSCs) contribute to an immunosuppressive TME.

   A. Tregs and MDSCs inhibit cytotoxic T cell responses and cytokine production, creating an immunosuppressive environment that allows tumour cells to evade immune attack.

6. In what ways does exercise alter cytokine signalling within the TME, and what are the potential implications for tumour behaviour?

   A. Exercise modulates cytokine profiles by increasing anti-inflammatory and decreasing pro-inflammatory cytokines, potentially reducing tumour-promoting inflammation.

7. What is the significance of cancer-associated fibroblasts (CAFs) in shaping the TME, and how might exercise modify their activity?

   A. CAFs remodel the ECM, support angiogenesis, and secrete tumour-promoting signals. Exercise may reduce their activation and reprogramme the TME to be less supportive of cancer, although this is a very understudied area.

8. How do adipokines secreted by cancer-associated adipocytes (CAAs) impact cancer cell behaviour, particularly in obesity-associated cancers?

    A. Adipokines like leptin and FABP4 promote cancer cell proliferation and invasion. In obesity, these are elevated, enhancing tumour progression.

9. Describe how exercise affects the secretory profile of adipose tissue and the downstream consequences for tumour progression.

    A. Exercise decreases pro-tumourigenic adipokines (e.g., leptin) and increases protective ones (e.g., adiponectin), improving insulin sensitivity and reducing systemic inflammation.

10. What are myokines, and which ones have been implicated in mediating anti-tumour effects of exercise?

    A. Myokines are cytokines released by skeletal muscle during exercise. IL-6, SPARC and irisin are known to suppress tumour growth and modulate immune responses.

11. Summarise how exercise-induced vascular normalisation might enhance immune cell trafficking into the tumour.

    A. Exercise improves vascular structure and function, reducing hypoxia and enabling better immune cell infiltration into tumours.

12. Explain how skeletal muscle functions as an endocrine organ. Which signalling molecules are involved, and what effects do they have on the TME?

    A. Skeletal muscle releases myokines during exercise that affect distant tissues, including tumours. These molecules can inhibit tumour growth and modulate immune activity.

13. How does exercise influence the viability and extravasation of circulating tumour cells (CTCs)?

    A. Exercise-induced shear stress reduces CTC viability. Changes in immune activity and endothelial signalling may also inhibit CTC migration and extravasation.

14. What are the key characteristics of cancer stem cells (CSCs), and what does emerging research suggest about how exercise might affect CSC behaviour?

    A. CSCs are capable of self-renewal and drive tumour growth. Exercise may reduce CSC numbers and impair their ability to form tumours, possibly through metabolic or immune mechanisms.

15. In what ways might exercise act as a primer for cancer therapies such as immune checkpoint inhibitors?

    A. Exercise enhances immune surveillance and may increase the efficacy of immunotherapy by improving T cell infiltration and reducing immunosuppression.

16. Discuss how obesity alters the adipose tissue microenvironment to support tumour growth. How can exercise reverse or mitigate these changes?

    A. Obesity leads to adipocyte hypertrophy, inflammation and altered adipokine secretion. Exercise reverses these effects, improving metabolic and immune function.

17. What role do extracellular vesicles (EVs) play in intracellular communication, and how might their cargo be modified by exercise?

    A. EVs transport small molecules, including proteins and RNA, between cells, influencing tumour behaviour. Exercise may alter EV content to promote anti-tumour signalling.

18. Exercise exerts both systemic and local effects on the tumour ecosystem. Summarise at least three different cell types that are influenced by exercise, describing the nature and consequences of these changes.

    A. Exercise enhances NK and T cell cytotoxicity, reduces MDSCs and Tregs, and may reprogramme CAFs and CAAs to suppress tumour progression.

Chapter 4 Test your understanding question bank with answers

A. Epigenetic regulation

1. How does exercise influence DNA methylation patterns in tumour suppressor genes, and why is this important for cancer control?

   A. Exercise reduces promoter hypermethylation of tumour suppressors, restoring gene expression and restraining proliferation.

2. Describe how AMPK activation affects histone acetylation and transcriptional regulation in both muscle and tumour cells.

   A. AMPK phosphorylates HDACs and promotes HAT recruitment, increasing histone acetylation and transcription of metabolic/anti-tumour genes.

3. Which exercise-responsive miRNAs are implicated in anti-tumour pathways, and what cellular processes do they regulate?

   A. miR-630, miR-5703, miR-16 and others regulate inflammation, apoptosis, cell cycle and Hippo signalling.

4. Explain how exercise-induced activation of p53 may occur, despite the lack of direct evidence linking exercise-modulated miRNAs to p53 in cancer.

   A. Exercise activates p53 indirectly via metabolic stress, AMPK, p38 and ROS-mediated checkpoint engagement.

B. *AMPK and metabolic stress pathways*

5. What triggers AMPK activation during exercise, and why is this relevant in the TME?

   A. Increased AMP:ATP during exercise; tumours under metabolic stress respond similarly.

6. Explain how AMPK inhibits mTOR signalling and how this may contribute to tumour suppression.

   A. AMPK phosphorylates TSC2 and Raptor suppresses mTORC1 limits anabolic signalling.

7. Describe the dual role of AMPK in regulating autophagy in cancer cells.

   A. AMPK can activate or inhibit autophagy, depending on ULK1 phosphorylation site and content.

8. How might AMPK activation increase tumour cell vulnerability to apoptosis or therapy?

   A. AMPK promotes p53/p21 signalling and increases sensitivity to metabolic or chemotherapeutic stress.

C. *MAPK signalling*

9. Why does the duration and pattern of ERK activation lead to different biological outcomes in cancer versus exercise?

   A. Exercise causes transient ERK activation (adaptive); tumours often have chronic activation (proliferative).

10. How might exercise-induced JNK activation contribute to anti-tumour immunity?

A. Exercise-induced JNK activation enhances cytokine production and immune recruitment.

11. Explain the context-dependent, dual roles of p38 MAPK in tumour suppression and progression.

    p38 can induce growth arrest/apoptosis or support inflammation/angiogenesis, depending on context.

12. How does improved vascular perfusion alter MAPK signalling within tumours?

    A. Improved perfusion reduces hypoxia-driven, pathological MAPK activation.

D. *Hippo-YAP/TAZ mechanotransduction*

13. What systemic signals during exercise lead to YAP/TAZ inhibition, and how is this mediated?

    A. Catecholamines β-adrenergic receptors LATS1/2 phosphorylation YAP/TAZ cytoplasmic retention.

14. How do mechanical cues from ECM stiffness support YAP/TAZ-driven oncogenic transcription?

    A. Stiff ECM increases Rho/ROCK activity actomyosin tension nuclear YAP/TAZ

15. Explain how exercise-induced ECM remodelling could reduce nuclear YAP/TAZ localisation.

    A. ECM softening and improved vascular/pressure dynamics reduce YAP nuclear localisation.

16. Why is YAP/TAZ signalling considered important for cancer stem cell maintenance and therapeutic resistance?

    A. YAP/TAZ maintain stemness, EMT, chemoresistance and metastatic traits.

E. *Myokines and exerkines*

17. Contrast tumour-derived IL-6 with exercise-induced IL-6 in terms of signalling and biological outcomes.

    A. Tumour IL-6 = chronic, pro-inflammatory; exercise IL-6 = acute, anti-inflammatory, AMPK-activating.

18. How does IL-15 support anti-tumour immune responses during exercise?

    A. IL-15 expands NK and CD8 T cells and enhances cytotoxicity.

19. Describe how SPARC exerts anti-proliferative effects in colorectal and prostate cancer models.

    A. SPARC induces apoptosis, ER stress, caspase activation.

20. Summarise the context-dependent effects of irisin on tumour proliferation and metastasis.

    Irisin can inhibit PI3K/Akt or stimulate proliferation depending on tissue context.

21. How might OSM contribute to the anti-tumour effects of exercise-conditioned serum?

    A. OSM in exercise serum promotes apoptosis and cell cycle arrest.

22. What roles do musclin and FGF21 play in cancer cachexia, and how is exercise involved?

    A. Musclin protects muscle in cachexia; FGF21 worsens atrophy when chronically elevated.

23. Explain how decorin may suppress tumour growth and modulate cachexia-related signalling.

    A. Decorin inhibits EGFR, TGFβ1, miR-21 and increases p21/53.

24. What is the role of myostatin and activin A in cancer cachexia, and how might exercise counteract these pathways?

    A. Myostatin/activin A promote atrophy; exercise reduces myostatin and increases antagonists like decorin.

25. How do exercise-induced extracellular vesicles (EVs) influence tumour metabolism or immune evasion?

    A. EVs carry anti-tumour miRNAs, metabolic enzymes or immunomodulatory factors.

F. *Cachexia and muscle-tumour crosstalk*

26. Why is chronic IL-6 elevation associated with muscle wasting, and how does this differ from exercise-induced IL-6 dynamics?

    A. Chronic IL-6 activates proteolysis pathways; exercise IL-6 is transient and anti-inflammatory.

27. Which exercise-responsive myokines show the strongest evidence for attenuating muscle loss in cancer?

    A. IL-15, decorin, musclin show strong protective effects.

28. How do myostatin/ActRIIB inhibitors reduce cachexia, and what is the link to exercise?

    A. ActRIIB blockade prevents Smad2/3-mediated atrophy; exercise naturally reduces myostatin.

G. *Metabolic reprogramming of tumour cells*

29. How does exercise-conditioned serum shift cancer cell metabolism away from the Warburg phenotype?

    A. Increased mitochondrial respiration, reduced GLUT1, higher ROS and cell cycle arrest.

30. What features of the obesogenic metabolic microenvironment promote tumour initiation and progression?

    A. Elevated leptin/IL-6/TNF-α, lipid transfer, hyperinsulinaemia, fuel abundance.

31. Describe how exercise remodels adipose tissue to decrease tumour fuel availability.

    A. Exercise reduces visceral fat, increases adiponectin, enhances beiging and FFA oxidation.

32. How does improved tumour perfusion alter hypoxia-driven metabolic signalling?

    A. Improved oxygenation reduces HIF-1α stabilisation and glycolysis dependence.

H. *Angiogenesis and vascular function*

33. What features of tumour vasculature distinguish pathological angiogenesis from physiological vascularisation?

    A. Tumour vessels = leaky, chaotic; physiological = stabilised, pericyte-covered.

34. How does exercise promote vascular normalisation in tumour tissue?

    A. Exercise increases shear stress, VEGF regulation, pericyte recruitment.

35. Explain how vascular normalisation improves drug delivery and immune infiltration.

    A. Normalised vessels improve drug penetration and immune cell access.

36. Why can VEGF and NO have both tumour-promoting and tumour-suppressive roles depending on context?

    A. Context determines NO/VEGF's role (chronic versus transient signalling).

I. ECM mechanics and interstitial pressure

37. How do ECM and interstitial pressure activate oncogenic mechanotransduction pathways?

    A. Stiff ECM activates integrins FAK Rho/ROCK YAP/TAZ

38. In what ways might exercise reduce ECM stiffness or solid stress in tumours?

    A. Exercise modulates MMP activity, reduces fibrosis, improves perfusion.

39. How could reduced mechanical barriers improve immune infiltration into tumour tissue?

    A. Reduced stiffness decreases physical barriers and improve T cell motility.

J. Systemic endocrine and hormonal modulation

40. How does exercise reduce insulin and IGF-1 signalling, and why is this important for cancer progression?

    A. Exercise improves insulin sensitivity lowers insulin/IGF-1 signalling reduces proliferation.

41. Explain how exercise affects oestrogen biosynthesis via adipose tissue and its implications for hormone-sensitive cancers.

    A. Reduced adiposity decreases aromatase activity lower oestrogen reduced risk in hormone-sensitive cancers.

42. Describe how chronic stress hormone signalling contributes to tumour progression and how exercise may reset these dynamics.

    A. Exercise restores cortisol rhythms reduces chronic stress signalling.

43. What changes occur in adipokine secretion with exercise, and how doe these shape the TME?

    A. Increase in adiponectin/omentin-1; decrease in leptin/IL-6/TNF-α

Chapter 5 Test your understanding question bank with answers

1. What are the primary physiological adaptations induced by aerobic exercise?

    A. Improvements in cardiorespiratory fitness (e.g., increased VO_2max), increased mitochondrial density and capillarisation, enhanced metabolic flexibility, reduced systemic inflammation and improved insulin sensitivity.

2. How does aerobic exercise contribute to reduced cancer recurrence risk?

    A. Through better metabolic regulation, reduced adiposity, improved immune surveillance (e.g., enhanced NK cell activity), and lower chronic inflammation.

3. Why is aerobic exercise considered beneficial during chemotherapy?

    A. It helps manage side effects such as fatigue, nausea and sleep disturbance; maintains cardiorespiratory fitness; supports treatment tolerance; and improves psychological wellbeing.

4. What distinguishes resistance training from aerobic training in cancer care?

    A. Resistance training focuses on strengthening muscles and bones, preserving lean mass and functional strength, while aerobic training primarily improves cardiovascular and metabolic health.

5. How can resistance training mitigate the effects of sarcopenia and cachexia?

    A. By stimulating muscle growth and maintenance, preserving lean mass, improving functional strength and counteracting catabolic processes associated with advanced disease or treatment.

6. What are the key considerations for prescribing resistance training to patients with lymphoedema?

    A. Use supervised, progressive loading; start with low intensity; monitor symptoms; emphasise proper technique; progress gradually. Evidence shows it is safe and beneficial when well-structured.

7. How does endurance training differ from general aerobic exercise in its goals and adaptations?

   A. Endurance training emphasises sustained effort, psychological resilience and long-duration performance, building stamina and mental toughness in addition to aerobic capacity.

8. What neurobiological mechanisms underpin the mental health benefits of endurance training?

   A. Increased endorphins and endocannabinoids, enhanced BDNF-driven neuroplasticity, improved emotional regulation, and reductions in stress and depressive symptoms.

9. In what ways might endurance training reduce cancer recurrence anxiety?

   A. By improving coping skills, reducing perceived stress, enhancing self-efficacy and providing a sense of mastery and control.

10. How does exercise improve sleep hygiene in cancer survivors?

    A. It helps regulate circadian rhythms, reduces anxiety and hyperarousal, improves sleep duration and quality and alleviates fatigue, all contributing to better sleep patterns.

11. Which forms of exercise are particularly helpful for managing chemotherapy-induced neuropathy?

    A. Combined aerobic and resistance training, balance and proprioceptive exercises, and lower intensity endurance activities, all improve sensory symptoms and functional mobility.

12. In what ways can group-based exercise enhance psychological wellbeing and social connection?

    A. It reduces isolation, fosters peer support, promotes shared experience, builds community, and enhances motivation, leading to better mood and emotional resilience.

13. What is NEAT, and why is it important in cancer prevention and survivorship?

    A. NEAT (non-exercise activity thermogenesis) refers to everyday movement outside structured exercise. It helps reduce sedentary time, supports metabolic health and lowers risk of weight gain and comorbidities.

14. Which everyday activities can contribute meaningfully to physical activity levels?

    A. Walking, gardening, housework, active commuting, carrying shopping, stair climbing and frequent movement breaks throughout the day.

15. How can NEAT benefit individuals unable to engage in structured exercise programmes?

    A. It offers a low-barrier way to stay active, supports mobility and mood, reduces inflammation and fatigue, and contributes to meaningful health improvements even at low intensities.

16. Why is self-monitoring an effective strategy for sustaining exercise behaviour?

    A. It increases awareness of activity levels, provides feedback, reinforces progress and supports goal setting, which are key drivers of long-term behaviour change.

17. What role do support networks play in exercise adherence for cancer survivors?

    A. They provide accountability, encouragement, shared experience and emotional support, all of which increase motivation and sustain engagement.

18. How can digital tools complement traditional behaviour change strategies?

    A. Apps and wearables facilitate self-monitoring, goal setting and feedback, and can offer remote coaching and create virtual communities that support persistence and adherence.

Chapter 6 Test your understanding question bank with answers

1. Which physiological parameter is considered the most accurate objective measure of exercise intensity?

    A. VO_2max

2. Explain the difference between exercise volume and intensity.

    A. Volume refers to the total workload (frequency x time x intensity), whereas intensity reflects the effort or metabolic demand per unit of activity

3. Which type of immune cell is most acutely mobilised in response to high-intensity exercise?

   A. Natural killer (NK) cells

4. What is the "J-shaped curve" in exercise immunology, and how does it apply to exercise oncology?

   A. It describes the biphasic relationship between exercise volume/intensity and immune function, where moderate activity improves immunity, while excessive or very low activity may impair it. In oncology, this suggests moderate intensity may support anti-tumour immunity, while very high intensity might increase metastatic risk under some conditions.

5. List two biological pathways activated by high-intensity exercise that may influence tumour biology.

   A. The Hippo pathway (via catecholamines) and suppression of Wnt/β-catenin signalling.

6. Name one potential risk associated with poorly recovered high-intensity exercise in cancer patients.

   A. Transient immunosuppression or increased circulating tumour cells (CTCs).

7. Describe one benefit and one limitation of using RPE (rating of perceived exertion) to measure exercise intensity in cancer patients.

   A. Benefit: It is subjective, accessible and useful when heart rate monitoring is unreliable (e.g., with beta blockers). Limitation: It can be influenced by mood, fatigue or cognitive changes.

8. What does the term "minimum effective dose" mean in the context of exercise oncology?

   A. The smallest amount of exercise required to elicit meaningful biological or clinical benefits.

9. What is meant by "precision exercise prescription"?

   A. Tailoring exercise interventions to individual factors such as cancer type, treatment stage, fitness level, and biological responsiveness.

10. What are some recommended features of a prehabilitation programme for cancer surgery?

    A. Endurance training (60–90% VO_2max for 20–35 mins) and resistance exercises using body weight or light resistance (0–40% of 1RM).

11. Why is warm-up considered essential before high-intensity exercise, particularly in cancer populations?

    A. To enhance vascular function, reduce endothelial stress and lower risk of tumour cell dissemination.

12. Summarise one mechanistic reason by moderate-intensity exercise is beneficial in suppressing tumour growth?

    A. It improves immune surveillance by enhancing mobilisation of CD8+ T cells and normalises tumour vasculature, improving oxygen and drug delivery.

13. What are some of the individual factors that may influence exercise response in cancer patients?

    A. Age, treatment status, comorbidities, baseline fitness, tumour immunogenicity, metabolic profile.

14. A patient undergoing chemotherapy reports severe fatigue. What intensity of exercise might be appropriate to recommend and why?

    A. Low-to-moderate intensity, as it maintains function without inducing excessive fatigue or physiological stress.

15. How might future exercise oncology trials integrate the concept of phenotyping?

    A. By stratifying participants based on fitness, tumour biology or treatment phase, and personalising intensity and volume accordingly to enhance efficacy and safety.

Chapter 7 Test your understanding question bank with answers

1. What are the two main physiological distinctions between acute and chronic exercise effects in cancer care?

    A. Acute exercise triggers transient systemic responses like catecholamine and cytokine release, while chronic exercise induces sustained adaptations such as improved mitochondrial function, insulin sensitivity and immune reprogramming.

2. Why is frequency an important variable in exercise prescription for cancer patients?

    A. Because it determines how often tumour-suppressive and immune-modulating responses are stimulated and influences adherence, treatment tolerance and cumulative benefit over time.

3. What does current evidence suggest is the minimum effective frequency of exercise for cancer survivors?

    A. Three sessions per week of moderate-intensity aerobic exercise are generally sufficient to yield improvements in fatigue, QoL, and treatment tolerance.

4. How does session duration influence biological and behavioural outcomes in cancer patients?

    A. Even short bouts (10–30 minutes) can trigger anti-tumour immune responses, while longer sessions may offer additional fitness benefits but risk overtraining and lower adherence during treatment.

5. In which phases of the cancer continuum might high frequency or longer-duration exercise be most appropriate?

    A. Pre-treatment (prehabilitation) and post-treatment (survivorship) phases, when patients typically have higher capacity and can safely accumulate higher training volumes.

6. How can exercise prescriptions be adapted during active treatment to support adherence and safety?

    A. By reducing duration, adjusting intensity and prioritising consistency through short, manageable sessions (e.g., daily 10- to 20-minute walks).

7. What are some patient-specific factors that influence how frequency and duration should be prescribed?

    A. Treatment phase, baseline fitness, comorbidities, age, sex, tumour type, psychosocial readiness, and individual preferences.

8. Why might shorter, more frequent exercise sessions be more beneficial than fewer longer sessions?

    A. They are often more sustainable, better tolerated during treatment and support habit formation and immune resilience without overburdening the patient.

Chapter 8 Test your understanding question bank with answers

1. What are the general WHO physical activity recommendations for adults, including those with chronic conditions such as cancer?

    A. 150–300 minutes of moderate-intensity aerobic activity or 75–150 minutes of vigorous intensity activity per week, plus muscle-strengthening activities on two or more days.

2. Name three key benefits of regular exercise for individuals undergoing cancer treatment.

   A. Improved physical function, reduced treatment-related side effects and enhanced psychological wellbeing.

3. What is the primary goal of prehabilitation in cancer care?

   A. To enhance physical and psychological resilience before treatment begins.

4. What does a symptom-led approach to exercise involve?

   A. Adjusting exercise intensity or duration based on daily symptoms such as fatigue or pain.

5. List two common barriers to exercise adherence among cancer patients.

   A. Cancer-related fatigue and lack of support or guidance from healthcare providers.

6. What principle supports the idea that exercise should be adapted to a patient's current energy and side-effect levels?

   A. Autoregulatory or symptom-led programming.

7. What type of training is recommended for post-treatment cancer survivors aiming to restore fitness?

   A. Gradual progression to 150 minutes per week of moderate aerobic activity and two strength training sessions per week.

8. What role do community exercise professionals play in cancer care?

   A. They support long-term exercise adherence and social engagement post-treatment.

9. Define "precision exercise oncology."

   A. An approach to exercise prescription that tailors type, intensity and duration based on individual tumour biology, treatment history and physiological responses.

10. What is the "2-day rule" in symptom-led programming?

    A. A principle where patients modify or rest from exercise if symptoms worsen for two consecutive days.

11. What behavioural strategies can enhance exercise adherence in cancer survivors?

    A. Goal setting, social support, motivational interviewing and embedding exercise into daily routines.

12. Why is patient preference important in exercise prescription?

    A. It increases the likelihood of adherence and long-term engagement by aligning with personal interests and lifestyle.

13. List two functions of cardiopulmonary exercise testing (CPET) in exercise oncology.

    A. Evaluating cardiorespiratory fitness and identifying safe, personalised exercise intensities.

14. In the context of exercise oncology, what is meant by "training periodisation"?

    A. A systematic scheduling of training loads to optimise physiological adaptation and avoid overtraining.

Chapter 9 Test your understanding question bank with answers

1. How does the concept of "every step counts" align with both the molecular mechanisms and population-level benefits of exercise discussed throughout this book?

   A. This phrase reflects the idea that even small amounts of physical activity can elicit beneficial biological responses (e.g., improved immune surveillance, myokine release, vascular remodelling) while also contributing to reductions in population-level cancer risk. Mechanistically, acute bouts of exercise can modulate circulating cytokines, glucose uptake and immune cell mobilisation. Epidemiologically, even modest increases in daily movement are associated with reduced cancer incidence and improved survivorship outcomes.

2. What challenges might a clinician face in implementing exercise as part of a standard cancer care pathway, and how could these be addressed at the system level?

   A. Challenges include lack of training in exercise prescription, time constraints, limited referral pathways, and patient concerns about safety. System-level solutions involve embedding exercise professionals in oncology teams, standardising referral systems, improving reimbursement models, and including exercise in clinical guidelines and electronic health records. Education for both patients and providers is key.

3. Why is it important to move from general exercise guidelines to precision exercise prescriptions? What tools or biomarkers might support this shift?

    A. Precision prescriptions allow for more effective and tolerable interventions tailored to tumour type, treatment stage, patient capacity and biological phenotype. Tools supporting this include wearable technologies, physiological monitoring, and in the future, perhaps biomarkers to guide dosage adjustments and track response to exercise in real-time.

4. What factors contribute to the underrepresentation of certain populations in exercise oncology research, and how can future studies become more inclusive?

    A. Barriers include socio-economic status, geography, language, cultural beliefs, and medical comorbidities. Underrepresentation of minority ethnic groups, older adults, rural populations and those with advanced cancers is common. Future studies should adopt inclusive recruitment strategies, community-based research, culturally sensitive programme design and remove logistical barriers (e.g., transportation, childcare, financial cost).

5. Compare the role of physical activity in prehabilitation versus survivorship. How do goals, barriers and outcomes differ across these phases of care?

    A. Prehab: Goal is to build physical and psychological resilience before treatment. Barriers may include short timelines or anxiety post-diagnosis. Outcomes include improved surgical recovery, fewer complications and faster return to baseline.

    Survivorship: Focus is on long-term function, reducing recurrence risk, managing chronic side effects and improving quality of life. Barriers may include fatigue, comorbidities and loss of structured support. Outcomes include improved physical fitness, mental wellbeing and secondary prevention.

6. What role might wearable technology and remote platforms play in shaping the future of exercise oncology delivery and monitoring?

    A. These tools can support personalised, adaptive exercise plans, enhance accessibility, and provide real-time feedback on physiological responses (e.g., heart rate, activity levels). They also enable remote supervision, improve adherence through gamification or behavioural nudges, and facilitate data collection for research.

GLOSSARY

1RM (1 repetition maximum) The maximum amount of weight that a person can lift for one complete repetition of a given exercise; used as a measure of maximal strength.

Acetylation A biochemical modification where an acetyl group is added to a molecule, often to histones or proteins, influencing gene expression and protein function.

Adjunct A treatment or intervention used in addition to the primary therapy to enhance its effectiveness.

Angiogenesis The formation of new blood vessels from pre-existing vessels; critical in tumour growth and metastasis.

Anoikis A form of programmed cell death triggered when cells detach from the surrounding extracellular matrix, preventing inappropriate cell survival and migration.

Apoptosis A form of programmed cell death involving or eliminating damaged or unnecessary cells.

Autophagy A regulated process by which cells degrade and recycle their own components, contributing to cellular homeostasis and survival under stress.

Biogenesis The process by which new cellular components, especially organelles like mitochondria, are formed within a cell.

Cachexia A complex syndrome involving weight loss, muscle atrophy, fatigue and weakness, often seen in advanced cancer.

Carcinogen A substance or agent capable of causing cancer by inducing genetic mutations or promoting tumour growth.

Cytokines Small proteins released by cells that have a specific effect on the interactions and communication between cells, especially in immune responses.

Cytoskeleton A dynamic network of protein filaments within cells that provides structure, shape and facilitates intracellular transport and cell movement.

Cytotoxic Refers to substances or mechanisms that are toxic to cells, often used to describe immune cells or drugs that kill cancer cells.

Endocrine Relating to glands that secrete hormones directly into the bloodstream to regulate bodily functions.

Epithelial-to-mesenchymal transition (EMT) A biological process in which epithelial cells acquire mesenchymal, migratory properties, often implicated in cancer metastasis.

Epigenetics The study of heritable changes in gene expression that do not involve changes to the underlying DNA sequence.

Exercise A structured, planned and repetitive form of physical activity performed with the objective of improving or maintaining one or more components of physical fitness, such as strength, endurance or flexibility.

Exerkines Exercise-induced signalling molecules released into circulation, affecting distant tissues and organs.

Exosome Small extracellular vesicles released by cells that carry proteins, lipids and nucleic acids, playing a role in intercellular communication.

Extracellular matrix (ECM) A complex network of proteins and carbohydrates surrounding cells, providing structural and biochemical support.

Extravasation The process by which cells, particularly immune or tumour cells, exit the bloodstream and enter surrounding tissues.

Fibrosis The thickening and scarring of connective tissue, often resulting from chronic inflammation or injury.

Histone A type of protein around which DNA winds, helping to package it into a compact, organised structure within the nucleus; histones are involved in regulating gene expression through chemical modifications such as acetylation and methylation.

Hypoxia A condition in which tissues are deprived of adequate oxygen supply, common in the tumour microenvironment and influencing cancer progression.

Immunoediting The process by which the immune system interacts with tumour cells, comprising elimination, equilibrium and escape phases.

Immunosurveillance The monitoring function of the immune system to detect and destroy transformed or cancerous cells.

Inflammation A biological response to harmful stimuli such as pathogens or damaged cells, often associated with cancer progression.

Insulin resistance A condition in which cells fail to respond normally to insulin, often associated with obesity and cancer.

Integrin A family of cell surface receptors involved in cell adhesion and signalling, playing a role in cell migration and survival.

Intravasation The process by which cancer cells enter blood or lymphatic vessels; a key step in metastasis.

Leukocytosis An increase in the number of white blood cells in the bloodstream, often a response to infection, inflammation or malignancy.

Mechanotransduction The process by which cells convert mechanical stimuli into biochemical signals, influencing cell behaviour.

Metabolic flexibility The capacity of an organism to adapt fuel oxidation to fuel availability, particularly relevant in exercise physiology.

Metabolism The set of life-sustaining chemical reactions in organisms that convert food into energy and building blocks for growth and repair.

Metabolic equivalent of task (MET) A unit used to estimate the amount of oxygen used by the body during physical activity; 1 MET is the energy expended at rest.

Metastasis The spread of cancer cells from the primary site to distant organs or tissues.

Methylation The addition of a methyl group to DNA or proteins, often influencing gene expression and cellular function.

Mitochondria Organelles known as the powerhouses of the cell, responsible for producing energy (ATP) through oxidative phosphorylation.

Mutation A change in the DNA sequence that may alter gene function and contribute to disease, including cancer.

Myokines Cytokines and peptides produced and released by muscle fibres that exert autocrine, paracrine or endocrine effects.

Neutropenia An abnormally low concentration of neutrophils (a type of white blood cell), often caused by chemotherapy.

Palliative care Specialised medical care focused on providing relief from the symptoms and stress of serious illness.

Phenotype The observable physical or biochemical characteristics of an organism, resulting from the interaction of its genotype with the environment.

Phosphorylation The addition of a phosphate group to a molecule, often regulating protein activity and signal transduction.

Physical activity Any bodily movement produced by skeletal muscles that results in energy expenditure.

Precision oncology A medical approach that tailors treatment based on genetic, environmental and lifestyle factors of an individual and their cancer.

Proliferation The rapid multiplication of cells; a process that is often dysregulated in cancer.

Sedentary behaviour Any waking behaviour characterised by low energy expenditure while sitting or lying down.

Stroma The supportive tissue surrounding tumours, including fibroblasts, immune cells and the extracellular matrix.

Transcription The process by which genetic information in DNA is copied into messenger RNA for protein synthesis.

Transdifferentiation The process by which one specialised cell type transforms into another without reverting to a pluripotent state.

Tumour microenvironment The environment surrounding a tumour including blood vessels, immune cells, fibroblasts, adipocytes, stem cells, signalling molecules and the extracellular matrix.

Vascular normalisation A therapeutic strategy aimed at restoring the structure and function of abnormal blood vessels in tumours.

INDEX

For Product Safety Concerns and Information please contact our EU representative GPSR@taylorandfrancis.com Taylor & Francis Verlag GmbH, Kaufingerstraße 24, 80331 München, Germany